When Abortion Was a Crime

When Abortion Was a Crime

Women, Medicine, and Law
in the United States, 1867–1973

Leslie J. Reagan

UNIVERSITY OF CALIFORNIA PRESS

Berkeley / Los Angeles / London

University of California Press
Berkeley and Los Angeles, California

University of California Press, Ltd.
London, England

First Paperback Printing 1998

Library of Congress Cataloging-in-Publication Data

Reagan, Leslie J.
   When abortion was a crime : women, medicine, and law in
the United States, 1867–1973 / Leslie J. Reagan.
      p.   cm.
   Includes bibliographical references and index.
   ISBN 0-520-21657-1 (pbk. : alk. paper)
      1. Abortion—United States—History.   2. Abortion ser-
vices—United States—History.   3. Abortion—Law and legislation—United States—History.   I. Title.
   HO767.5.U5R378   1997
   363.4'6'0973—dc20   96-22568

Printed in the United States of America

9 8 7 6 5 4 3 2 1

The paper used in this publication meets the minimum require-
ments of American National Standards for Information Sciences—
Permanence of Paper for Printed Library Materials, ANSI
Z39.48–1984.

Some material in the introduction and chapter 4 previously ap-
peared in Leslie J. Reagan, "'About to Meet Her Maker': Women,
Doctors, Dying Declarations, and the State's Investigation of
Abortion, Chicago, 1867–1940," *Journal of American History* 77
(March 1991): 1240–1264. Reprinted courtesy of the Organization
of American Historians.

To my mother, Susan Gardner,
*   for her strength and creativity.*

To my father, Phil Reagan,
*   for his sense of adventure.*

Contents

LIST OF ILLUSTRATIONS   ix

ACKNOWLEDGMENTS   xi

Introduction   1

1
An Open Secret   19

2
Private Practices   46

3
Antiabortion Campaigns, Private and Public   80

4
Interrogations and Investigations   113

5
Expansion and Specialization   132

6
Raids and Rules   160

7
Repercussions   193

8
Radicalization of Reform   216

Epilogue: Post-*Roe*, Post-*Casey*   246

NOTE ON SOURCES   255

LIST OF ABBREVIATIONS   258

NOTES   259

BIBLIOGRAPHY   343

INDEX   367

Illustrations

Plates

1. "It Comes down the Ages"   51
2. Perforation of the uterus   78
3. "One of the Reputable Physicians"   86
4. "One of the Abortionists"   87
5. "The Quack House, the Victim, the Agency"   103
6. "The D.A.'s Peeping Toms"   227

Figures

1. Coroner's investigations of abortion-related deaths, Chicago, 1878–1931   117
2. Therapeutic abortion cases, New York City, 1943–1962   205
3. Therapeutic abortion, by race, New York City, 1943–1962   206
4. Abortion cases admitted annually to Cook County Hospital, 1921–1963   210
5. Women's deaths resulting from abortion, New York City, 1951–1962   211

6. Deaths resulting from abortion, by race, New York
   City, 1951–1962   212
7. Percent of total maternal mortality resulting from
   abortion, 1927–1962   213

Acknowledgments

It is a pleasure to take a few moments and remember all of the enthusiastic support and assistance that I received as I worked on this book. Friends, family, teachers, colleagues, and many others have sustained me through the process.

I was fortunate to be part of the women's history program at the University of Wisconsin at Madison. This program, founded by Gerda Lerner, brought together an energetic and creative group of graduate students and faculty. Two excellent advisors, Judith Walzer Leavitt and Linda Gordon, encouraged and challenged me every step of the way. I am grateful for their guidance and friendship. I appreciate too the counsel of Gerda Lerner, Hendrik Hartog, Ronald Numbers, Vanessa Northington Gamble, and Carl Kaestle. Morris Vogel, Steve Stern, and the late Tom Shick encouraged me at an early stage.

Graduate students in the Wisconsin history department created an invigorating intellectual climate, which nurtured me and this project. Furthermore, their commitment to both outstanding scholarship and progressive activism is one I cherish. For all of their support, I thank Kathleen Brown, Eve Fine, Joyce Follet, Colin Gordon, Roger Horowitz, Nancy Isenberg, Marie Laberge, Nancy MacLean, Earl Mulderink, Edward Pearson, Leslie Schwalm, Doris Stormoen, and Susan Smith. I am particularly grateful to Kathy Brown, Joyce Follet, Leslie Schwalm, and Mary Odem, who remain engaged with my work, even by long distance telephone and often on short notice.

I appreciate the comments and encouragement of Allan Brandt, Anna

Clark, Mary Fissell, Judith R. Walkowitz, and Danny Walkowitz. I am grateful to my colleagues in the Social History Group at the University of Illinois and to Diane Gottheil, Karen Hewitt, Evan Melhado, Jean Rhodes, Dorothee Schneider, Paula Treichler, Kathy Oberdeck, and William Munro for their suggestions on various phases of this project. I thank my research assistants, Lynne Curry, Mark Hemphill, and Rose Holz, for aiding me in the final stages of research.

Of critical importance are the librarians and archivists who facilitated my research. I thank Bob Bailey and Elaine Shemoney Evans at the Illinois State Archives, Lyle Benedict at the Municipal Reference Collection in the Chicago Public Library, Micaela Sullivan-Fowler, formerly at the American Medical Association, and Cathy Kurnyta, formerly at the Cook County Medical Examiner's Office. Jackie Jackson gave me a delightful home away from home when I did research in Springfield. Kate Spelman graciously offered legal advice. I thank the University of Illinois staff in history and medicine for their timely and friendly assistance. Editors and anonymous reviewers at the University of California Press, the *Bulletin of the History of Medicine,* and the *Journal of American History* have all offered helpful advice to make this book a better one. Jim Clark, Eileen McWilliam, Dore Brown, and Carolyn Hill at the University of California Press have been especially encouraging.

Many women and men, from clerks to professionals, volunteered their own abortion stories when they learned of my project and told me firmly that this was a book we "needed." Their belief in this project has always been important to me. I thank Susan Alexander and Sybille Fritzsche for sharing their memories of their legal effort to overturn the Illinois abortion law. It has been a pleasure getting to know them. I thank Peter Fritzsche for introducing me to his mother.

I have had the good fortune to have been granted vital financial support for the research and writing of this book. I am grateful to the Department of the History of Medicine of the University of Wisconsin Medical School for the Maurice L. Richardson Fellowships, the University of Wisconsin, Madison History Department, the American Bar Foundation, and the Institute for Legal Studies at the University of Wisconsin, Madison for crucial support as a graduate student. The Institute of the History of Medicine and the Department of History at Johns Hopkins University provided postdoctoral support. Since coming to the University of Illinois at Urbana-Champaign, I have received funding for research assistance from the UIUC Research Board; a semester as a Fellow at the Center for Advanced Study gave me time to write; and both of my departments, the Department of History and the Medical Humanities and Social Sciences Program in the College of Medicine, graciously granted leave to research, write, and complete my book. A National Institutes of Health, National Library of Medicine grant (grant number R01 LM05753), supported the final revisions of the manuscript. This book's contents do not necessarily represent the official views of the National Library of Medicine.

The support of family has been special. I deeply appreciate the interest that all members of all sides of my diverse family—Gardners, Reagans, Schneiders, Edwards, DeJarnatt, Goodman, Kanefield, Spelman, and Brillinger—have shown in my book. Recently, it has been a pleasure to talk of the delights and difficulties of writing with Billy, David, Mom, and Dad. Zola and Irv helped me by sharing their thoughts. My late grandparents, Mercedes Philip Gardner and William Irving Gardner, had an abiding belief in the importance of higher education and conveyed their belief in me and my chosen intellectual challenges. I am sorry they cannot see this book.

I met Daniel Schneider as I was about to head for Chicago to do research. He has always been interested in this project, from hearing about my discoveries in crumbling legal records to discussing the book's structure. Daniel has generously read many drafts, given excellent editorial advice, and produced all of the figures for this book. For his enthusiasm, his thoughtfulness, and his help, I am deeply grateful.

At the time that abortion was becoming legal in this country, I'm not sure that I even knew what it was, but I remember a moment in the kitchen when I asked my mom about it. Her response, though of few words, and perhaps a bit embarrassed, firmly imparted the belief that women had to be able to control their reproduction and that, sometimes, they had to be able to have abortions. That brief, dimly recalled conversation, I have since learned from my research, was like many others that mothers and daughters, friends and family members had about abortion through the twentieth century.

Introduction

There would be no history of illegal abortion to tell without the continuing demand for abortion from women, regardless of law. Generations of women persisted in controlling their reproduction through abortion and made abortion an issue for legal and medical authorities. Those women, their lives, and their perspectives are central in this book. Their demand for abortions, generally hidden from public view and rarely spoken of in public, transformed medical practice and law over the course of the twentieth century.

This book analyzes the triangle of interactions among the medical profession, state authorities, and women in the practice, policing, and politics of abortion during the era when abortion was a crime. As individual women consulted with doctors, they made them understand their needs. Sympathy for their female patients drew physicians into the world of abortion in spite of legal and professional prohibitions. Indeed, it was physicians and lawyers who initiated the earliest efforts to rewrite the abortion laws. Ultimately, women's pressing need for abortion fueled a mass movement that succeeded in reversing public policy toward abortion in the 1960s and early 1970s.

Public policy made at the national and state levels deserves to be examined where it was carried out: at the local level, in one-on-one interactions and on a day-to-day basis. Understanding the impact of abortion law requires analyzing the actual practice of abortion and the state's enforcement of the criminal laws. The stunning transformation in law and public policy regarding abortion and women's rights was rooted in the declining conditions of abortion under the criminal law and built on generations of women demanding abortions—and getting them.

This is the first study of the entire era of illegal abortion in the United States. Most scholarship on abortion has focused on two moments of legal change: when abortion was criminalized in the mid–nineteenth century, and when it was decriminalized a hundred years later in the mid-1960s and early 1970s.[1] The century of illegal abortion is typically treated as obscure and unchanging. I find, however, that the history of illegal abortion was dynamic, not static.

This book joins a growing literature that interrogates and reconceptualizes the relationship between the public and the private. The nineteenth-century ideology of "separate spheres" bifurcated the world into the "public sphere," the world of politics and business in which men lived, and the "private sphere," the domestic world of women and children. The concept of separate spheres proved to be fruitful for women's historians and produced an abundance of important new insights and knowledge.[2] Recently, however, women's historians have questioned the idea of separate spheres both because it excluded the majority of women who were working class or women of color and because it inaccurately described white middle-class life. The worlds of men and women no longer appear to be as exclusive and separate as once thought: men lived in the private sphere too, and women walked on public streets, participated in business, worked for wages, and intervened in political life; indeed, women created issues of national political importance.[3] Of recently renewed theoretical interest to a variety of scholars is the public sphere itself. Here, attention has been on the nature of the public sphere, its membership, democratic discourse, citizenship, and the formation of public opinion and debate.[4]

This book challenges the dichotomy between public and private in another way. It looks more toward the private sphere and finds interaction between what have been assumed to be two distinct spheres. The relationship between public and private is dynamic; it is not just that the public has invaded private life or that excluded, politically unrecognized groups, including women, have found ways to move into public life. Rather, during the period of this study, the private invaded the public. Abortion is an example of how private activities and conversations reshaped public policy. The words and needs of women had the power to change medicine, law, and public debate. The public sphere, moreover, was not the only place where crucial communication and spirited debate occurred. They occurred in "private" arenas such as the home and the medical office. Those conversations, generally designated "private" and thus irrelevant to public discourse, impacted debates in the public sphere and eventually changed public policy. For over a century, women challenged public policy and altered medical thinking and practice through their conversation and activity in private arenas. I use the terms *private* and *public,* but with a sense of their ambiguity and interaction.

Analysis of public policy should examine how policy has been implemented and by whom, rather than be narrowly restricted to federal legislation or agency activity. Looking at statutes alone, or the actions of legislators or the judiciary, inhibits our view of how law works, how public policy is made, and who acts on behalf of the state to enforce the law. Abortion serves as a case study for rethinking the nature of the state in the United States. Much of the regulation of abortion was carried out not by government agents, but by voluntary agencies and individuals. The state expected the medical profession to assist in enforcing the law. It may be more accurate to think of the state apparatus not as the government, but as consisting of official agencies that work in conjunction with other semiofficial agencies. State officials, this history and others show, have often relied on "private" agents to act as part of the state.[5]

Feminist scholars in the 1970s tended to see the medical profession as the source of the regulation of female sexuality and reproduction, but the medical profession's role was more complex.[6] This book shifts attention to the state's interest in controlling abortion and the alliance between medicine and the state. It would have been virtually impossible for the state to enforce the criminal abortion laws without the cooperation of physicians. State officials won medical cooperation in suppressing abortion by threatening doctors and medical institutions with prosecution or scandal. Physicians learned to protect themselves from legal trouble by reporting to officials women injured or dying as a result of illegal abortions. By the 1940s and 1950s, physicians and hospitals had become so accustomed to this regulatory stance toward women and abortion that they instituted new regulations to observe and curb the practice of abortion in the hospital. The medical profession and its institutions acted as an arm of the state.

Yet the medical profession's position was contradictory. While physicians helped control abortion, they too were brought under greater control. State officials demanded that the profession police the practices of its members. The duty of self-policing and physicians' fears of prosecution for abortion created dilemmas for doctors who at times compromised their duties to patients in order to carry out their duties to the state.

Furthermore, plenty of physicians provided abortions. This book points to the power of patients, even female patients, to influence and change medical practice. The widespread practice of abortion by physicians attests to both the ability of patients to communicate their needs to physicians and the ability of physicians to listen. Physicians' practices were shaped by the experiences and perspectives of private life, not only by professional antiabortion values. The physician-patient relationship was often more close than distant. This was particularly true in the early twentieth century, but became more class stratified as medicine became increasingly specialized and hospital oriented. Medicine was more of a negotiated terrain between physicians and patients than has been realized.[7]

The peaks of the medical profession's public hostility to abortion have obscured the depth of medical involvement in abortion. The antiabortion stance of organized medicine should not be mistaken for an accurate representation of the views and practices of the entire profession. This study views the medical profession as complex and composed of competing groups with opposing views and practices rather than as a unified whole. The medical profession was not monolithic, but divided in its attitude toward abortion and in its treatment of patients. This book differentiates between organized medicine and individual physicians. By "organized medicine," I mean medicine's institutional structures, such as the American Medical Association (AMA) and other medical societies, medical schools, and hospitals that produced the official, public image of the profession and acted in concert with the state. Furthermore, this study distinguishes between prescriptive commentary about medical practices, as found in the medical literature, and actual practice by physicians. These official and instructional materials reveal the thought, and perhaps the practice, of only a few. Finally, attention to specialization is crucial. Specialists played critical public roles in the history of abortion; their interests and those of general practitioners were not identical.

This book is the first to chart the nation's enforcement of the criminal abortion laws. To understand the power of law in the lives of the masses of Americans requires that one take seriously the experiences of ordinary people caught in criminal investigations. Thus it is necessary to analyze the processes and routine procedures of the legal system that shape those experiences. Most historians of crime and punishment have focused on police and prisons, while historians of women and the law have focused mainly on marriage and property rights, not crime.[8] Surprisingly little historical work has examined the relationship between medicine and law.[9] Few have studied law in practice.[10] Analysis of the day-to-day workings of the legal system, rather than statutory changes, judicial rulings, or the volume of cases, reveals how the law intervened in the lives of ordinary citizens to regulate reproductive and sexual behavior.[11]

Punishment for violation of the law and sexual norms has been gendered. In abortion cases, the investigative procedures themselves constituted a form of punishment and control for women. Publicity and public exposure of women's transgressions further served as punishment. This form of punishment served, in Michel Foucault's words, as "a school." The shame of public exposure was for all of "the potentially guilty," not only the individual who had been caught. This eighteenth-century mode of punishment, thought to have been replaced by the surveillance of the prison,[12] persisted in the state's response to women and their sexual crimes. Without analyzing gender, we cannot fully understand the systems of punishment.

Even as the abortion statutes remained the same through this period, the meaning of the law and the legality and illegality of abortion changed over time.[13] Law is not fixed, but fluid. The criminal abortion laws passed in every state by 1880 made exceptions for therapeutic abortions performed in order to save a woman's life. Because the laws governing abortion did not precisely define what was criminal and what was not, this had to be worked out in practice, in policing, and in the courts. The complexity of defining "legal" and "illegal" abortions for medical practitioners and legal authorities alike, the gray and ever-shifting nature of "criminality," is an important theme in this book. Nor was medical understanding of therapeutic abortion stable. Medicine too is interpretive and changing. Throughout the period of illegal abortion, physicians disagreed on the conditions that mandated a therapeutic abortion and on the methods: there was no consensus.[14] Changes in medicine influenced legal definitions of crime; at the same time, the law shaped medical thinking and practice. The medical profession and the legal profession each looked to the other to define the legality of abortion practices. Therapeutic abortion became increasingly important in the 1930s; by the 1960s the practice (and nonpractice) of therapeutic abortion was at the very heart of the campaign to reform and repeal the criminal abortion laws.

The illegality of abortion has hidden the existence of an unarticulated, alternative, popular morality, which supported women who had abortions. This popular ethic contradicted the law, the official attitude of the medical profession, and the teachings of some religions. Private discussions among family and friends, conversations between women and doctors, and the behavior of women (and the people who aided them) suggest that traditional ideas that accepted early abortions endured into the twentieth century. Furthermore, through the 1920s at least, working-class women did not make a distinction between contraceptives and abortion. What I call a popular morality that accepted abortion was almost never publicly expressed but was rooted in people's daily lives. Americans have a long history of accepting abortion in certain situations as a necessity and as a decision that, implicitly, belongs to women to make. This popular attitude made itself felt in the courts and in doctors' offices: prosecutors found it difficult to convict abortionists because juries regularly nullified the law by acquitting abortionists,[15] and few physicians escaped the pressure from women for abortions. Throughout the period of illegal abortion, women asserted their need for abortion and, in doing so, implicitly asserted their sense of having a right to control their own reproduction.

I am not suggesting a "gap" between people's beliefs and their ability to live up to them, but different, even oppositional, moral perspectives. The values expressed by ordinary people deserve to be taken seriously rather than categorized and dismissed as sinful or mistaken. Though some felt guilt about abortion and found ways to justify their behavior, others never held the official antiabortion views. Prescribed morality and popular morality may not be identical. Analysis of women's practices and ideas—popular behavior and belief—rather than exclusive focus on the statements of male theologians and philosophers suggests that it is incorrect to conclude that hostility to abortion is "almost an absolute value in history."[16] The reverse may be more accurate.

Although this book takes note of religious teachings and the religious background of women who had abortions, it does not focus on religious opinion. Organized religion had little interest in abortion until it entered the public, political arena in the late 1950s and early 1960s.[17] There was no reason to energetically fight abortion when, for nearly a century, abortion was a crime and no social movement suggested otherwise. From the 1920s on, however, there was much religious interest in, and division over, another method of reproductive control: contraception. Birth control became a topic of interest because a movement advocated women's right to reproductive control.[18] Further, it is incorrect to assume that the Catholic Church has always organized against abortion or that all Catholics subscribe to the views of their church leaders. Indeed, many Catholics shared what I have described as a popular ethic accepting abortion. A good history of religion and reproductive control would examine not only theology and sermons, but also the attitudes and actions of the congregations, with particular attention to women.

Women who had abortions did so within a context of illegality and religious disapproval, but the prohibitions were ambiguous. Christian traditions had tabooed abortion since antiquity, but the acceptance of abortion in order to save the life of a pregnant woman had a long tradition as well. Until the mid–nineteenth century, the Catholic Church implicitly accepted early abortions prior to ensoulment. Not until 1869, at about the same time that abortion became politicized in this country, did the church condemn abortion; in 1895, it condemned therapeutic abortion. Protestant churches accepted abortion when pregnancy threatened a woman's life, a view shared by the medical profession and written into the nation's laws. Jewish tradition clearly viewed the woman's life as primary. The Mishnah, a code of ancient Jewish law that guided later rabbinic thought, required abortion when childbirth threatened a woman's life, for "her life takes precedence over its life."[19]

This study points to the importance of studying the social history of sexuality as well as the medical and legal discourse about it. These discourses regarding abortion are important because they introduced new meanings of abortion and shaped people's views (and fears) of abortion and sexuality. I analyze the language women used to describe abortion and the production of stories about abortion in the press and in the courtroom. Yet exclusive attention to professional or even popular discourse about abortion would result in a distorted picture of that history. Medical discourse has convinced some scholars that physicians did not perform abortions in the period of illegal abortion,[20] and most press coverage of abortion in the early twentieth century gives the misleading impression that abortion was universally condemned and generally fatal. These conclusions are not correct. Analysis of discourse alone would miss the ongoing medical practice of abortion in total contradiction of official medical mores. As others have pointed out, Foucault's theory concerning the production of sexuality through discourse ignores differences in the power of individuals and social groups to enter and shape discourse.[21] The publicly articulated and published discussion of abortion rarely included the voices or perspectives of women who had abortions, except to provide shocking examples of depraved womanhood. Women who had abortions did not intervene to explain themselves, but instead, in other nonpublic arenas, made their perspectives known and acted to obtain a much-needed method for preventing births. More tolerant attitudes toward abortion, rooted in material experiences, persisted in the face of a public discourse that denounced it. The history of sexuality and reproduction demands a combined analysis of ideas and practice.

Common Law and the Criminalization of Abortion

Abortion was not always a crime. During the eighteenth and early nineteenth centuries, abortion of early pregnancy was legal under common law.[22] Abortions were illegal only after "quickening," the point at which a pregnant woman could feel the movements of the fetus (approximately the fourth month of pregnancy). The common law's attitude toward pregnancy and abortion was based on an understanding of pregnancy and human development as a process rather than an absolute moment. Indeed, the term *abortion* referred only to the miscarriages of later pregnancies, after quickening. What we would now identify as an early induced abortion was not called an "abortion" at all. If an early pregnancy ended, it had "slipp[ed] away," or the menses had been "restored."[23] At conception and the earliest stage of pregnancy before quickening, no one believed that a human life existed; not even the Catholic Church took this view.[24] Rather, the popular ethic regarding abortion and common law were grounded in the female experience of their own bodies.

Colonial and early-nineteenth-century women, historians have learned, perceived conception as the "blocking" or "obstructing" of menstruation, which required attention. The cessation of the menses indicated a worrisome imbalance in the body and the need to bring the body back into balance by restoring the flow. This idea of menstruation corresponded with medical and popular understanding of sickness and health. The body was a delicate system of equilibrium that could easily be thrown out of balance—by a change in weather or diet, for example—and that then needed to be restored through active intervention. A disruption in the healthy body, in the worldview of patients and physicians, required a visible, often violent, physical response to treatment in order to restore equilibrium. This theory underlay eighteenth- and nineteenth-century regular medical practice, which emphasized heroic measures—bleeding, blistering, purging, and puking—in response to sickness. The response to the blocking of the menses was part of this shared understanding of the body: women took drugs in order to make their menses regular and regarded the ensuing vomiting and evacuation as evidence of the drugs' effective action.[25]

Restoring the menses was a domestic practice. The power of certain herbs to restore menstruation was widely known. One colonial woman who feared pregnancy had "twice taken Savin; once boyled in milk and the other time strayned through a Cloath." Savin, derived from juniper bushes, was the most popular abortifacient and easily acquired since junipers grew wild throughout the country. Other herbs used as abortifacients included pennyroyal, tansy, ergot, and seneca snakeroot. Slave women used cottonroot. Many of these useful plants could be found in the woods or cultivated in gardens, and women could refer to home medical guides for recipes for "bringing on the menses."[26]

Both of these concepts, blocked menses and quickening, must be taken seriously by late-twentieth-century observers. Blocked menses cannot be dismissed as an excuse made by women who knew they were pregnant. Quickening was a moment recognized by women and by law as a defining moment in human development. Once quickening occurred, women recognized a moral obligation to carry the fetus to term. This age-old idea underpinned the practice of abortion in America. The legal acceptance of induced miscarriages before quickening tacitly assumed that women had a basic right to bodily integrity.

By the mid–eighteenth century, the most common means of inducing abortion—by taking drugs—was commercialized. The availability of abortifacients was so well-known that a common euphemism described their use. When Sarah Grosvenor, a Connecticut farm girl, confided to her sister in 1742 that she was "taking the trade," her sister understood.[27] That Grosvenor successfully conveyed her meaning to her sister in three metaphoric words tells us a great deal about the world of mid-eighteenth-century New England. Many New Englanders, including these sisters, knew of the possibility of inducing an abortion by purchasing and ingesting drugs. The need for a euphemism tells of the difficulty of speaking openly about sex and reproductive control and of the need for secrecy. Yet it reveals an awareness that women could and

did regulate their own fertility through abortion. Furthermore, abortifacients had become a profitable product sold by doctors, apothecaries,
and other healers.

The first statutes governing abortion in the United States, James
Mohr has found, were poison control measures designed to protect
pregnant women like Grosvenor by controlling the sale of abortifacient
drugs, which often killed the women who took them. The proliferation
of entrepreneurs who openly sold and advertised abortifacients may have
inspired this early legislation, passed in the 1820s and 1830s. The 1827
Illinois law, which prohibited the provision of abortifacients, was listed
under "poisoning."[28]

It is crucial to recognize what these early-nineteenth-century laws
did not cover: they did not punish women for inducing abortions, and
they did not eliminate the concept of quickening.[29] Even as poison
control measures, they said nothing about growing the plants needed
in one's own garden or mixing together one's own home remedy in
order to induce an abortion. The legal silence on domestic practices
suggests that the new laws were aimed at the commercialization of this
practice and, implicitly, retained to women the right to make their own
decisions about their pregnancies before quickening.

By the 1840s, the abortion business boomed. Despite the laws
forbidding the sale of abortifacients, they were advertised in the popular press and could be purchased from physicians or pharmacists or
through the mail. If drugs failed, women could go to a practitioner
who specialized in performing instrumental abortions. Advertisements
and newspaper exposés made it appear that what had been an occasional domestic practice had become a daily occurrence performed for
profit in northern cities. Madame Restell, for example, openly advertised and provided abortion services for thirty-five years. Restell began
her abortion business in New York City in the late 1830s; by the mid-
1840s, she had offices in Boston and Philadelphia and traveling agents
who sold her "Female Monthly Pills." Restell became the most infamous abortionist in the country, but she was not the only abortionist.[30] The clientele of these busy clinics were primarily married, white,
native-born Protestant women of the upper and middle classes.[31]

In 1857, the newly organized AMA initiated a crusade to make abortion at every stage of pregnancy illegal. The antiabortion campaign grew
in part, James Mohr has shown, out of regular physicians' desire to win
professional power, control medical practice, and restrict their competitors, particularly Homeopaths and midwives. "Regular," or "orthodox,"

physicians, practitioners of "heroic" medicine, had come under attack in the 1820s and 1830s as elitist. They faced competition from a variety of practitioners from other medical sects, collectively known as "Irregulars." Through the 1870s, regular physicians across the country worked for the passage of new criminal abortion laws. In securing criminal abortion laws, the Regulars won recognition of their particular views as well as some state control over the practice of medicine.[32]

Though professional issues underlay the medical campaign, gender, racial, and class anxieties pushed the criminalization of abortion forward. The visible use of abortion by middle-class married women, in conjunction with other challenges to gender norms and changes in the social makeup of the nation, generated anxieties among American men of the same class. Birth rates among the Yankee classes had declined by midcentury while immigrants poured into the country.[33] Antiabortion activists pointed out that immigrant families, many of them Catholic, were larger and would soon outpopulate native-born white Yankees and threaten their political power. Dr. Horatio R. Storer, the leader of the medical campaign against abortion, envisioned the spread of "civilization" west and south by native-born white Americans, not Mexicans, Chinese, Blacks, Indians, or Catholics. "Shall" these regions, he asked, "be filled by our own children or by those of aliens? This is a question our women must answer; upon their loins depends the future destiny of the nation."[34] Hostility to immigrants, Catholics, and people of color fueled this campaign to criminalize abortion. White male patriotism demanded that maternity be enforced among white Protestant women.

The antiabortion campaign was antifeminist at its core. Women were condemned for following "fashion" and for avoiding the self-sacrifice expected of mothers. "The true wife," Storer declared, did not seek "undue power in public life, . . . undue control in domestic affairs, . . . [or] privileges not her own."[35] The antiabortion campaign was a reactionary response to two important efforts of the nineteenth-century women's movements: the fight to admit women into the regular medical profession and the battle to make men conform to a single standard of sexual behavior. The antiabortion campaign coincided with the fight by male Regulars to keep women out of their medical schools, societies, and hospitals. Boston and Harvard University, Storer's hometown and alma mater, were key sites of struggle over women's place in medicine, and Storer was personally engaged in the battle against female physicians.[36] Advocates of women in medicine argued that women doctors would protect women patients from sexual violation.[37] Regular male doctors degraded female physicians by accusing them, along with midwives, of performing abortions.

The relative morality of men and women was of crucial importance to this campaign. For the specialists, whose interest in the female reproductive system raised questions about their sexual morality, the antiabortion campaign was a way to proclaim their own high morality in contrast to their competitors, their female patients, and even the ministers who tolerated abortion.[38] It was at the same time a backlash against the women's movement's critique of male sexual behavior and feminist claims to political power. Nineteenth-century feminists expressed their anger with male sexual domination and promiscuity in a number of movements, including the campaigns against prostitution and slavery and the fight for temperance. All sections of the women's movement advocated "voluntary motherhood," a slogan that addressed both men's sexual violation of their wives and women's desire to control childbearing. Women saw themselves as morally superior and urged men to adopt a single standard—the female standard of chastity until marriage, followed by monogamy and moderation.[39] The campaign against abortion challenged this feminist analysis of men by condemning women for having abortions. Indeed, Storer compared abortion to prostitution and, in so doing, called into question all claims made by middle-class nineteenth-century women on the basis of moral superiority. "There is little difference," he proclaimed, "between the immorality" of the man who visited prostitutes and the woman who aborted.[40] The nineteenth-century women's movements never defended abortion, but activist women and women doctors were blamed for the practice of abortion nonetheless.

The antiabortion campaign attempted to destroy the idea of quickening. As physicians targeted quickening, they discredited women's experiences of pregnancy and claimed pregnancy as medical terrain. "Quickening," as Storer described it, "is in fact but a sensation." A sensation that had emotional, social, and legal meaning was thus denigrated. Quickening was based on women's own bodily sensations—not on medical diagnosis. It made physicians, and obstetricians in particular, dependent on female self-diagnosis and judgment. Quickening could not be relied upon as an indicator of fetal life because, Storer argued, it did not occur at a standard moment. "Many women never quicken at all," he joked about women's perceptions, "though their children are born living."[41] Storer's propaganda aimed to erase the distinctions between earlier and later stages of pregnancy, thereby redefining the restoration of the menses. What had previously been understood as a blockage and a restoration of the menses prior to quickening was now associated with inducing a miscarriage after quickening by labeling it abortion. Furthermore, Storer equated abortion with infanticide.[42]

Regular medical men had entered the debate about sexual politics by attacking the female practice of abortion as immoral, unwomanly, and unpatriotic. In giving abortion new meaning, the Regulars provided a weapon that white, native-born, male legislators could use against the women of their own class who had been agitating for personal and political reform. Regular physicians won passage of new criminal abortion laws because their campaign appealed to a set of fears of white, native-born, male elites about losing political power to Catholic immigrants and to women. Class privilege did not protect middle-class white women from public policy designed to control them. Although the criminalization of abortion was aimed at middle-class white women, it affected women of every class and race. The new laws passed across the country between 1860 and 1880 regarded abortion in an entirely different light from common law and the statutes regulating abortifacients. In general, the laws included two innovations: they eliminated the common-law idea of quickening and prohibited abortion at any point in pregnancy. Some included punishment for the women who had abortions.[43] The "Comstock Law" passed in 1873 included abortion and birth control in federal antiobscenity legislation; states and municipalities passed similar ordinances.[44]

The antiabortion laws made one exception: physicians could perform therapeutic abortions if pregnancy and childbirth threatened the woman's life. A bill criminalizing abortion unless done for *"bona fide* medical or surgical purposes" passed the Illinois state legislature unanimously and was signed into law in 1867. A few years later, Illinois passed another law prohibiting the sale of abortifacients but made an exception for "the written prescription of some well known and respectable practicing physician." Physicians had won the criminalization of abortion and retained to themselves alone the right to induce abortions when they determined it necessary.[45]

Through the antiabortion campaign, doctors claimed scientific authority to define life and death. In so doing, they claimed the authority of religious leaders. In leading this moral crusade and thoroughly criticizing the ministry's lack of interest in abortion, regular doctors set themselves above religious leaders as well as above the general populace. The medical profession's claim to moral purity and the authority of the clergy was a stepping-stone to greater social authority. Regular physicians won an important victory when they persuaded the nation's states to criminalize abortion. Physicians entered a new partnership with the state and won the power to set reproductive policy. In the process, women's perceptions of pregnancy were delegitimated and women lost what had been a common-law right.

Periodization: Changing Patterns of Illegal Abortion

During the more than one hundred years that abortion was illegal in the United States, the patterns, practice, policing, and politics of abortion all changed over time, though not always simultaneously. I trace the history along several lines at once, according to the location, practice, and availability of abortion as well as its regulation. Abortion was widely available throughout much of the era when abortion was a crime. Yet periods of tolerance were punctuated by moments of severe repression. At some points the changing structure of medicine brought about crucial changes in the history of abortion; at others, changes in women's lives or the political and economic context came to the fore.

In the nineteenth century, abortion came under attack at a moment when women were claiming political power; in the twentieth century, it came under attack when they claimed sexual freedom. Abortion, like contraception, means that women can separate sex and procreation— still a controversial notion. Antiabortion campaigns developed when women asserted sexual independence, as during the Progressive Era and since the 1970s. When abortion was most firmly linked to the needs of family rather than the freedoms of women, as during the Depression, it was most ignored by those who would suppress it. Periods of antiabortion activity mark moments of hostility to female independence.

The epoch of illegal abortion may be broken down into four periods. The first covers the time from the criminalization of abortion state-by-state, accomplished nationwide by 1880, to 1930. This period, covering fifty years, is heavily marked by continuity. As other historians have also found, the reproductive lives of most women and the day-to-day practice of most physicians changed slowly.[46] In this period, abortion was widely accepted and was practiced in women's homes and in the offices of physicians and midwives. The diversity of practitioners, the privacy of medical practice, and the autonomy of physicians in the late nineteenth and early twentieth centuries made the widespread medical practice of abortion possible. A crackdown on abortion occurred between 1890 and 1920 as specialists in obstetrics renewed the earlier campaign against abortion, and the medical profession was drawn into the state's enforcement system.

The structural transformation that occurred during the 1930s, the second period, was crucial for the history of abortion. Abortion became more available and changed location. As the practice moved from private offices and homes to hospitals and clinics, abortion was consolidated in medical hands and became more visible. The changes wrought by the Depression accelerated the pace of change in the coming decades, particularly in the methods of enforcing the criminal abortion laws.

The third period was marked by increasing restrictions on abortion by state and medical authorities and intensifying demand for abortion from women of all groups. This period begins in 1940, when the new methods of controlling abortion were first instituted, and continues through 1973, when they were dismantled. In reaction to the growing practice of abortion as well as apparent changes in female gender and reproductive patterns, a backlash against abortion developed. 1940 marks a dividing line as hospitals instituted new policies, and police and prosecutors changed their tactics. The repression of abortion was part of the repression of political and personal deviance that took place in the 1940s and 1950s. Yet even in this period, the practice of abortion expanded in new directions in response to relentless demand. The new repression of abortion, however, was devastating for women. A dual system of abortion, divided by race and class, developed. During the postwar period, the criminalization of abortion produced its harshest results.

A new stage in the history of abortion, the movement to legalize it, overlaps with the third period. The movement to decriminalize abortion began in the mid-1950s and arose out of the difficult experiences resulting from the repression of abortion in the 1940s and 1950s. In the 1950s, a handful of physicians began to challenge the very abortion laws their profession had advocated a century earlier. The progress of that challenge attests to the continuing power of the medical profession to make public policy regarding reproduction. As legal reform moved forward, a new feminist movement arose, which radically transformed the movement for legal change. When the women's movement described abortion as an aspect of sexual freedom, they articulated a new feminist meaning for abortion; when they demanded abortion as a right, they echoed generations of women.

The structure of this book follows this periodization. The first half of the book uncovers the history of abortion from the late nineteenth century through the 1920s. Chapters 1 through 4 each cover different aspects of abortion, from women's lives to practice to politics to enforcement, during the first half-century of illegal abortion. The changes of the 1930s, both medical and social, precipitated other changes. The second half of the book traces the history of abortion in chronologically ordered chapters concluding with the U.S. Supreme Court decisions that ended the era of illegal abortion.

Women's history of abortion needs to be examined both as a commonly felt need to control reproduction, arising from women's biological capacity to bear children and social relations that assign childbearing to women, and in terms of differences among women. This book differentiates among women by class, race and ethnic identity, and marital status. Though class did not absolutely determine access to or safety of abortion, class position helped define when a woman felt she needed an abortion and affected the type available to her. In general, urban women had greater access to abortion than rural women, though some rural women located abortionists in their areas or traveled to cities for abortions. Race played a less obvious role in access to abortion, though the grim statistics of the postwar period show the connection between discrimination and death. I have made a specific effort to locate sources related to African Americans in order to learn more about black women's use of abortion and how race shaped the history of abortion.[47] Evidence concerning women of color is meager, however, until the 1930s, when medical and sociological studies began separating their findings by race. Before then, contemporary observers tended to focus their attention on the differences among many (white) foreign-born ethnic groups.

This book integrates a national analysis of the history of abortion with a local study. The advantage of this approach is that it connects everyday life and local medical and legal practice to national policy. It examines that relationship rather than assuming that all the public policy action takes place on the federal level without reference to local and "private" events. I select a major metropolis in order to uncover the nature of both abortion practices and police enforcement of the criminal abortion laws. Chicago, the second largest city in the nation, is the focus of my local study. Chicago, the city in "the heartland" that has often served as a metaphor for the spirit of America, was also known as an important medical center (the home of the AMA) and as a regional center for abortion.[48] Trains brought European immigrants, men and women migrating from farms to the city, African Americans moving from the South to the North, all going to live and work in Chicago. The same trains brought women looking for abortions. Directing my attention to one city enabled me to uncover the nitty-gritty details of the practice and regulation of abortion.

Though much of my analysis of the history of abortion draws on Chicago as a case study, sources verify that my findings hold true for other cities, large and small. Throughout I present national data and trends as well as regional ones and take note of patterns elsewhere. The book moves back and forth from a national overview of abortion practices and politics to a close look at events in Chicago. As medical practice became more standardized in hospitals, the story becomes a more national one and key events take place in other cities: New York, Detroit, Baltimore, Philadelphia, San Francisco, Washington, D.C., and elsewhere. This is primarily a study of abortion in urban areas, where abortion was concentrated. I comment occasionally on practices in rural areas, but the history of reproductive control and abortion is likely to be somewhat different there.

Legal records, most notably lower-level court and criminal trial records, and medical literature make up the foundation of my research. I have also surveyed other government documents, newspapers, popular periodicals, hospital records, and manuscript collections. Using these materials, I have delineated how medical thinking and state regulation have changed over time. Yet this is more than a study of prescriptive literature or policy. I have uncovered the circumstances of hundreds of actual induced abortions and reconstructed changing abortion practices.[49] This study periodizes the history of abortion for the first time.

This book presents the lives of many women and their abortions in rich detail in order to convey the variety and intricacy of the situations that made abortion necessary for women. It is in the minutiae of women's lives that we can discover why women had abortions and how they won sympathy from physicians who belonged to a profession dedicated to fighting abortion. Abortion was a moment in a woman's reproductive life. It cannot be separated from sexual relations or reproduction as a whole. Women themselves did not separate them, nor should we, whether analyzing abortion in the past or present. This book deepens our understanding of the female experience of reproduction and the connections between sexuality, contraception, pregnancy, and childbirth.[50] At its most fundamental, a policy that restricts abortion is one that forces women into maternity. Without contraceptives and abortion, most women in heterosexual relationships will become pregnant and bear children, whether they want to or not. When women sought abortions, they often revealed the texture of heterosexual relations and the rest of their lives. Many situations made enduring pregnancy unbearable to women. In using abortion, women rebelled against the law and asserted their sense that the decision to carry a pregnancy to term or to abort was theirs to make. A few expressed in words as well as in action the view that abortion was their right. The experiences of women's private lives and private practices over the course of one hundred years altered medical thinking and reshaped public policy. Despite the fact that women's abortion narratives are part of our own contemporary discourse, the stories told here have long been hidden.

CHAPTER I

An Open Secret

Her period was late. She had two children, one sixteen years old, one six. She was thirty-four. Frances Collins knew she was pregnant. She told her husband she had "missed." This had happened before and she had taken care of it before. Mrs. Collins talked to a "lady friend" about her problem. Her friend suggested Dr. Warner: "Go over and see him," she said, "he might be able to fix you up." In the first days of April in 1920, Mrs. Collins went to Dr. Warner's office on the West side of Chicago to have "her womb opened up," something, she commented later, she had "done many times." After the doctor inserted an instrument into her womb, she returned to her home at 4338 W. Congress. She called her husband away from his work as a master printer and told him, as he later recalled, "I am unwell." He asked her, "'Natural?' And she says no. That is all." Jerome Collins knew what she meant. When later asked at the inquest into his wife's death whether she told him any details about the abortion and where she had gone, Jerome answered, "No, she did not outright, she just said 'I had it done,' that is all." His wife lay down and rested. She seemed fine, but by the end of the month, she was "sick again"—the term commonly used for menstruation—"and she started to flow pretty hard." At that point, her husband called his mother-in-law to care for her. Finally, as things further declined and his wife was vomiting and getting chills, she told him to call the doctor who had performed the abortion. Dr. Warner visited her at home two or three times to care for her. At the end of April, Mrs. Collins's family doctor, Dr. Joseph T. Woof, saw her and hospitalized her. Dr. Woof had attended her in childbirth and knew that she had "had several abortions, against [his] advice."[1]

This vignette of Frances Collins's abortion suggests that abortion was not an unusual feature of married life in the early twentieth century. Both Mr. and Mrs. Collins seemed to take a matter-of-fact attitude toward abortion. They did not talk about it at length, but Jerome Collins was not surprised when his wife told him in few words that she had "had it done." He understood her meaning because she had done the same before. The Collins couple tacitly agreed on abortion as the means to avoid adding another child to the family. Her doctor, who had cared for her family for ten years, knew that she had had "several abortions created," though, as he said, "against my advice." Nonetheless, Dr. Woof described Mrs. Collins as "a very grand woman, one of the grandest little women the Lord ever created." Her abortions did not detract from her doctor's high opinion of her.[2]

Despite the criminalization of abortion nationwide, abortion continued, and despite the efforts of Dr. Horatio Storer and his antiabortion allies, the thinking of ordinary Americans about early pregnancy had not been transformed. Abortion was widely tolerated. Many ordinary Americans at the turn of the century had not adopted the idea that there was a rigid dividing line between menstruation and conception, but continued to think of menstruation and early pregnancy as related. Abortion continued to be an important method of birth control, particularly for working-class, married women like Collins.[3] Early-twentieth-century women's use of abortion was part of a long tradition among women to control and limit their childbearing.

In the past twenty-five years feminists have often used the metaphor of "silence" to describe the subordination of women. Describing women as silent and silenced brought attention to the dominance of the masculine voice in politics, law, medicine, and the media and the near absence of women's words and perspectives in these public political forums. The powerful metaphor's provocative image of the silenced woman—unable to speak, ignored and unheard—reverberated with women's experiences and encouraged women to be bold and to speak of their lives. In the late 1960s, an important tactic of the movement to legalize abortion was getting women to tell of their abortions at "speak-outs" and thus discover their shared experiences and shared oppression.[4] However, the metaphor of silence has limitations, for it has at times obscured women's historical experiences by portraying women as more isolated, helpless, and victimized than they felt.[5]

Within the limitations imposed by a sexist society in general and the laws forbidding reproductive control to women in particular, women found ways around the restrictions to obtain what they needed. Instead of visualizing women as gagged and silenced, it is more helpful to envision them talking about abortion as a "secret." It is notable that Frances Collins spoke of her abortion with others, including her husband, her "lady friend," and her doctor. Her friend understood her situation and helped her by naming a doctor who might perform an abortion. Although women could have abortions without anyone knowing about it at the turn of the century, many, like Mrs. Collins, talked about their abortions and relied upon friends, relatives, or partners to help them carry out their abortion plans. Thinking of abortion as cloaked in "secrecy" emphasizes the point that it was a topic of conversation while suggesting that those who spoke of abortion did so discreetly and selectively.

The metaphors of "silence" and "speaking" implicitly refer to women's ability to speak in specific forums from which women have been excluded. The speech that has been privileged is political speech in national and local civic institutions controlled by men. Emphasizing the "silence" surrounding abortion inaccurately represents the history of abortion and ignores what women did say in other arenas; women talked about abortion often. We need a more nuanced understanding of the ability of women to voice their concerns and of the limits on women's speech. They did not proclaim their abortions in open, political forums, but they did speak of their abortions among themselves and within smaller, more intimate spaces. Women talked about abortion in "private" spaces, at home, and in the semiprivate, semipublic spaces of medicine such as drug stores, doctors' and midwives' offices, hospitals, and birth control clinics. Discussion of abortion, like other female experiences of reproduction, was part of female life and conversation. These shared experiences, rooted in biology but socially created and culturally understood, helped forge the bonds of gender within social groups.[6] In some circumstances abortion might have been openly discussed with close friends; in other instances, it was, at most, whispered about.

The evidence shows that many American women and their friends and family accepted abortions. The widespread acceptance of abortion, expressed in word and deed during the era of its illegality, suggests the persistence of a popular ethic that differed from that of the law and the official views of medicine and religion. This popular acceptance of abortion took into account women's sense of their own bodies, the particular situations in which women found themselves, and the material reality that made women and men need reproductive control. This finding suggests the need to refine our thinking about morality. Neither legal statutes nor the words of priests, ministers, or rabbis can be assumed to represent the moral thinking of the citizenry or congregations. Instead of assuming universal agreement on the immorality of abortion as expressed in the law and insisted upon by regular medical leaders, we might think of gradations in moral thinking or the existence of multiple moralities. The behavior and beliefs of ordinary people in daily life deserve serious attention. Abortion was part of life.

Frances Collins died following an attempted illegal abortion.[7] If she had been successful, a friend and her husband would have known about her abortion; perhaps a few relatives and other friends would also have learned her secret—but I would know nothing of Frances Collins and her abortion. I know of her strategy for getting rid of her pregnancy only because she died and because her death reached the attention of the Cook County coroner who conducted an inquest into it. At the inquest, witnesses described Collins's life, her pregnancy, her efforts to abort, and her death. A court reporter recorded their testimony. A transcript of these proceedings has been preserved as a public record in the Cook County Medical Examiner's Office in Chicago. The records generated by the coroner's office during inquests were produced for specific legal tasks, but because of the structure of an inquest, much more informal than a trial, they contain a great deal of information about individuals and, at the same time, permit the observation of patterns of abortion. Analysis of inquests into women's deaths resulting from illegal abortions are crucial for my analysis of abortion from the late nineteenth century through the 1930s. Many of the details of early-twentieth-century abortion practices and the most intimate stories of women and their relationships are drawn from these public records. These stories can be painful to read because the women died as a result of their illegal abortions, but their deaths allow us to learn about the lives of women, particularly immigrant and working women, who were most likely to appear in legal records. In studying these texts closely, this book honors the lives of these women who died trying to control their reproduction. Their deaths, however, were unusual. Most women survived their abortions and never had to tell anyone unless they chose to do so.

Mrs. Collins was one of hundreds of thousands of women who had abortions every year. Some late-nineteenth-century doctors believed there were two million abortions a year.[8] In 1904, Dr. C. S. Bacon estimated that "six to ten thousand abortions are induced in Chicago every year." As one physician remarked in 1911, "Those who apply for abortions are from every walk of life, from the factory girl to the millionaire's daughter; from the laborer's wife to that of the banker, no class, no sect seems to be above . . . the destruction of the fetus."[9] As early-twentieth-century reformers investigated abortion, they produced and preserved knowledge of the business. Their reports, themselves evidence of the growing scrutiny of female sexual and reproductive behavior, show that a significant segment of the female population had abortions. A study of ten thousand working-class clients of Margaret Sanger's birth control clinics in the late 1920s found that 20 percent of all pregnancies had been intentionally aborted. Surveys of educated, middle-class women in the 1920s showed that 10 to 23 percent had had abortions.[10] Anecdotal information, patient histories collected at maternity and birth control clinics, and mortality data show that women of every racial and religious group had abortions.[11] A more comprehensive survey conducted by Regine K. Stix of almost one thousand women who went to the birth control clinic in the Bronx in 1931 and 1932 found that 35 percent of the Catholic, Protestant, and Jewish clients alike had had at least one illegal abortion.[12] By the 1930s, Dr. Frederick J. Taussig, a St. Louis obstetrician and nationally recognized authority on abortion, estimated that there were at least 681,000 abortions per year in the United States.[13]

Most of the women who had abortions at the turn of the century were married. Tracking changes in the demographic characteristics of those who had illegal abortions is difficult, but evidence shows that abortion continued to be a practice of mostly married women until after World War II.[14] Yet the image of the seduced and abandoned unmarried woman dominated turn-of-the-century newspapers and popular thinking. The image of the victimized single woman spoke to fears of the city and the changing roles of women in the same way that visions of married women aborting had expressed mid-nineteenth-century anxieties. Newspapers, physicians, and prosecutors highlighted the abortion-related deaths of unwed women.[15]

When women themselves spoke of abortions they usually did not use the medical word *abortion*. Their language gives insight into women's perspectives on pregnancy and its termination. The term *abor-*

tion was a foreign and formal word, part of the jargon used by professionals, not an ordinary word used by ordinary people. Discovering the vernacular for an illegal practice is difficult, but the phrases used by women and men appear occasionally in turn-of-the-century abortion reports. One woman told a New York doctor, "I have missed twice, but I am going to bring my courses on," and a Chicago doctor sold pills to one woman to "bring her around."[16] These phrases tell of the persistence of older notions that perceived early pregnancy as a menstrual problem. Mrs. Collins used few words to indicate that she had had an abortion; she "had it done." Other women declared that they wanted to be "fixed up," just as Mr. Collins reported that his wife's friend had named a doctor who might "fix" her.[17] One woman reported that she had gone to a doctor twice "to be put straight."[18] Once the period was back on schedule and the pregnancy ended, her crooked, out-of-kilter body had been put straight and realigned. The words these women used suggests they perceived their bodies as out of order. When women declared that they wanted to "get rid of" it, their language more frankly admitted the presence of a pregnancy.[19] Yet it also suggested that there was something foreign inside the woman's body, that perhaps she had been invaded and needed to "rid" herself of it. One man recalled his wife telling him of going to a midwife "to get rid of the child."[20] This phrase more explicitly equated pregnancy with a live human being and echoed the language of the physicians, officials, and reformers who argued that once conception occurred, the embryo was equal to a child. A dispensary nurse reported in 1918 that when she visited a pregnant patient who had never returned to the clinic, the patient smiled and said, "Thank the Lord, I have been relieved."[21]

I have used the term "abortion" throughout this book to refer to the purposeful ending of pregnancies at every stage. I am using the term promulgated by medicine and law since the mid–nineteenth century and one that Americans today take for granted, but it is somewhat of an anachronism for the early twentieth century. We have all adopted the medical term "abortion" to describe the efforts to get the period back on schedule and to end extremely early pregnancies, but in the early twentieth century the attempt to redraw the line at a different point in the reproductive process, at conception, was a point of cultural struggle. It is crucial to keep these changing and contested understandings of pregnancy and abortion in mind.

We know of some of the talk among women about abortion because doctors described women's conversations. Physicians were privy to everyday female conversations about reproduction in general, which at times included the topic of abortion. Some medical men were surprised by what they heard of women's attitudes toward reproduction and remarked on it. For example, in response to newspaper exposure of doctors who did abortions in 1888, Dr. Truman W. Miller defended his profession by exposing female conversation and activity. "I am sure there is no comparison between the number of abortions committed by doctors and the number committed by women themselves," he charged. "They talk about such matters commonly and impart information unsparingly." Thirty years later, another physician observed a "matter of fact attitude" about abortions among "women of all ages and nationalities and . . . of every social status." [22]

At professional meetings and in medical texts, physicians told their colleagues of women's attitudes toward abortion and detailed the methods women used. The reports in some cases were no more than a sentence or two in an article about another issue or a remark made during the discussion of a paper presented at a meeting and later published. Physicians presented information about women's abortions as interesting anecdotes, as patient "history" and prelude to their own medical innovation, or as part of a medical discussion on abortion. As medical researchers learned statistical methods, they collected data on dozens or hundreds of cases in order to answer questions about maternal mortality and morbidity or to test and argue for particular treatments in abortion cases. Physicians who acted as reporters of abortion practices for other physicians and the public, whether shocked, sympathetic, or scientific, appear throughout this book. From these different types of medical reports, I glean medical perspectives and practices and read these sources against the grain to grasp the perspective of women having abortions.

To the dismay of medical leaders, the public still believed that quickening marked the beginning of life. The practice of abortion persisted nationwide. "Many otherwise good and exemplary women," Dr. Joseph Taber Johnson reported in 1895, thought "that prior to quickening it is no more harm to cause the evacuation of the contents of their wombs than it is that of their bladders or their bowels." [23]

Women's critics found it provoking that women did not appear to be ashamed about their illegal abortions, but freely discussed them, advised each other in the methods for inducing abortions, and referred their friends to abortionists. One physician observed in 1891 that leading ladies of the community "not only . . . commit this crime, but talk about it very unconcernedly, or engage in disseminating a knowledge of the work among friends as earnestly as they would work for a supper for the benefit of a hospital, kindergarten, or the far-distant heathen."[24] The scene sketched by this doctor implicated well-to-do, respected women active in voluntary and charitable activities in the crime of abortion and criticized them for treating the subject lightly. It may be fruitful to read the doctor's comparison literally: control over their own reproduction was as important to women as building a hospital or caring for the needy. Indeed, women's involvement in charitable and reform activities made the ability to control childbearing necessary, and that control made voluntary activities possible.

A Massachusetts doctor told his colleagues of a trick he played on a patient, which points to how women told each other of their abortions. A "young wife" had come to him seeking an abortion, and he had tried unsuccessfully to dissuade her. So, "thinking a little delay might bring about a better reasoning" on her part, the doctor finally gave her a placebo. The woman miscarried after a train accident but believed it was thanks to his help. "She showed her gratitude," the doctor recalled, "by sending to me one after another of her friends, I think seven in number, who insisted in having the same prescription that I had given Mrs. X." Another doctor remarked on abortion as a way to argue against making birth control information available to "laymen." Women who had illegal abortions, he remarked, were "not . . . secretive about the matter when it comes to passing this knowledge on to some sister who is also in trouble." In the same way, he warned, women would pass information about contraceptives. Physicians' recollections make clear that female dialogue included talking about abortions.[25]

Women shared with one another very specific knowledge about how to induce abortions. Female sharing of abortion techniques was both part of the routine exchange of knowledge about how to treat illnesses of all kinds and a continuation of earlier traditions when women traded recipes for abortifacients.[26] "The older ladies of the community are prolific in advice," one Chicago physician remarked in 1900. "Hot drinks, hot douches and hot baths are recommended. Violent exercise is suggested and jumping off a chair or rolling down stairs is a favorite procedure. Certain teas are given . . . and the different emmenagogue pills are too easily procurable."[27]

"Older ladies" shared the traditional techniques known to them; younger women shared more modern and scientific information. The information women gave each other changed over time along with changes in medicine. When a turn-of-the-century physician warned a young married woman of septic infection, the woman answered, " 'My friend told me to boil my catheter before using it.' "[28] Medical precautions against sepsis, this report suggests, had entered popular knowledge. Armed with medical wisdom and personal experience, these patients dismissed warnings and vexed their doctors. Barbara Brookes has found that early-twentieth-century English women "helped" each other induce abortions. American women did the same. In 1920 a nurse reported the story of a married, working-class woman, "Annie K.," who had induced three abortions already and, if pregnant, planned to do so again. When warned of the dangers of abortion, "Annie laughed and said: 'Oh! it's easy.' And . . . added: 'I have told lots of women how to do it.' "[29]

Women also aided each other in finding someone else to do an abortion. Female relatives often helped find and pay for abortions. Helping daughters, sisters, and nieces obtain abortions was, like attending deliveries and giving advice on child rearing, part of the maternal role and sibling relationship. The nature of familial relationships would determine to which relative, whether older or a peer, individuals turned. The willingness of female relatives to obtain abortions for their kin cut across class, from the wealthiest to the poorest families. A New York physician told of a patient, "the mother of many children, a lady of considerable wealth," who sought an abortion for her daughter-in-law.[30] In 1917, when Ellen Matson, a very poor, second-generation Swedish woman, had an abortion, her mother, sister, and aunt knew of it. Matson's mother and sister visited her at the doctor's home after the abortion; her aunt loaned her five dollars from her meager funds.[31] Twenty-one-year-old Mary Colbert did not ask her aunts to help her obtain an abortion, but the aunt who raised her wished she had. After her niece's death as a result of abortion, Annie Cullinan mournfully recalled having asked her, "Mamie, why did you not tell me, and I would get a good doctor."[32]

Parents, especially mothers, often played a crucial role in the effort to obtain an abortion when their daughter was unwed. Reflecting the sympathies and training of gender, daughters generally turned to mothers for help when faced with a pregnancy out of wedlock. In the late nineteenth century, Joan Jacobs Brumberg has argued, illegitimacy became a "traumatic event" for middle-class families, which threatened the reputations of both the unmarried women themselves and their families.[33] Many parents had a strong interest in protecting their daughters and themselves from the shame associated with single mother-hood. In late-nineteenth-century New York, one woman approached a female doctor about an abortion for her daughter, whose fiancé had fled. "Death before dishonor," the mother reportedly declared, "my daughter is not going to be disgraced all her days, and the man to go scot-free."[34] The mother's words succinctly summarized the sexual double standard: she knew that bearing an illegitimate child would stigmatize her daughter for life while the boyfriend could experience sexual pleasures without hurting his honor. If fathers were apt to over-react to their obvious inability to control the sexuality of their daugh-ters, daughters and their mothers might collude to keep the man of the house ignorant. In 1914, when Mrs. Julia Reed's eighteen-year-old daughter's period did not arrive, Mrs. Reed took her to two people to find out whether she was pregnant, bought pills to induce an abortion, and, when that did not work, took her daughter to another doctor, whom she paid for an abortion. Throughout the entire episode, neither mother nor daughter told the father of the family for fear he would kick the daughter out of the house. In contrast, both of Emma Alby's par-ents responded to their single daughter's supposed pregnancy as a fam-ily problem and tried to solve it by finding an abortionist.[35] However, not everyone could assume that their female relatives would help or sympathize with their need for abortions. One woman reminded her sister that abortion was a "sin." Some parents, outraged at discovering the pregnancy of an unmarried daughter, threw their daughters out of the familial home.[36]

To avoid the social disaster of single motherhood, turn-of-the-century physicians and women's charity groups urged unwed women to bear their children in maternity homes. Some homes arranged for adoption of the illegitimate infants; others insisted that the new moth-ers keep them. *The Journal of the American Medical Association* viewed these homes as a way "to combat the crime of induced abortion."[37] Yet many homes refused African American women. One African American physician established a hospital in Louisville, Kentucky, in order to pro-vide a place where unmarried African American women could deliver their babies and give them up for adoption instead of having abor-tions.[38] The policies of unwed mother's homes could be oppressive. Maternity homes expected mothers to repent and required them to stay long periods of time, perform domestic tasks, and participate in re-ligious services. State agencies and private charities required the women, whether keeping or giving up their newborns, to breast-feed for several months.[39] Some women surely concluded that an abortion, though illegal, could be a simpler solution to a pregnancy out of wedlock. Regina Kunzel has found that many women in maternity homes had tried but failed to abort their pregnancies. One maternity home inmate gave her new friends at the home valuable information for the future: she described how to do their own abortions.[40]

The economic difficulty of rearing children as a single woman helped push the pregnant and unmarried to have abortions. Working women earned wages half those of men and inadequate for a woman by herself, let alone with dependent children. A 1908 study of Chicago's store and factory workers found that more than half of the women living alone earned less than a subsistence wage. Although real wages increased in the 1920s, the average female worker in manufacturing still earned below subsistence. African American women, who were segregated into domestic service jobs, were paid less than white coworkers.[41] Furthermore, single working mothers risked losing their children as a result of being charged with child neglect by reformers and officials.[42]

Female friendship at times included participating in abortions.[43] Female work companions could prove to be good friends indeed. When Mary Schwartz told Marie Hansen, a coworker at the Illinois Meat Company in Chicago, of her "condition" and asked for her help, Hansen immediately accepted this duty of friendship. "I will try and help you the best I [can]," Hansen recalled telling her friend. Mary Schwartz depended upon Hansen from beginning to end. Schwartz asked for help on a Monday and that day Hansen took her to Dr. Justin L. Mitchell's office at 79th and Halsted, south of Chicago's meatpacking district where they worked. Three years earlier, Hansen had gone to Mitchell for an abortion; now they told him that Schwartz "wants to get fixed up" and negotiated with him to drop his price from fifty dollars to thirty. Schwartz got a loan for twenty-five dollars, for which Hansen co-signed, and Hansen personally loaned her five dollars "in dimes" to pay for the abortion. The next morning Hansen brought her friend to Dr. Mitchell's again, waited outside the office while he operated, and took her to her own home to recuperate. When Schwartz fell ill that evening, Hansen called the doctor and "told him that she was bad sick." Hansen followed the doctor's orders and gave Schwartz castor oil and placed warm towels on her stomach to stop her pains, but her friend "kept on suffering." She took her to the doctor on Thursday evening and again on Friday morning for a second operation. Hansen reminded the doctor to perform the medical procedure properly:

"Don't forget to scrape her. . . . and do a good job." At 4 A.M. Saturday morning, a very worried Hansen called Schwartz's lover to come get Mary, "because she was real bad sick." Joe Hejna, who worked as a foreman at the Illinois Meat Company, drove over, picked up Mary, called in his own doctor, and rushed her to a hospital. Schwartz leaned on her friend every step of the way and her loyal friend was at her side throughout the entire abortion process. This is all we know about the quality of the women's friendship: when Mary Schwartz asked Marie Hansen for help, she helped. The grief that Hansen must have felt when she testified at her friend's inquest was muted. The only hint of her feelings is that she had to be told to "talk up a little louder."[44]

Women's daily lives could include all aspects of reproduction and its control—from delivering babies to ending a pregnancy. In 1928, while Catherine Beyer visited a friend who had just given birth, another friend, Catherine Mau, asked Beyer to accompany her to the office of a Chicago midwife for an abortion. Beyer later recalled that Mau had explained to the midwife that "she had three children and her husband was out of work and she could not support another one, and that her husband was sickly." The midwife took her patient into another room and inserted a catheter while Beyer waited outside in a rocking chair. The two friends left the midwife's office to return to their homes, children, husbands, and dinner duties.[45]

Women helped friends and relatives who had abortions by nursing them and by assuming their domestic duties. Beyer visited Mau two days after the abortion to help the midwife "wash her out" and put her to bed. Then Beyer fed Mau's children.[46] When Collins became feverish, her husband called in her mother to care for her. Another woman's friend nursed her at home and cooked special soups for her. Elsie Golcher arranged for a friend and a sister-in-law to watch her children while she was away from home during her abortion. When concern about Carolina Petrovitis's well-being reached a crisis point after her abortion, the women attending her intervened. Carolina's sister and female neighbors consulted and decided to call in a doctor whom they trusted, not the one called by her husband. The group telephoned a doctor who had successfully taken care of a lady across the street who had been "sick in the same condition."[47]

Caring for the sick, especially for women during pregnancy, was a social responsibility shared by neighboring women. Female friends and relatives determined when the situation had become an emergency, when to call in a doctor, and which doctor to call. Though cities encouraged anonymity, a sense of community persisted. These women lived in an immigrant neighborhood of one of the largest industrial cities in the world, but their sense of collective responsibility for women during pregnancy echoed the assumptions and actions of midwife Martha Ballard and the neighborhood women of rural eighteenth-century Hallowell, Maine.[48]

Many counted on female friends and relatives to see them through the entire process of abortion—from locating the abortionist, to raising money to pay for it, to accompanying them to the abortionist's office and observing the procedure, to nursing them during their recovery and taking over household duties for them. Expressing understanding and giving material assistance during abortions, as during childbirth and other female life events, was for many a part of the fabric of female friendship.[49] The expectations women had of their female friends and relatives at these times were only rarely preserved in print, but we have observed the ways in which women depended upon each other at crucial moments. Female friendship meant being able to rely upon each other in time of need.

Women also counted on men. Lovers often helped women obtain abortions. Men and women in unmarried couples shared assumptions about what should be done in the event of pregnancy: women had abortions; men paid for them. Male assumption of financial responsibility fit heterosexual dating norms, which required men to cover the costs of entertainment and often to pay for other living expenses as well. Records of early-twentieth-century Cook County coroner's inquests into women's abortion-related deaths reveal working-class boyfriends acting on this assumption and paying for their "sweethearts'" abortions. A survey of 1,300 college students found that elite couples had the same expectation in the event of an unwanted pregnancy.[50]

Some men were more actively involved in the abortion than simply paying for it. Boyfriends hunted for the names of abortionists and made the initial contact.[51] When Ellen Matson told Charley Morehouse that her period was late and taking quinine "did not bring it on," he arranged an appointment for her with a doctor. He went to the doctor with her and paid for the box of "brown pills," which she took every hour every day for over two weeks. When those failed, he got the name of another doctor and gave her the money for an abortion. Afterwards, he picked her up and took her home.[52] In some instances, men accompanied their lovers to the offices of abortionists.[53] John Harris, a waiter who had little money, agreed to pay the costs of a private hospital and a $100 operation to care for his sweetheart after her abortion. When the woman's physician ordered wine "to wet her lips," Harris ran out to purchase it.[54] After one woman's abortion, her male friend remained with her at the nurse's flat and talked with her all night trying to calm her fears.[55]

A remark made by one young man implies that he assumed that his lover would make her own decisions about her pregnancy. Edward Dettman related that when Mary Colbert told him she had missed her period, she asked him, "What can be done?" He responded, "I don't know, that was up to her." Colbert had indeed made up her mind. She refused his offer of marriage. She told her lover that she did not want to marry in "disgrace"; instead he took her to Dr. Emil Gleitsman for an abortion. Her boyfriend had offered to marry, Colbert told her aunt, but she chose a different path. "She did not want to get married then," her aunt recalled being told. "She did not want to marry anyone."[56]

It is useful to examine this particular episode further to interrogate assumptions about the motivations of unmarried men involved in illegal abortions and the desires of unmarried women. In the analysis of nineteenth- and early-twentieth-century feminists, abortions occurred because of male sexual exploitation and pressure. Feminists believed that unmarried women had abortions because they had entered a sexual relationship on the understanding that sex was a prelude to marriage; if pregnancy resulted, women expected to marry. If a woman had an abortion, it meant, to feminists and others, that she had been abandoned by her lover, who refused to marry. Feminist interpretation of abortion did not admit the possibility of female sexual independence, only female victimization. Other possible explanations for abortion— that the woman did not want to marry, or that both parties in the relationship viewed the potential child and the potential marriage as impossible, or that some women, like men, participated in sexual affairs that they had no intention of concluding in marriage—were not acknowledged. It was difficult for turn-of-the-century feminists to recognize alternative explanations for the situation of young, single women when only a few radicals and birth controllers were beginning to talk about female sexual pleasure. Nonetheless, Joanne Meyerowitz has found that by the 1920s some reformers realized that the young women were not all victims.[57]

As we reach the end of the twentieth century, it is problematic to employ nineteenth-century feminist assumptions that all unwed women who got pregnant were victims, that their boyfriends were villains, and that abortions were evidence of victimization.[58] After all, the turn of the century was a time when heterosexual dating norms were changing and women increasingly experimented with (hetero)sexuality and challenged older sexual norms. In part, some feminists still emphasize female victimization because one segment of contemporary feminism views heterosexual relations as inherently oppressive.[59] That an unmarried woman had an abortion does not necessarily mean that her hopes of marriage had been dashed and she had been abandoned by an irresponsible young man. Nor does it necessarily mean she "chose" abortion because she chose freedom from marriage. We cannot make either of these assumptions about every case; the interpersonal relationships and their meanings are more complex and difficult to get at. In the Colbert case, *she* decided to get rid of the pregnancy, and he helped her. Exactly what prompted her actions, what her feelings were, we cannot know (we cannot even assume that she knew), but there are some hints. She told her lover she did not want to marry and have it known in her family that she had married in "disgrace." She told her aunt something a bit different; she did not want to marry anyone. Why did she have the abortion? The answer probably lies in both of the reasons she gave: she did not want to marry, and she did not want to marry in this situation, and, perhaps, she did not want to marry this particular man. The point is, her boyfriend did not refuse to marry, did not abandon her, never to be seen again, and did not coerce her into an abortion; he followed her wishes.

Furthermore, the independence achieved through earning wages gave some women the freedom to turn down undesirable marriages. One turn-of-the-century physician believed that "the emancipation of the modern woman" helped explain the ubiquity of abortion. He reported that one modern, wage-earning woman said that she "was not going to give up a hundred-dollar place for a fifty-dollar man."[60] The meaning of abortion for unmarried women at the turn of the century is not clear-cut, but ambiguous. We need nuanced, not facile, analysis of the intimacies of heterosexual relationships and the reasons for abortion.

In questioning the assumption that when single women had abortions they had been wronged by their lovers, I do not deny that some men treated their lovers badly. Some women were seduced and abandoned; some were raped. The stories of Milda Hoffmann and Edna Lamb in Chicago in 1916 and 1917 fit the dominant ideology about abortion and female victimization. Seventeen-year-old Milda Hoffmann was the classic "woman adrift." She left the home of her mother and stepfather in Milwaukee for Chicago, where she worked as a "chamber maid" and lived alone in one room. No one knew her seducer, and her mother knew little of her life.[61] Edna Lamb had several boyfriends, but her girlfriend believed that the one "responsible" for Lamb's pregnancy was a traveling man with whom, she had heard, Lamb had gone to a hotel. Lamb told her doctor she could not marry because the man was dead. Perhaps.[62]

Although it was unusual for husbands to be as involved as many boyfriends were in their sweethearts' abortions, some men supported their wives' plans to have abortions or helped them find abortionists. The boyfriends' active involvement grew out of the circumstances in which these pregnancies occurred—outside of marriage. Pregnancy made the lovers' illicit affair visible, and both unmarried men and women had an interest in covering up the affair. Though husbands might support abortions, their wives often took care of this matter themselves. Carolina and George Petrovitis, an immigrant couple with children, discussed and agreed that they did not want more children: "We both did not want it—we want to take a rest." She found a midwife to help her on her own, however.[63] The relative noninvolvement of husbands compared to boyfriends during abortions paralleled the role of husbands during childbirth. Childbirth was a female event, and husbands stayed out of the birthing room. Nonetheless, husbands had specific duties during deliveries: they ran to get the midwife or doctor and paid the bill. They generally did not pick up the domestic tasks that a new mother could not perform, such as cooking and watching the children; instead, a female relative or neighbor usually helped out with those chores.[64] In the same way, female relatives, neighbors, and friends were more important than husbands in assisting married women having abortions.

Although husbands tended to play a minor role when their wives had abortions, some tacitly agreed with the plan to avoid bearing a child. Husbands often became involved in abortions only late in the process, when they called in other women and doctors as their wives' health deteriorated. Jerome Collins called in two doctors and his mother-in-law to care for his wife when she took a turn for the worse. Frank Mau, another Chicago husband, knew his wife was pregnant in 1928 and that "she wanted it taken away." He knew nothing more about it until one February night at 2 A.M. when his wife told him to call the midwife and she miscarried at home. Like Collins, Frank Mau called in a physician about two weeks later when his wife was in great pain. Both women died of peritonitis, infections following their abortions.[65] Though their deaths were shocking, neither husband appeared to be shocked by his wife's abortion.

Some husbands tried to control their wives either by forbidding abortions or by insisting on them. A native-born farmer's wife with one child told Dr. Anne Burnet in 1889 that "she would like to have a family but her husband objected," and so she had five or six abortions. She had first gone to a doctor for the operations, but after her husband acquired an instrument from the doctor, she induced the abortions herself because "it cost less."[66] Nineteenth-century feminists often blamed husbands for married women's use of abortion. Husbands, in feminists' analysis, abused their wives, first in bed and again when they forced them to undergo abortions.[67]

Q: When was Mrs. Projahn first taken ill or consulted a Doctor . . . ?
A: On September 7. . . .
Q: What induced you to go to him on this occasion, your family was growing too large?
A: That's the way the wife figured it.
Q: She didn't want any more children?
A: No.

Earnest Projahn answered the questions put to him by the deputy coroner during the inquest into his wife's death.[68] On a Friday night in September of 1916, Projahn had taken his wife to a doctor for an abortion. During the inquest, Mrs. Emily Projahn's determination to limit the number of children in her family became evident. To a hospital intern she explained, "My husband and my self came to the conclusion that we had enough children and wanted something done so we would not have to support another." The Projahns had four living children; two others had died. She did not want another child and felt her husband's salary as a fireman could not support one. Her husband later claimed that he opposed the abortion and "spoke against it all the time." Though he may have made this statement in the hopes of avoiding further legal trouble for his role in the abortion, his remark, "That's the way the wife figured it," suggests that he followed her lead in this matter, however reluctantly. Mr. Projahn eventually came around to his wife's way of thinking and performed the male role of locating the abortionist and accompanying her to the doctor's office.[69]

Mrs. Projahn explained why she wanted to abort her pregnancy in the new language of the birth control movement. They could not "af-

ford" another child.[70] The birth control movement, supported by socialist movements, had been actively promoting the idea that the size of
working-class families could be controlled and that childbearing could
be linked to family finances. Birth controllers advocated the use of contraceptives as revolutionary and spoke to several concerns at once. The
working class, they claimed, could use birth control in their fight
against class oppression by refusing to produce wage workers and soldiers. It was a method, neo-Malthusians promised, by which the poor
could rise above poverty. Emma Goldman, Margaret Sanger, and feminists added to this radical working-class argument the idea that birth
control would free women. It would free (married) women from the
oppression of compulsory motherhood and allow them to enjoy sex.
The rise of the early-twentieth-century birth control movement marked
an important change in feminism as the birth controllers rejected the
old strategy of abstinence and declared the legitimacy of female sexual
pleasure.[71]

Though working-class and immigrant couples like the Projahns in
Chicago seemed to have readily adopted the language of the birth control movement to describe their desire to limit their number of children, the method they used to achieve family limitation—abortion—
was condemned by the birth control movement. The birth control
movement not only promoted the use of contraceptives and a new way
of thinking about reproduction and the family, it also generated its own
abortion discourse. The birth control movement struggled to teach
people that, first, contraception and abortion were different and, second, that one was morally acceptable and the other not. The birth control movement's rejection of the attitude that treated discussion of reproduction, sex, and reproductive control as shameful, its acceptance of
female sexual desire, and its claim that using contraceptives was moral
were all radical steps. Yet the movement did not break with nineteenth-
century feminist thought on abortion. Birth controllers contrasted the
danger of abortion to the safety of contraceptives and argued strenu-
ously against abortion.[72] Though some women adopted the birth controllers' negative opinion of abortion and used the medical term for it
by the 1920s, they still had abortions. But they reported feeling "guilty"
about their actions.[73]

Reeducating the public on abortion was not going to be an easy
project. Birth controllers explained over and over again in their literature and in speaking with their clients at clinics that birth control did
not mean abortion. Yet, despite their emphatic denials and careful
definitions of birth control, women still came to birth control clinics

looking for abortions. In 1927, Chicago's clinics, which had been telling women for several years that they did "not approve of or perform abortions," turned away 201 patients, or 16 percent of their clientele, because of pregnancy.[74] The importance of abortion to poor women in the tenements, from Jews to Italian Catholics, can be seen in Kate Simon's memoirs of growing up in a post–World War I immigrant neighborhood in the Bronx. As an adult, Simon learned of her mother's thirteen abortions, which, her mother informed her, was "by no means the neighborhood record."[75]

The *Birth Control Review* became a forum in which this struggle between the movement and its followers was recorded. The movement used abortion to bolster its claims for the morality of contraception by differentiating between the two and claiming that contraception could combat abortion. As part of the campaign to legalize and legitimate birth control, Margaret Sanger and the *Review* reprinted verbatim heart-wrenching letters received from women around the country. Many wrote thinking that Sanger's advocacy of birth control meant she could help them prevent births by ending pregnancies. When the *Review* published these letters, however, it editorialized that this was not birth control. At the beginning of one collection of letters from women telling of their abortions the magazine commented, "There is no commoner misapprehension concerning Birth Control than that which identifies it with abortion."[76] The more well-off leaders and workers in the birth control movement never defended abortion or discussed their own need for it, but they did express sympathy for women who faced motherhood against their wishes. Birth controllers blamed not women, but the laws that banned contraceptives and the physicians who refused to provide them. Abortions, therapeutic and criminal both, could be avoided, they argued, through the use of contraception.[77]

Because of the friction over the meaning of "birth control" between the leaders of the birth control movement and the poor women they meant to serve, I use the *Birth Control Review* (*BCR*) to gain insights into the thinking and lives of poor women who had abortions (or wanted them), a group given less attention in medical journals. Each woman's reasons for aborting were rooted in the particularities of her own life. The writers assumed that one had to know the details of daily life, typically regarded as mundane, in order to understand and see the necessity of abortion. As women beseeched a public figure who might be able to assist them but did not know them, they wrote of the intricacies and intimacies of their lives.

The power dynamics in heterosexual relationships influenced birth control practices and effectiveness. If a woman's husband refused to use any method of birth control and regarded sex as his pleasure to be had at will, she had a harder time avoiding pregnancy. As one writer to Sanger remarked in 1918, "My husband says he wants no more babies but I have come to believe he cares more for his passion than he does for me for he won't do anything to keep me from getting pregnant." For these women, abortion was particularly important. Women in more companionate marriages avoided this abuse, but not the fear of pregnancy. Couples who wanted to limit their family size but knew nothing about how to prevent conception sometimes agreed to avoid sexual relations in order to protect women from the dangers of another pregnancy. Women with husbands who agreed to leave them alone were comparatively lucky, but the fear of pregnancy destroyed more than one loving relationship. Moreover, this was a difficult agreement to keep, and a woman could, after months of abstinence, still end up pregnant and searching for a way to end it.[78]

Just about every woman in a sexual relationship with a man had pregnancy on her mind. Married and unmarried women alike often worried about the results of sleeping with husbands or lovers. When their periods were late, they noticed and watched. "I have missed my monthly sickness once and I am afraid I am pregnant as I never miss unless I am," related Mrs. C. M. C. in 1918. Another mother wondered if she was "not regular" and feared she might be "caught again." Both hoped for help if it turned out they were pregnant.[79] As Ellen Ross noted about London's poorest women at the turn of the century, these women, who lived "in a culture that was not very conscious of time, . . . nonetheless kept close track of their menstrual periods."[80]

"They tore me, and I didn't heal back right," wrote one poor Kansas woman about her daughter's birth. "Walking through hundred[s] of miles of fire could not have been as bad as what I suffered for her. I am afraid now to give birth to another." She almost died giving birth and now regularly took drugs to avoid pregnancy.[81] The dangers of childbirth drove married women to use contraceptives and abortion. Judith Walzer Leavitt has found that nineteenth- and early-twentieth-century middle-class women approached childbearing with foreboding. They remembered relatives and friends who had died during childbirth and knew of the debilitating injuries and illnesses women suffered due to childbearing.[82] Letters to Margaret Sanger in the 1910s and 1920s document the same fear of death during delivery among working-class and immigrant women. An immigrant mother of eleven children worried she was pregnant again. She hoped for a way out because, she said, "my last baby almost cost my life."[83] Another reported that the hospital doubted she would survive the delivery of her first child and during the agony of her second she prayed to die. She had had two abortions since, but feared she was "slowly killing [her]self."[84]

For many women, the need for abortion grew out of their concern for the well-being of their existing children. Most of the women who had abortions in the early twentieth century were married and already mothers.[85] Today, having abortions and having children are often set against each other as though to do one is to oppose the other. This is a false opposition that gives us an incorrect picture of how abortion fits, then and now, into women's lives.[86] Mothers often explained their abortions in terms of the family's scarce resources: another sibling would take food away from the children they already had and loved. For poor families, more children might mean that an older daughter or son would have to leave school to work for the family.[87] In richer families, it would be harder to send children to college. Even unmarried and childless women who had abortions may have thought in terms of the potential child, as they do today.[88] Perhaps they did not want their child to be ridiculed as a bastard or knew they could not raise it. This is not to suggest that women did not seek abortions for reasons of their own or that women's personal needs were inappropriate reasons. For some with visions of good jobs or education, having an abortion could be an assertion of control over their own destiny. For the poorest, whose lives seemed controlled by fate, abortion was not associated with personal freedom, but with family needs.

Mothers worried about their children when they had abortions. One New York mother of six said of her most recent abortion, "I know I am running an awful risk and do not care to leave my brood motherless. But what can I do?"[89] Women spoke of their children on their death beds. When told she was near death, Mrs. Mau "said that would be terrible, 'What will my children do?'" Several weeks later Mrs. Mau's three children lost their mother.[90]

In the early twentieth century, many children became orphans when their mothers died during childbirth or during abortions. The Cook County coroner counted the number of orphans created as a result of abortions; in 1918 and 1919 "a total of 215 children [were] left motherless" in the county.[91] We know little about these children whose mothers died due to illegal abortions. Some have given painful accounts of losing their mothers, of never being told why their mothers died, of lives and families torn apart. As adults, these orphans still grieve for their mothers.[92]

Family finances played an enormous role in women's decisions to abort. One outlined her family's meager budget and her grocery list when she wrote to Margaret Sanger. She described their meals: "We never have meat or fresh fruit or vegetables . . . many times we go two days at a time on only bread and coffee." She and her husband were "lovers of children," but, she explained, she could not feed her existing baby, let alone another. She was "behind" on her periods and looking for help.[93] Another woman sought birth control for her three daughters, each of whom had two children and periodically had abortions in order to avoid more. She feared for their lives, but they told her, *"They don't care for they will be better dead than to live in hell with a big family and nothing to raise them on"* (emphasis in original).[94] When a mother of nine on New York's east side delivered her tenth child, she "groan[ed]," the attending nurse reported, "Oh God! another mouth to feed."[95] Others literally could not afford to bear a child. Margaret Winter's doctor was suing the Winters for fees owed him for delivering their baby nine months earlier. She went to a midwife for an abortion instead.[96]

Poor women sought abortions because they were already overburdened with household work and child care and each additional child meant more work. A baby had to be nursed, cuddled, and watched. A baby generated more laundry. Young children required the preparation of special foods. Mothers shouldered all of this additional work, though they expected older children to pick up some of it.[97] A new child represented new household expenses for food and clothing. In 1918, a twenty-two-year-old mother of three despaired when she suspected another pregnancy. Her husband had tuberculosis and could barely work. They had taken in his five orphaned brothers and sisters, and she now cared for a family of ten. She did "all the cooking, housework and sewing for all" and cared for her baby too. The thought of one more made her "crazy," and she took drugs to bring on her "monthly sickness."[98]

Most women who had abortions, like these and like Mrs. Projahn, tended to bear children in the early years of marriage and to abort later pregnancies. They were reaching the end of their reproductive life cycles and, in some cases, the end of their ropes. In contrast, some upper-class women and their husbands tended to avoid childbearing in the earlier years of marriage (while in college) and aborted first pregnancies rather than last ones. Upper-class couples were having babies and beginning families as working-class couples finished their childbearing and began aborting pregnancies.[99]

Class affected birth control use as well. Middle-class married couples had greater access to contraceptives than did the poor or unmarried.

They could afford douches and condoms and had family physicians who more readily provided middle-class women with diaphragms. The birth control movement regularly condemned doctors who refused to give poorer women information about how to avoid pregnancy. (Such refusals were not always a result of conscious hostility; many doctors were themselves ignorant about birth control).[100] Even if poor women obtained contraceptives, the conditions in which they lived made using those contraceptives difficult. For women living in crowded tenements that lacked the privacy they might want when inserting diaphragms and the running water they needed to clean the devices, using a diaphragm would have meant another chore that only the most determined could manage.[101] For the poor, withdrawal was certainly a cheaper and more accessible method, if the husband chose to use it.

Some women sought abortions because they were afraid of being beaten by husbands who reacted with rage when they learned that another child was on the way. "I am a poor married woman in great trouble," began one woman's letter begging Sanger to "take pity" on her and help her end a pregnancy. She had two children, a toddler and an infant, and wrote, "I['']m in the family way again and I['']m nearly crazy for when my husband finds out that I['']m going to have another baby he will beat the life out of me." Desperation permeated this woman's letter; she would "rather jump in the river" than have another baby. Whether she wanted a baby or not is unknowable; the wife beating made her "want" an abortion. She promised to pay for help received: "I [would] rather starve a couple weeks or months and get enough money . . . so I wouldn't have another baby."[102]

Like many women, this one quite logically thought that "birth control" and "family limitation" included preventing birth through abortion. The popular tradition of women did not make a distinction between contraception and abortion, but saw them as part of the same project—a way to avoid unwanted childbearing. An asterisked editorial note in *BCR* reminded readers of the birth control movement's definition of birth control and where it drew the line in responding to women's needs for reproductive control. "The tragedy of such cases," the editor commented, "is that the victims so often write in after it is too late for birth control to help them."[103]

Medical warnings to women about the danger of pregnancies prompted some to seek abortions. A Nebraska woman had two abortions during her sixteen-month marriage because her husband was "'diseased' and our doctor told us it was for the best not to have any [children]." On his advice, she had used a douche, but still conceived.

Then her doctor gave her medicines. Now, she said, "I use drugs every month to start my menstrual period and I know that I cannot live long, constantly taking these awful drugs." An Illinois woman who suffered from varicose veins had been told by her doctor after her first child not to have more or she might "never be able to walk again." Since then, she had been to a physician twice "to be 'put straight'" and feared "serious internal injury" if she went again. She sought birth control in order to avoid future abortions.[104]

Women's reasons for abortion were many and their need urgent. They found many ways to obtain abortions. A Chicago doctor presented a case that reveals some of the methods women used to induce their own abortions at home. Beginning in August of 1893, a married woman and mother of two realized her period was late. She "used steam and hot water, sitz baths, douches, much and various medication," Dr. Frank A. Stahl reported, "all without the hoped for result. Growing desperate, two weeks after [her] regular period a buttonhook was employed." Although she went to doctors for help, the woman's periods still did not return, and she resorted to another traditional method, "lift[ing] heavy chairs, boxes and weights." Not until December, five months after she had begun trying to get rid of her pregnancy, did her physician "empty the uterus."[105]

An abortion induced at home by the woman herself was the most invisible to observers at the time and remains so to the historian now. In cases where women successfully restored their menses at home, it is difficult for anyone to discern the difference between a regular period and one that was assisted. Most of the information we have about self-induced abortions is a result of unsuccessful cases coming to the attention of physicians who later reported them to their colleagues. As Dr. Stahl's report indicates, the eighteenth- and nineteenth-century domestic tradition of inducing early abortions continued after the criminalization of abortion. It illustrates as well women's escalating attempts to abort. When one method failed, another was tried. This woman followed the same pattern followed by colonial women: she began with folk remedies and drugs, then turned to instrumental means, invading her own uterus with a readily available tool used at home. Because she finally went to a professor of obstetrics, her strategies are known to us.

In the early twentieth century, many women who aborted their pregnancies did so themselves at home. There is no way to track the number of self-induced abortions, but my sense is that this practice declined over time as people increasingly turned to doctors for all forms of health care. The practice was concentrated in the groups with the least resources: the poor, African American, rural, and unmarried. Self-induced abortions were always dangerous, but the relative danger compared to childbirth was less in this period when maternal mortality rates were high than it was after the 1930s when maternal mortality finally fell. When domestic efforts to produce an abortion failed, pregnancies progressed and the danger of later instrumental abortions increased. Many women ended up in hospital emergency rooms. Some ended up in morgues. Dr. Maximillian Herzog, a professor of pathology at the Chicago Policlinic, asserted in 1900 that "by far the largest number of criminal abortions" were induced by women taking abortifacients, which caused hemorrhaging. Some women mixed their own home remedies. One Chicago woman told of applying a mustard plaster to her abdomen to induce an abortion. Women employed a wide array of instruments found within their own homes to induce miscarriages, including knitting needles, crochet hooks, hairpins, scissors, and button hooks. One physician testified that patients at Cook County Hospital in Chicago used hairpins and cotton balls to irritate the cervix and induce abortions. A domestic servant resorted to using a bone stay out of her corset to induce a miscarriage. A farm woman used a chicken feather.[106] Dr. G. D. Royston, who interviewed patients at a St. Louis dispensary in 1917, reported that "introduction of catheters, crochet needles, etc., by the patients themselves are first in frequency."[107]

Some evidence suggests that black and white women may have relied upon different methods to induce their abortions. Royston suggested that black and white women in his 1917 St. Louis study used different techniques to induce abortion, though his analysis was based on interviews with only four black women, compared to forty-seven white women. The black women, he found, "pinned their faith on drugs. Two attributed their successes to the ingestion of blueing and starch or gunpowder and whiskey." These items could all be found in homes. In contrast, almost half of the white women's abortions were induced by a physician or midwife and very few by drugs. A Cook County Hospital physician remarked of slippery elm that, "the colored folks used that a great deal."[108] If African American women were more likely than white women to self-induce their abortions, it had less to do with cultural differences than with lack of access to doctors and midwives, for reasons of poverty and discrimination.

Further evidence of early-twentieth-century women's self-reliance in performing abortions is recorded in business transactions. While some women creatively used whatever could be found around the house to induce abortions, others purchased abortifacients or other implements at a commercial institution located in their own neighborhoods and throughout the city—the drugstore. By 1889, there were over one thousand druggists in Chicago.[109] The pharmacist, not the doctor, was often the first health professional consulted by the sick or by women caring for ill family members. Pharmacists offered on-the-spot diagnoses and suggested remedies;[110] some advised their patrons on abortion methods. Druggists sold the rubber catheters, slippery elm, and orange sticks women used to induce their own miscarriages, as well as "Chichester's Diamond Brand Pills" and "Pennyroyal pills" to induce abortions.[111] One annoyed doctor wrote to the AMA after having been called late one evening to care for a woman who had a "severe attack of 'Cramps.'" He sent along a box of "Tansy and Pennyroyal Compound Pills" that a Detroit druggist had sold his patient; the druggist had "assured her that it would produce an abortion."[112]

Fairs and other mass public events that made up city life were places where women could learn of abortion remedies. At the 1922 Pageant of Progress in Chicago, Young Ling passed out printed business cards advertising medicine for "Ladies." The card listed in bold type, "Curing Ladies Stomach Sick and No Menses Every Month Medicine . . . 1 ounce for $25.00." One lady, who was not pleased to receive this bit of advertising, sent the card to the AMA.[113]

In addition to the pharmacists and others who sold devices and drugs that women used to induce abortions at home, numerous individuals offered abortions for a fee. Many women found midwives or physicians who performed needed abortions. This side of the abortion business is the focus of the next chapter.

The historical record clearly shows that generations of women desired and needed abortions, and neither law nor church nor taboo could stop them. In their conversations and behavior, women expressed their sense that abortion was morally acceptable, and through their actions they asserted a "right" to make moral decisions about reproduction and to use abortion. They did not use the language of civil rights to express their views, but simply assumed that the decision to avoid childbearing, through the use of contraceptives and abortion, was theirs to make. Their success in obtaining abortions, however, should not obscure the difficulties and dangers they faced or the degree to which they felt compelled to have abortions because of social mores, economic pressure, or male coercion. The risks and the illegality of abortion could not suppress the socially created and gendered need for abortion felt by women.

The involvement of a wide variety of people in abortion and their discussion of abortion at home, in the doctor's office, and in the arenas of family and friendship demonstrate a popular acceptance of abortion. The historical record offers, on a rare occasion, explicit statements that suggest not only that abortion was tolerated, but also that there was a persistent, implicit, popular belief that having an abortion was what we would now call a woman's "right." In 1929 one Chicago man, serving as a juror at a coroner's inquest into a woman's death due to abortion, expressed this popular ethic during a discussion of the legality of abortion. He asked with surprise, "But the fact that she does not want any more children does not make any difference?" The deputy coroner answered him, "No, not a bit." Then he and the physicians on the jury stressed that abortions for any reason except to save the woman's life were illegal. The juror said no more. We do not know whether he learned that he was wrong to assume it a woman's right to control her reproduction or whether he learned to keep quiet when surrounded by authorities.[114]

The evidence of people's behavior—the persistent use of abortion by women of all social groups, and the sympathy of many men and women for their doing so—suggests the existence of an alternative popular morality in conflict with the law. The popular attitude toward abortion viewed it as an appropriate response to an unwanted pregnancy in specific situations. A large segment of the female population had one or more abortions at some point in their lives, and many of those women gained support—material and emotional—from their male partners, female friends, and relatives. The antiabortion views written into statutes nationwide and asserted by the leaders of medicine not only did not reflect reality, but were hostile to the attitudes and behavior of many Americans.

In 1920, one medical commentator asked rhetorically, did "public opinion in the United States sanction abortion?" and concluded that it did indeed. "The United States," he argued, "tolerates abortion done within the bounds of discreet secrecy." Abortion was widely practiced, openly discussed, and accepted by many people, but only within small groups—between couples, inside families, and among groups of female friends. Only a few people articulated this popular but proscribed view in print. Even the commentator who argued that the public accepted abortion said so anonymously. Instead of acknowledging the prevalence of abortion, the public overlooked it and treated it, said "A. B. C.," as "an open secret."[115]

CHAPTER 2

Private Practices

"I can not take your case," Dr. E. W. Edwards told the nervous young woman seated in his office. "But," he added, "I have given your friend the address of a physician I can recommend for that. I know him to be safe or I would not send you to him." He comforted the woman by patting her hand and gave her and the young man with her Dr. John B. Chaffee's address. It was 1888, and the couple had approached a physician near Chicago's Opera House in search of an abortion. They followed his directions to 527 State Street, the heart of Chicago's downtown business district, and climbed upstairs to Dr. Chaffee's office. There, the young man first spoke quietly to the doctor, who immediately agreed to "do the work" and called the patient to a private room, ready to begin. Frightened, she asked about the danger. "It is perfectly safe," he replied. "I would not endanger your life. You will feel perfectly well after it, and no one, not even a physician, could ever tell there had been anything the matter with you." The doctor explained the abortion procedure in an effort to reassure his patient. Nonetheless, she was not prepared to begin that day, and her companion took over the negotiations. "Doctor," he asked, "do you often have cases of this kind—is there much of this abortion practice going on?" "Lord, yes, thousands are doing it all the time. The only thing to do when one gets into trouble is to get out again." When the young man asked where she could stay during the abortion, Dr. Chaffee gave the woman a business card with the name "Mrs. Pierce" on it, recommending this individual as one from whom she could expect "ex-

46

cellent care . . . and motherly treatment." Armed with this information, the pair walked to 1616 Wabash Avenue to arrange a room and nursing during the doctor's "treatments." Mrs. Pierce welcomed the woman warmly and again reassured her of the operation's safety: "Dr. Chaffee . . . is one of the best in the city. He is very careful, takes plenty of time, guards against inflammation, and is entirely safe to trust one's self to under such circumstances." The fees for nursing, room, and board were $15 per week.[1]

Finally, after hunting through the city, this couple had successfully located a physician, a nurse, and a room in which the young unmarried woman could safely and secretly have an abortion—her reputation preserved. They were pleased. Both were reporters for the *Chicago Times.* She was not the desperate unmarried woman she seemed, and he was neither her brother nor lover. Rather, the pair played these roles as part of their investigation of the abortion business in Chicago. They reported their discoveries in a month-long series of "revelations." The story began on December 12, 1888, and stayed on the front page every day through Christmas.[2] In the method of the New Journalism forged in the 1880s, these investigative journalists had gone undercover and underground, into the "social cesspool," to expose the underworld and elite hypocrisy and, thus, inspire social reform.[3]

The 1888 *Times* exposé is the earliest known in-depth study of illegal abortion. The investigation showed abortion to be commercially available in the nation's second largest city despite the criminal abortion law. The reporters retold their conversations with the hundreds of practitioners whom they had approached. They made the private practice of abortion public. As the newspaper published numerous, seemingly confidential conversations with Chicago's practitioners, it described the abortion underground. Abortionists, the journalists found, were drawn from the city's physicians and midwives. Furthermore, as the reporters' meeting with Dr. Edwards indicated, practitioners who did not perform abortions themselves had ties to those who did. Finally, the investigators discovered a widespread sympathy for the plight of unmarried, pregnant women. Doctors Edwards and Chaffee and nurse Pierce, the journalists observed, all seemed to understand a young woman's declared need for an abortion. This chapter begins by analyzing this late-nineteenth-century report on abortion and the creation of a popular story about abortion in the press. It ends by reconstructing the abortion methods and routines followed by physicians and midwives in actual abortion cases in early-twentieth-century Chicago.

The 1888 exposé is an excellent example of an important finding: the medical profession's relationship to abortion was laden with contradictions. The regular medical profession led the campaign to criminalize abortion around the country and publicly opposed abortion, yet numerous individual physicians responded to women's requests for abortion and participated in its illegal practice. Despite outward appearances of unanimity, the profession was divided. Official standards were not accurate depictions of the profession in the past.

The structure and location of health care, particularly in the turn-of-the-century city, provided the conditions in which abortion could flourish. Health care was not a unified system, but diverse, divided, and decentralized. Sectarianism divided physicians into Irregulars and Regulars; education, specialization, class, ethnicity, and sex further divided them. The diverse and decentralized character of health services contributed to the accessibility of abortion. In a city like Chicago with so many competing health care practitioners, those who sought illicit services could always appeal to someone else.[4] The unobserved nature and domestic location of medical practice further enhanced the availability of abortion by keeping it hidden. Most health care, including abortions, took place in patients' homes, practitioners' offices, or sometimes other nonhospital settings such as Mrs. Pierce's.[5] Physicians generally practiced alone, and no one scrutinized their decisions or practices; they enjoyed the privilege of autonomy. Midwives also practiced alone, though they faced growing intervention from various investigators during this period. Each of these structural features of turn-of-the-century medicine contributed to the thriving abortion trade.

The ongoing practice of abortion in spite of the criminal law, particularly by physicians, attests to women's ability to explain their lives and their need for reproductive control. Women found ways to communicate their needs to practitioners, both male and female, doctors and midwives, and gain their sympathy and aid. Medical involvement in abortion contradicts the assumption that doctors did not practice abortion. More generally it shows physicians to have been responsive, not impervious, to patient demands. Furthermore, the ability to respond to women's expressed need for controlling their fertility was not restricted by gender. Numerous male physicians, like Doctors Edwards and Chaffee, comprehended the lives of their female patients to such an extent that they helped them obtain abortions.

Some of the tensions around abortion evident at the turn of the century related to the issue of money and medicine and the profession's desire to separate itself from the market. Medicine was a private business. I use the terms *private* and *business* deliberately. Physicians and patients regarded their interactions as private and confidential. Medicine seemed private since it was unobserved and often took place behind closed doors and in domestic spaces. In these intimate settings doctors heard women's words and learned from them. Yet it was a semi-public relationship, since the state monitored medical practice through licensing requirements and the profession attempted to regulate itself. Furthermore, medicine was a business, though physicians preferred to think of themselves as independent professionals who worked for the greater good. "Fee for service," and the tendency to advertise despite professional ethics forbidding it, pointed to the commercial aspects of medicine.[6] The newspaper exposé made the private commercial practice of abortion public.

Women in rural Illinois and elsewhere in the Midwest, along with women in Chicago, had access to Chicago papers and abortion stories. By the end of the nineteenth century, Chicago was a national printing capital, and numerous newspapers competed for readers' attention. Dailies, weeklies, and a thriving foreign language press sold papers throughout the city for a few pennies each.[7] Newspapers were an urban phenomenon that described and constructed the idea of the city for their readers.[8] Chicago attracted people from the region and around the world. Many came for the entertainment and the commercialized sex industry for which the city was known.[9] The city also attracted women looking for abortions.

The *Chicago Times*'s vivid and detailed report on the prosperous business of abortion offers an extraordinary opportunity to reconstruct the abortion underground at the turn of the century. Yet this rich story does more than "reveal" reality—it is the product of a particular breed of journalists with their own assumptions and goals. In exploring the underside of the city and exposing it in order to bring about social improvement, these "new journalists" combined exciting writing with moral fervor and an eye to selling papers. The *New York World* and London's *Pall Mall Gazette* have been credited with creating this new style of journalism, but the *Chicago Times* was also recognized as a leader in this investigative, "realistic" mode of reporting. The abortion exposé is a typical example of the "stunts" carried out by reporters of the time, who went in disguise to expose crime and corruption. Two of the most famous reports were Elizabeth Cochran's exposure of the insane asylum on Blackwell's Island for the *New York World* and W. T.

Stead's exposé of London's sex trade in virgins in the *Pall Mall Gazette*. Reporters intended the facts to arouse outrage and stimulate reform and, as Judith R. Walkowitz's analysis of the Stead case shows, stories about the sexual underground stimulated excitement and voyeurism as well.[10]

Not only was the *Times* well-known for its scandalous style, it was a defender of the immigrant masses and loyal to the Irish Catholics of the city.[11] The *Chicago Times*'s investigative report about abortion helped construct social divisions along class and ethnic lines at the same time that it constructed an abortion narrative. As the paper pointed to the hypocrisy within the medical profession, the Protestant clergy, and church-going ladies, it suggested that a specific class—the city's native-born, Protestant elite—was most in need of reform. According to the *Times*, the medical profession should kick out "malpractitioners" like Chaffee instead of pursuing doctors who advertised; the State Board of Health should revoke the licenses of those who agreed to perform abortions; ministers should focus on the immoral behavior of their congregations instead of the dangers of Sunday newspapers; and ladies should do their duty and bear children. The poor, in contrast, were cast as honorable: only they obeyed God's law to "perpetuat[e] the human race." Protestants compared unfavorably to Catholics, who, the paper asserted, almost never turned to abortion.[12] Although the paper praised Catholics, it occasionally struck a contradictory note when it appealed to the racial fears of white, native-born Protestants. "Is the Anglo-Saxon-American race to be driven out by the healthy sons and daughters . . . of Celtic, Teutonic, and Latin origin?" it asked. Like Horatio Storer, the *Times* implied that abortion threatened Yankee political power.[13] Readers added their own interpretations through letters to the editor. The story of abortion in Chicago, as it rolled off the presses day after day, did not get told in a linear fashion, but shifted as it presented alternate accounts.

The series ran under the headline "Infanticide." It began by describing the problem in Paris of single women from the country coming to the city, where they delivered and then killed their babies in order to avoid the humiliation of having to give their names to government officials. When the story moved to Chicago, however, the investigation did not focus on infanticide, but on abortion. The charge that infanticide was rampant in the city was frightening, for it called up images of murdering cherished babies, an image that editorial cartoons of babies and toddlers reinforced. (The use of illustrations was another modern

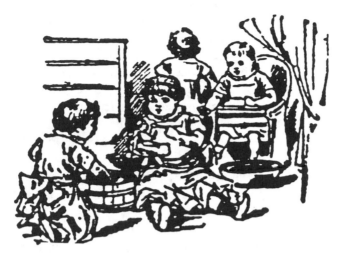

Plate 1. "It Comes down the Ages." The *Times* exposé helped equate abortion with infanticide by including sketches of children. *Chicago Times*, December 22, 1888, p. 4.

technique characteristic of the New Journalism.[14] See plate 1.) *Child-murder*, another term the paper used, constructed abortion as the active killing of children, rather than a means for bringing on the menses. These words and sketches erased the difference between abortions early in pregnancy, long before quickening, and the murder of living individuals. While this language expressed the horror some felt about abortion (as shown in letters to the editor), it taught others a new way to think about abortion. It denied the view held by many that abortion was a necessary and tolerable practice, an attitude that the paper's own investigation uncovered. Using the word *infanticide* invited ugly images and avoided terms that suggested sexuality and the female reproductive organs. Although the reporters used the word *abortion*, they treated it as a dirty word; the newswoman was surprised that Chaffee did not "take offense" when her partner used the term.[15]

The paper played to the voyeuristic interests of everyone in Chicago as the journalists constructed their stories in a manner intended to sell newspapers as well as to bring about reform. The "Infanticide" series began on a Wednesday with charges that Chicago harbored immorality equal to that of Paris and promises that incredible "revelations" about Chicago would begin the following day.[16] The newspaper began by naming midwives willing to perform abortions and alluded that physicians would be named as well.[17] On Saturday, the exposure of physicians, including Doctors Edwards and Chaffee, began. The paper promised that 10,000 extra copies would be printed for the Sunday edition and a few days later boasted that circulation had surpassed previous records.[18]

The *Times* began its exposé of the commercial underworld of abortion by going into the neighborhoods of midwives. Headlines tempted people to read, "How the Midwives Look upon Abortion and with What Ease They Can Be Hired to Perform It." The male reporter began by describing the "neatly painted, two-story frame house" in front of which hung a sign that said "Mme. Karl, Midwife" and invited his readers into her sitting room with him as he made the midwife's acquaintance. He told Mme. Karl of "a young lady relative [who] must be saved from the disgrace that must fall upon her . . . if she were permitted to become a mother." Could she help? The "plump" and "good-looking woman," as he described Karl, questioned him about how he got her name and remarked, "That is a very risky business." She needed to speak to the woman herself, but, she assured him, "It will be no trouble to get rid of it." Once she examined the patient, she would arrange for a doctor to perform the operation. After finishing his report on Karl, he described his visits to other midwives. Mme. M. Schoenian lived above a store and had a tin sign that advertised her midwifery services in German and English. "A stout, very stout, dumpy woman," Mme. Schoenian agreed to perform the abortion herself and promised safety. "I don't need any doctor," she explained. "I charge from $15 to $30, according to how long it takes."[19]

In this way, the reporter described the appearance of midwives and their homes, their cleanliness or lack thereof, and their accents, along with recording his conversations with them about abortion. These descriptions told readers that many of the midwives were immigrants and lived in poorer neighborhoods. The paper published the names and addresses of sixteen midwives who either agreed to perform abortions or gave the male relative, a reporter in disguise, a referral. The city's midwives, he concluded, were "all willing to perform the work necessary if . . . no exposure would result."[20]

Yet some midwives had refused to do abortions and offered to deliver the baby and arrange for its adoption instead. Midwives clearly provided a variety of reproductive services, from abortion to attending deliveries to arranging adoptions. When the journalist asked Mrs. Elizabeth Pemmer about an abortion for his unmarried "sister," she exclaimed, "Ugh! My God! I can not do that, but I will keep her until the child is born and then for $25 will get it into a good foundling house." Pemmer took unwed women into her home, cared for them up to the time of delivery, and promised secrecy. Mrs. Mary E. Thiery reacted the same way. (When the reporter pressed them, one finally offered an abortifacient; the other named a midwife.)[21]

The reporter, he noted in print, felt at "a disadvantage" as a lone man; he needed a woman at his side to present a more convincing show and to uncover the medical side of the abortion business. Midwives spoke of physicians whom they called for assistance, but would not give him their names. Eventually, "a young woman of intelligence, nerve, and newspaper training"—"the girl reporter" as the newspaper dubbed her—was added to the team. Both remained anonymous. When the (male) reporter introduced his new partner to his readers, he remarked that he was "in charge" of the investigation.[22]

The "girl reporter" stole the show nevertheless as she added a new dimension to the story: gender. Her reports showed how gender shaped her feelings in ways different from her male partner's. She told of feeling ashamed as she declared her own sexual impurity, even though the story was false. The girl reporter soon became a topic of interest herself and the object of speculation, adulation, and condemnation.[23]

The "girl reporter" discovered that some of the most eminent men in the medical profession were willing to participate in illegal abortion. Dr. George M. Chamberlain, one of Chicago's prominent physicians, agreed to "relieve her," but Dr. Chamberlain first asked who sent her to him, a question that, in the reporter's view, immediately revealed his guilt. Chamberlain was a staff member at St. Luke's Hospital and a member of both the AMA and the Illinois State Medical Society. The reporter pointedly remarked that this physician had gained his hospital position through his connections with "aristocratic ladies."[24] Perhaps, she implied, he had helped some of these ladies out of predicaments similar to the one she pretended. Dr. Milton Jay, dean of the Bennett Medical College of Eclectic Medicine and Surgery, also consented to perform an abortion.[25]

In concluding her day's report, the girl reporter mused as to a diary, "Tonight as I write this I am sick of the whole business." This personal writing style made the story intimate and interesting. It was a rare pleasure for readers to have the sensation of sharing a young woman's diary. It also consciously broke up the format of newspaper articles as it moved from reports to a more reflective style. "I did not suppose there was so much rascality among the 'reputable' people. I am sick of it," she continued, "because two or three of the physicians who expressed their entire willingness to take up my case were men I had heard the highest praise of." The elite doctors did not seem to be any better than the quacks from whom they distinguished themselves.[26]

The *Chicago Times* had a particular interest in exposing the respectable doctors; the girl reporter had remarked that she had been "commissioned only to see the physicians of the better class." She realized that "the dark and dirty stairways" of Clark Street probably led to innumerable physicians willing to perform the deed, but ferreting out the practitioners already believed to be the worst in the city was not the purpose of the investigation.[27] The city's reporters, elite, and medical profession expected to find illegal practices in the city's neighborhoods already labeled poor and criminal and populated by foreigners. What was unexpected and damaging to those who enjoyed the privileges of the upper classes was showing that men of the "better class," as well as their inferiors, participated in the illegal business of abortion. Poking at the hypocrisy of members of the class that regarded itself better than the immigrant masses was the paper's goal. And, not unimportant, it was a good way to sell papers to both the common people and high society.

Physicians' responses to women's requests for abortion can be broken down into four groups. On one end was the physician who refused to perform an abortion or help a woman in any way; the *Times* quoted a number of these physicians whom it congratulated. Next were the physicians like Dr. Edwards who did not do abortions themselves, but referred women to other physicians who would. These doctors played a crucial role in aiding women seeking abortions. This was the most common form of medical involvement in abortion throughout the era of illegal abortion. Then there were physicians, like Dr. Chamberlain, who occasionally performed abortions for their own patients. The majority of physicians probably fell into these last two categories. Finally, a few, like Dr. Chaffee, performed abortions regularly; they were the so-called professional abortionists.[28]

The *Times* investigation made it obvious that physicians were an important source of abortions and that abortion was part of regular medicine. The paper named forty-eight doctors who, when approached by an unwed woman seeking an abortion, agreed to help her. Thirty-four doctors agreed to perform the abortion themselves. Thirteen refused the girl reporter's request, but referred her to someone else who would; all but one sent her to a doctor. One sold her a box of pills and referred her to another doctor. Two-thirds of the doctors who agreed to perform an abortion were Regulars, several of whom belonged to the AMA. Many belonged to a national or local medical society.[29]

When the journalists, posing as sister and brother, approached Dr. James H. Etheridge about an abortion, he refused their request. "I don't handle such cases," he told them. "There are enough ways in this state for a man to get into the penitentiary without taking a crowbar and prying his way in." Yet Dr. Etheridge, like many others, relented and offered helpful information. He suggested they visit another office at Wabash Avenue and Harmon Court, where they might "find a man who would get the lady out of trouble." Two days after this account the paper reported that Etheridge had "emphatically indorsed this exposure." He praised the series and promised that doctors exposed as abortionists by the *Times* "will be promptly handed over to the judiciary committee of the Chicago Medical Society, who will handle them without gloves." Dr. Etheridge signed the letter as president of the Chicago Medical Society.[30]

The newspaper asked President Etheridge to explain himself. Etheridge offered a different interpretation of his conversation with the reporters. Although he might look like a "go-between," he told the reporter, he had some ideas of his own about how to capture abortionists. He had sent the couple to a known abortionist, figuring that if anything happened to the woman, he would be able to track the abortionist. His story echoed a contemporaneous cultural phenomenon of middle-class explorers of the underground who, when the murders of prostitutes by "Jack the Ripper" grabbed London's fears and fantasies, joined the police in detective work in poor neighborhoods.[31]

Etheridge was not the only doctor who supported the *Times*'s antiabortion crusade; the medical profession as a whole gave the newspaper "a hearty response." Medical men and women—both Regulars and Homeopaths—hastily joined the battle against abortion and the criticism of Chicago's women, midwives, and professional abortionists. The Chicago Medical Society held mass meetings and the national journal of the AMA commented on the investigations. Scores of physicians, in response to the *Times*' solicitation to put themselves "on record," wrote in support.[32] The Medico-Legal Society promised "moral and financial support to bring these abortionists to justice," and the *Times* gave its evidence to the society to help convict the abortionists. Medical students added their own drama to the story by saluting professors found to be honorable by surprising them with speeches and flowers. Students applauded the brave investigative work of the "girl reporter" as well: homeopathic medical students sent her flowers, and dental students sent her a gold pen. She thanked them and promised to use the pen's "pointed sharpness . . . to prick the sham and pretense" that sustained "social evil." [33]

The reaction of the city's regular medical association, the Chicago Medical Society, to the *Times's* accusations points to hypocrisy in medical support for the newspaper's antiabortion campaign. The charges against reputable physicians put the city's Regulars in an uncomfortable position since regular doctors had led the campaign to criminalize abortion and regarded themselves as superior, medically and morally, to other practitioners. The paper had accused several members of the Chicago Medical Society, including its president, of agreeing to help the woman who wanted an abortion. On December 17, 1888, the society met in a room "crowded to its utmost capacity" with 130 members and visitors to discuss the charges. Society members denounced the paper's investigation and defended their associates. One physician suggested that the society should conduct its own internal investigation. The purpose, however, would not be to expel colleagues, but to "exonerat[e] the members named." Dr. Jacob Frank's comments revealed his hostility to women working as journalists. He urged the society to defend its members against any charges "made by any woman . . . who went sneaking around like a snake, trying to make a reputation." Two journalists, one male and one female, had reported on abortion in Chicago, but she alone was the object of name calling. The group voted "to investigate the charges against three of its members, Drs. Thurston, Stanley and Silva." [34] The society did not investigate President Etheridge. Dr. Etheridge claimed that he planned only to gather evidence against the abortionist and that he trusted the community would understand for he was "well enough known" to be above suspicion. Etheridge relied upon his stature to protect him from blame, which it did. The society unanimously passed a motion "express[ing] its confidence in the professional integrity of its president." [35]

In the end, the Chicago Medical Society protected its members. The society applauded its president, exonerated one physician, failed to investigate others, and expelled only one, Dr. Thurston, for reasons unexplained in their own minutes. The *Times* claimed that Thurston had been expelled as a result of its exposé, though the society denied it. [36]

The 1888 exposé revealed the commercial world of abortion in Chicago at the precise moment that Chicago was gaining national recognition as a major medical center. As the city expanded and business boomed, medicine thrived as well. By the 1880s, Chicago had a national reputation as a nucleus of medical education, institutions, and organizations and had gained fame as a leader in connecting the laboratory and bacteriology to medicine. The city was a center of both regular and irregular medicine, with four outstanding regular medical schools, two homeopathic colleges, and an eclectic school, as well as proprietary medical schools, pharmaceutical colleges, and nursing and midwifery schools. The AMA's headquarters was located in Chicago. Two postgraduate clinics for training surgeons and other specialists, over two dozen hospitals, twenty dispensaries, and numerous medical societies and journals added to the pride of the city's medical establishment.[37] The exposure of the medical practice of abortion in Chicago suggested corruption at the center of medicine, belying medicine's pure and scientific exterior.

The exposure of medical involvement in abortion threatened the profession's identity as morally pure and trustworthy, thus jeopardizing its legal privileges and social authority. The physician-abortionists named in the exposé, an editorial in the *Journal of the American Medical Association* (hereafter referred to as *JAMA*) declared, "have blackened the good name of our noble profession." The claim that the profession could be trusted to be morally upright underpinned physician claims to independence in decision making and practice. The AMA had initiated the crusade to criminalize abortion thirty years earlier and had its headquarters in Chicago, yet could not patrol its own members. As an Indianapolis physician noted, "the medical profession must have felt embarrassed and humiliated" by the disclosures. The doctor, according to *JAMA*, "is supposed to be *more intelligent,* to be actuated by higher and *more noble* principles" (emphasis added).[38] Medical professional identity had become tied to a sense of moral superiority.[39]

Association with abortion threatened the medical profession in general, but it was especially threatening for physicians whose status was more precarious. Because they had long been disparaged as abortionists by male doctors and by the press, women physicians particularly needed to distance themselves from abortion.[40] Female physicians complained of the number of women who expected them to induce abortions out of feminine sympathy. Dr. Odelia Blinn reported in a letter to the *Times* that in one year more than three hundred women had asked her for an abortion. When the reporter approached Dr. Sarah Hackett Stevenson, nationally famous as the first woman admitted to the AMA, Dr. Stevenson refused to provide an abortion, advising her instead to marry. One woman physician agreed to perform an abortion.[41] Female physicians, who had trouble gaining respect from male colleagues, could not afford to be associated with abortion.

The *Times*'s representation of the women who had abortions was mixed. On the one hand, the use of a reporter playing an unmarried woman to learn about the abortion trade suggested that it was this type of woman who most used abortion. On the other hand, the reporter expressed her surprise that it was married "society women," more than desperate unwed women of the lower classes, who patronized abortionists. Physicians confirmed in letters to the editor that married women had abortions. The class identity of the woman who sought abortions was more consistent: she was rich. The reporters told their contacts many times that money was no object. According to the *Times,* upper-class women patronized abortionists. Their access to abortion was another form of class privilege. "The doctors who were ready to comply with my request had an extensive practice among the best class of people," the female journalist reported. "Their fees were high" and few "shop-girls and the servant girls," she informed her readers, could have been "applicants for the succor which I claimed to be so much in need of."[42]

These images of society women having abortions echoed mid-nineteenth-century ideas that "frivolous" women avoided their maternal duties by having abortions in favor of careers or social activities. "Sisters of Chicago," the newswoman asked, "are our own morals, the health and morals of the next generation to be sacrificed that we may not lose a winter's round of receptions and dances?" According to her description of contemporary marriage, young husbands imagined "a happy fireside and family," but their wives dreamed of "society" and "elegant entertainment." The idea that middle-class men and women both might want to limit family size did not enter her musings. The women the reporter described could be condemned by men of their own class for abandoning motherhood and by working-class women and men for their class privileges.[43]

The paper's coverage of the women who sought abortions sparked a gender struggle over the cause of abortion and the moral quality of the sexes. A handful of letters from women physicians and other female writers injected into the local discourse the nineteenth-century feminist analysis of abortion and demands for changes in male sexual behavior. The double standard, marital rape, and male sexual immorality were at the root of abortion, they argued. The cause of abortion, "Justitia" argued, could be found in the marriage bed, where "'marital' (or husband's) rights are claimed from reluctant wives as continually and habitually as the sun sets or the tides flow." When conception resulted, the writer bluntly pointed out, it had taken two, but husbands blamed their wives for pregnancies. Wives of drunkards, she said, suffered even more knowing their children would be damaged as a result of their fathers' sins. Dr. Odelia Blinn recalled the hundreds of women who had asked her for abortions. "The vast majority," she observed, "were married women," who sought abortions because of their husbands. The doctor urged a single standard of sexuality and teaching men, like women, chastity. "Has it ever occurred to *The Times* to investigate what men are doing while women are committing infanticide?" demanded Dr. Blinn. The paper should investigate prostitution, she suggested; then the other sex would "feel the blow" of being publicly charged with immorality.[44]

As women criticized the representation of women in the *Times,* men used those same representations to attack women and feminine concern about male alcohol abuse and sexual immorality. Instead of charging men with immorality, they recommended that women better themselves. Abortion "is a more degrading evil than drunkenness," argued one downstate Illinois paper, "but women will shamelessly commit this crime who roll their eyes in holy horror at a man who sells or a man who drinks whisky." The *Times* quoted an Iowa physician who had remarked at an AMA meeting, "Our young men are properly taught the evil effects of alcoholic excess—why should not young women be warned of the nature and results of feticide?"[45]

Medical men criticized the paper for using a journalist who represented herself as an "unwed" woman whose desperation evoked their sympathy. Their complaints reveal both paternalistic and antagonistic attitudes toward women. "It was hardly fair," observed one medical journal, "to enlist the sympathy of the doctor and to tempt him by the relation of a story that necessarily appealed to the heart of every father. How many of these guilty ones would have been tempted had the female reporter stated that she was a married woman and did not wish to bear children?" The writer suspected only one would have agreed. This medical observer viewed young female patients as daughters, as dependents who had been seduced and abandoned, who deserved his compassion. For a married woman avoiding what he regarded as her wifely and feminine duty, however, he had no sympathy. The *Journal of the AMA* similarly felt that the profession had been wronged by the paper's use of a "presumably captivating young woman," who told her story "with many a pearly tear trembling on her pretty little eyelids."[46] Doctors who aided her, this last commentator's remarks suggest, had responded to the woman's physical, as well as her emotional, appeal. Pretty young women apparently tempted men both sexually and professionally. This language hinted at the links between abortion and forbidden sexuality.

Angered at how the profession had been besmirched by the exposé, the AMA turned on women who sought abortions. *JAMA,* which had initially urged the prosecution of abortionists, switched to recommending prosecution of women. When women solicited abortions from doctors, an editorial advised, doctors should dispense with "moral lectures . . . [and] hand them over to the police." The journal's editor now felt "pity" for the physician "whose weak sympathy leads him to commit crime to prevent disgrace to an unfortunate young woman," but not for the desperate woman. "Let us condemn the other party to the act," he suggested.[47]

An anonymous physician offered a more sympathetic perspective when he revealed his distress in facing an unmarried woman seeking an abortion. For this physician, the paper's use of an unmarried woman raised moral ambiguities rather than angry defenses. In a letter to the *Times,* the doctor told of an incident when he refused to help an unmarried woman, who "knelt before me and prayed of me with uplifted hands to relieve her." Two days later she committed suicide. If he had been visited by the "unwed" reporter, the doctor admitted, he might not, remembering his earlier patient, have refused her. "It is our duty to preserve life whenever possible," he asserted, and asked, "Did I do it?" Medicine and law allowed the physician to sacrifice the fetus to save the life of the mother. As this doctor introduced a layer of ethical complexity to the discussion, he introduced scientific-sounding language that treated pregnancy as a developmental process. He called the fetus "an unconscious, imperfect germ," in contrast to the *Times*'s labeling the fetus a "child." The *Times* avoided the difficult question posed by this doctor; in a subheading it answered, "He Did His Full Duty," and reiterated, "Abortion is Not Justifiable under Any Circumstances."[48]

The exposure of abortion in Chicago embarrassed the AMA and the city, but abortion services could be bought from physicians in many other cities as well. The *Times* likened several American cities to London, where, it reported, abortionists "prosper." San Francisco, New York, Philadelphia, Cincinnati, and St. Louis were all "lesser Londons." The paper's readers informed the *Times* that abortion thrived elsewhere in the Midwest, including Wisconsin, Iowa, and the small towns of Illinois.[49] "The chief responsibility for the prevalence of criminal abortion rests upon the medical profession," declared Nebraska physician Inez Philbrick in 1904. "In every community," she remarked, "members of the profession live by its induction." Others concurred and charged that physician-abortionists belonged to their medical societies.[50] Chicago was not unique. The character of social relations and commerce in the city facilitated abortion.

The Legal Loophole: Therapeutic Abortions

The underlying structure of medicine and the law at the turn of the century fostered the practice of abortion everywhere. When the *Chicago Times* focused on the business of abortion, it ignored the exception in the state criminal abortion law that allowed physicians to perform therapeutic abortions. The law itself contributed to the medical practice of abortion. The Illinois abortion statute exempted "any person who procures or attempts to produce the miscarriage of any pregnant woman for *bona fide* medical or surgical purposes." What constituted a bona fide reason, however, was left undefined.[51] The Illinois Supreme Court did not rule on the indications for therapeutic abortion until the 1970s.[52] Physicians could legitimately, according to the law and medical ethics, perform therapeutic abortions in order to save the life of the pregnant woman.

Determining when an abortion was necessary—and thus legal—was left to the medical profession. The medical discourse on abortion (neglected by the *Times*) centered on the medical "indications" that required therapeutic abortion. Medical texts gave physicians guidance about the conditions that indicated a therapeutic abortion and taught them which instruments and techniques to use in performing therapeutic abortions. Prescriptive texts did not, however, provide definite answers about when a physician should perform an abortion. Instead, the literature reveals disagreement and conflicting attitudes toward abortion and medicine within the profession. This professional discussion was not produced for public consumption, but was a semiprivate discourse within and for the profession only. Within these protected, professional venues, doctors could express disagreement.

These ongoing debates among doctors were, on the most obvious level, about medical knowledge and proper treatment; no one wanted women to endure unnecessary therapeutic abortions or to die because one had not been performed. They concerned larger issues than proper medicine, however. The discourse was an effort to mark out a territory for physicians where abortions were unquestionably legitimate and create a clear line that differentiated this area from the area of criminality. Yet, for all the efforts of antiabortion physicians and specialists in obstetrics, who claimed therapeutic abortion as their procedure, legal therapeutic abortion resisted definition, and the line between legal and illegal was always vague.

The legal loophole provided a space in which doctors and women could negotiate and allowed physicians to perform abortions in the privacy of their own offices or homes. Since physicians customarily reached medical diagnoses and decisions independently and practiced alone, they might determine that a therapeutic abortion was medically indicated and perform one without anyone ever knowing of it. Disagreement within the medical profession about when a therapeutic abortion was indicated gave doctors flexibility. They could, whether in conscious collusion or unconscious sympathy, use the legal loophole to provide wanted abortions. The medical indications for this procedure left room for social reasons and personal judgment as well as for "real" reasons, but there is no way to distinguish among them. Indeed, medical diagnosis and therapeutics always implicitly, if not explicitly, included a social and cultural component.[53]

The medical profession as a whole assumed the legitimacy of performing therapeutic abortions. The most vehement of the antiabortion physicians had always insisted on the principle that if pregnancy threatened a woman's life, her life was primary and the fetus had to be sacrificed. On rare occasions physicians explicitly voiced their belief in the morality and necessity of therapeutic abortion. They usually did so only because they had been challenged by someone presenting the Catholic Church's position, which opposed *all* abortions, including those to save the life of the woman. At a 1904 symposium on abortion sponsored by the Chicago Medical Society, Dr. Charles B. Reed defended the morality of therapeutic abortions after listening to the comments of a Catholic priest. The Reverend O'Callaghan had explained

Catholic doctrine and argued that an abortion could not be justified even "when absolutely necessary to save the mother." In response, Reed began his talk by stating that with "the advance of moral feeling, the opinion has developed that . . . where the lives of both mother and child are imperiled and one can be saved, the child should be sacrificed, since the value of the mother to the State is far greater than that of the unborn babe." As one Minnesota physician remarked on the issue, the "reasoning that may satisfy the conscience of a theologian does not satisfy the conscience of the physician." At Milwaukee's Catholic Marquette University School of Medicine, the differences between Jesuit trustees and medical school faculty over therapeutic abortions exploded and led to mass resignations by the school's professors.[54]

Medical discussion of therapeutic abortion revolved around precisely when the medical situation demanded that a therapeutic abortion be performed, not its legitimacy. Turn-of-the-century physicians accepted a series of physical and disease indications for abortion.[55] "Probably the most common reason," reported one Illinois doctor in 1899, was hyperemesis gravidarum, or excessive nausea and vomiting, which dehydrated and starved the woman. Excessive vomiting as a result of pregnancy was "a serious emergency," which could kill a woman. According to one doctor, the nineteenth century recorded many deaths due to excessive vomiting during pregnancy, but as physicians increasingly did abortions, the number of these deaths fell. Advances in medicine eventually eliminated vomiting as an indication for therapeutic abortion, but change progressed unevenly. Although physicians reported a cure for vomiting during pregnancy in 1925, physicians continued to disagree, and some still advised abortion for vomiting a decade later.[56] Tuberculosis became a leading indication for abortion by the 1910s, but physicians debated this indication through the 1940s.[57]

Excessive vomiting was the most important indication for abortion and one which allowed women and their doctors room for maneuvering. Vomiting was common during pregnancy; how much was "excessive"? The ambiguity of an indication such as vomiting allowed it to be used to justify an abortion that might be desirable on personal as well as medical grounds. Physicians who knew their patient wanted a way out of a pregnancy might determine that the vomiting was dangerous and induce an abortion to protect her. The doctor might have knowingly stretched the "truth" to accommodate his patient or might simply have reached the conclusion the patient desired; there is no way to know. Furthermore, it was an easy symptom for women to self-induce.

Resourceful women learned to feign the symptoms of pernicious vomiting in order to obtain the therapeutic abortions they wanted, and as a result, some medical leaders urged students and colleagues to distrust their female patients' descriptions of their disorders. The legal status of abortion injected distrust into the relationship between physicians and female patients. Dr. Joseph B. DeLee advised in his 1916 textbook on obstetrics, "A word of warning: Let the inexperienced physician beware of simulated disease. A woman will read up on some disease which she knows sometimes gives the indication for abortion, and will try to impress the doctor that she is deathly ill." Pregnant women, according to Dr. E. A. Weiss, "purposely simulate[d] and prolong[ed] the vomiting and distress" in order to win wished-for therapeutic abortions. Physicians, however, were not just tricked by their patients. Weiss believed that there was an "increasing tendency on the part of the laity as well as the profession to take advantage of the law and [medical] teaching," which allowed therapeutic abortion. Dr. Walter Dorsett, chairman of the AMA section on obstetrics, charged that these "fad doctors," who were willing to find reasons to perform therapeutic abortions, were popular among women.[58]

Therapeutic abortion was a contested subject in medicine, as manifested in the question and answer section of *JAMA*. The correspondence between AMA members and medical advisers makes it evident that physicians did not always agree with or follow the official line. It bears repeating that scholars cannot take official medical texts as accurate descriptions of medical belief or practice, but must read them carefully as prescriptive literature written by leaders of the profession, who hope to shape medicine in particular ways. In this case, the texts point to disagreement among doctors. Query letters from physicians to *JAMA* asking for advice on therapeutic abortions show both the more conservative prescriptive advice given by the AMA and the more liberal interpretation of the abortion law by physicians in practice.

Physicians induced abortions for eugenic and other social reasons, though these were officially proscribed. For example, in 1902 a doctor asked whether it was justifiable to perform a therapeutic abortion in a case where the woman was "mentally unsound" and "the child," he was sure, "would be a degenerate." The doctor explained that the "husband is a neurasthenic with a bad heredity; her mother has paranoia and has been in the asylum for 35 years; her father was an inebriate." *JAMA* tersely answered: "It would be criminal." Two weeks later another correspondent suggested that some doctors disagreed with the journal's position. The Indiana doctor wrote, "There are tens of thousands of intelligent people in and outside of the medical profession who join with me in asking you why it would be a crime?" *JAMA* answered shortly, "Because the laws . . . make no exceptions for such conditions," and concluded, "We do not care to discuss the propriety of modification of the law."[59] The AMA's objection was based not on the need for consent and the danger of coercion, but on its narrow interpretation of when the law allowed physicians to perform abortions.

JAMA's answer to a query about the possibility of performing an abortion when the pregnancy resulted from rape simultaneously demonstrates the AMA's role in teaching doctors its interpretation of the law and suggests that some did perform abortions for rape. When a physician asked whether an abortion could be justified when pregnancy followed the drugging and rape of a sixteen-year-old girl "of unquestionable reputation," the editor answered firmly in the negative. The physician had confirmed the young woman's moral purity and performed a medical examination and microscopic examinations of her clothing and "vaginal contents" before concluding that a rape had occurred. Nonetheless, *JAMA*'s response exhibited age-old doubts about the veracity of women when they charged rape. The editor asked the doctor to remember "that pregnancy is rare after *real* rape, and that the fright may easily cause suppression of menstruation and other subjective symptoms." "The enormity of the crime of rape," *JAMA* judged, "does not justify murder. This is law." *JAMA*'s answer to this letter was more explicit than the laws, which did not specify what justified therapeutic abortions.[60]

When the journal listed the social reasons that did not indicate a therapeutic abortion, it simultaneously described some of the reasons for which physicians performed abortions. According to *JAMA*, state statutes usually "tolerate" only abortions performed "to preserve the life of the mother from some impending danger. The danger must be real; the bare possibility of death is not sufficient." Furthermore, the medical adviser warned, "under no conditions can an abortion be lawfully induced for the sole purpose of preserving a woman's reputation, or of contributing to her comfort or pleasure, or because of the patient's financial circumstances." These caveats revealed that physicians performed abortions out of concern for their patients: in order to hide the pregnancies of unwed women, because of poverty, and because their patients wanted them.[61] Though not officially approved, abortions were performed by physicians when women expressed their anxieties about pregnancy.[62]

Sometimes, even *JAMA* admitted, physicians had to grant women the right to make decisions about their own pregnancies. A 1902 discussion about contracted pelvis, a physical deformity that prevented a woman from delivering a baby vaginally, demonstrates the complexity of medical decision making and the active role played by patients themselves. A Florida physician wrote of a patient with contracted pelvis, who had had a therapeutic abortion previously. He had "urged and insisted" upon a cesarean section, "but both Mr. and Mrs. R. reject the idea as too dangerous and too expensive." He feared having to perform abortions every few months. The *JAMA* editor admitted that a woman and "her husband have some right" to decide between a dangerous operation to save the fetus or an abortion to save the woman. But the editor limited this right to women who became pregnant "in ignorance" of their pelvic condition. For this woman, who knew of her condition, "her right to a choice in the conduct of the case is undoubtedly much lessened." The advising physician assumed that the woman's pregnancy was her fault and, therefore, in his eyes, she had a less compelling right to make decisions about her own health and body. How the woman was supposed to avoid pregnancy he did not mention, but the medical profession had opposed the teaching of birth control. The *JAMA* editor favored convincing the couple to agree to a cesarean section, even though the operation was often fatal.[63]

Nonetheless, the advisor acknowledged that the couple might be able to win an abortion despite the doctor's preference and propaganda. The patient deserved the best advice, and, he continued, "sometimes this is not accepted, and we must be content with an alternative." The editor finished by reminding the doctor to call a consultant before performing an abortion. The contradictory answer indicates that the editor realized that many would be unable to convince patients to risk death with a cesarean section and physicians would have to perform abortions. In these types of cases, physicians let women decide the course of action.[64] Different women no doubt weighed their desire for children and the dangers of surgery differently.

Physicians responded to the problem of contracted pelvis with different procedures over time. Therapeutic abortion, induced early in a pregnancy, was an advance over the nineteenth-century method of performing craniotomies, when at the time of delivery the physician punctured the fetal head and pulled out the fully-formed fetus piece by piece in order to preserve the woman's life. By 1920 cesarean sections had replaced therapeutic abortion as the preferred response to the problem of contracted pelvis, though a c-section was still dangerous and probably more dangerous than an early abortion. The profession decided for women that it preferred to perform surgery that resulted in babies, even if it endangered women's lives. As medical knowledge and skill advanced, women lost their place in making decisions about whether or not they would undergo a more dangerous operation. For some, the increasingly safe c-section was a boon; for those who wanted to rid themselves of a pregnancy, however, they no longer had a legitimate out.[65]

The economics of medicine at the turn of the century gave women power in their relationship to doctors. If necessary, a well-to-do woman could threaten to end the doctor's relationship with her entire family. Affluent women, who saw private physicians regularly and often selected the family doctor, had the greatest ability to pressure physicians into providing abortions. For the doctor, losing a family's medical business could mean losing years of fees for child deliveries, children's illnesses, and injuries. The threat of losing—or the promise of winning—a family's business often proved effective. According to medical commentators, these threats worked especially well with young doctors. The competition in the profession, the problem of "overcrowding" as doctors called it, helped make doctors willing to respond to patient demands. Some general practitioners, noted one doctor in 1909, fell into doing abortions after "los[ing] family after family because of their stand against performing abortions." Milwaukee physician E. F. Fish painted a dreary picture to account for the practice of abortion by "young men in the profession." After refusing requests for abortions, the young doctor, "finally, hungry, penniless, his clothing threadbare, his rent due . . . yields to temptation—because he needs money."[66]

The 1888 exposé, the medical discussion about therapeutic abortion, and police reports all point to the readiness of many physicians to help women obtain abortions. Some agreed to do abortions; many more assisted women in an essential way by giving them the name of an abortionist. The evidence of city or regional medical networks underscores the depth of medical involvement in abortion. In one 1929 case in New York, prosecutors found checks showing that the abortionist paid kickbacks to fifty or sixty area physicians.[67] JAMA regularly reported on physicians convicted of abortion.[68]

Law and economics contributed to the practice of abortion, but legal loopholes and money alone do not explain the evident willingness of doctors to perform abortions or refer patients to others who would. Why did doctors help women who sought what was known as the "illegal operation"? Part of the explanation for physicians' capacity to sympathize with women's requests for abortion lies in the nature of medical practice at the turn of the century. Medical practice embedded physicians in family life and female lives. Physicians practiced in the home. There, they primarily interacted with the woman of the house. She called in the doctor for help when her own knowledge and nursing failed and was there when he attended any member of her family. She talked with the doctor about the illness or injury for which he had been called and consulted with him on treatment. It was she who carried out (or not) his orders to feed, bathe, and medicate the patient and continued to care for the sick in her family after he left. (A few families hired nurses, but even then the woman of the household supervised the nurse.) One of the main duties of family practice for any doctor was attending women during childbirth, which, for most women, still took place in the home. This event often first brought the doctor into a family. A physician who succeeded in attending a delivery had a good chance of being called again. Success meant more than delivering a baby, however; it meant developing a working relationship with the birthing woman and her female friends and relatives who attended the delivery along with the physician. Family doctors had to be able to get along with the women in the family. As a result, physicians tended to know women, and, since physicians observed the family in its home while caring for its illnesses, doctors tended to be familiar with their female patients' worries, financial difficulties, household and child-rearing burdens, as well as their fears and physical injuries related to childbearing and general health. Medical practice itself created new understandings in doctors, and medicine may have attracted men who knew how to communicate across gender lines.[69]

Middle-class women were not the only ones to benefit from medical understanding of the female condition. Physicians who cared for many women and many families could have insights into a woman's life without knowing an individual woman well. When women told doctors of their lives, explaining the particularities that made an abortion necessary, many doctors understood. They knew that women's bodies had been weakened from childbearing and wearied from housework, and they had observed the hardships of rearing several children in a poor household. For example, Kate Simon tells of a much-respected Dr. James who performed abortions for poor immigrant women in a Jewish-Italian neighborhood of the Bronx in the 1920s. When he was occasionally arrested, other doctors came to his defense.[70] In short, medical practice sensitized many doctors to the lives of women.

Though urban areas like Chicago provided a favorable environment for the business of abortion, it was not solely an urban phenomenon. It may have been common among rural physicians to perform abortions as part of their family practices. A Milwaukee doctor reported hearing a "country" doctor say, "We all do that kind of work when it is in a nice family and a girl has to be protected."[71] As this physician's comment reveals, the woman's status affected whether a physician sympathized with her and would perform an abortion. The doctor judged whether a pregnancy out of wedlock was to be expected of a particular "girl" or whether it could be excused and aborted as a mistake. The occasional abortion for a deserving patient would never be known by anyone other than the doctor, his patient, and her family. Several long-time, respected, small-town doctors were prosecuted, however, for abortion when patients died. Doctor John W. Aiken, for example, had been the eminent and only physician for over thirty years in Tennessee, Illinois, when he was prosecuted for murder by abortion in 1899. Small towns could lose their only physician in cases like these.[72]

Not every doctor listened and agreed to perform abortions. Many lived up to their profession's rules and refused women's requests. When these doctors reported their experiences, they highlighted their own noble characters while confirming that plenty of others did not share their antipathy to abortion. Physicians who refused to do abortions grimly reported losing patients. In 1900, after observing medicine in Chicago since the 1860s, Dr. Denslow Lewis, a professor of gynecology and president of the Attending Staff of Cook County Hospital, remarked that prominent citizens and physicians regarded abortion "as a matter of routine." He knew of one married woman whose family physician had performed eleven abortions for her. Lewis himself had "lost the patronage of well-known society women" when he refused to perform abortions for them. A prominent gentleman remonstrated Dr. Mary Dixon-Jones of New York when she would not perform an abortion for his wife. "Any doctor who wanted a good practice should take care of his families," the gentleman told her. "This was the physician's duty, and it was done by the best." Another doctor told a familiar tale of being asked to induce an abortion. "For promptly refusing," he recalled, "she dismissed me."[73] These patients knew they could find more responsive practitioners elsewhere.

The 1888 *Times* exposé provided a handy list of abortionists. Ironically, as the newspaper advertised its intention to suppress abortion, it also stimulated it. Furthermore, not only did abortion information appear on the front page of newspapers, it appeared in the advertising pages in the back. Dr. Rudolph W. Holmes charged in 1904 that Chicago's "daily papers, magazines, and even some so-called religious papers are most fruitful means of disseminating the knowledge concerning the means for producing abortion." Almost every daily paper in the city, he maintained, carried advertisements with information about abortion, though they were not listed under that word. Sellers of abortifacients caught women's attention by advertising their products as "ladies' safe remedy." Physicians and midwives who advertised themselves as specialists in the "diseases of women" sometimes agreed to induce abortions.[74]

Patterns of Practice

Historians have generally treated midwives and doctors separately, but these two groups of practitioners did not practice in two separate worlds.[75] It is important to see the similarities and connections between them as well as their differences. Midwives and doctors provided reproductive health care services in an era when health care was practiced primarily in the practitioner's office or the patient's home rather than in a hospital. Because of the location and structure of care at the turn of the century, their style of practice shared certain characteristics. The *Times* uncovered the availability of abortion in Chicago; other records of actual abortion cases in the Chicago area, drawn from legal records and newspaper accounts, permit a closer examination of actual turn-of-the-century abortion practices.[76]

The abortion practice, like other obstetrical practices, seems to have been split between doctors and midwives. In 1915, midwives delivered about half of Chicago's babies,[77] and the available evidence suggests that midwives and doctors performed abortions in approximately equal numbers at the turn of the century as well. A 1917 study of women who came to the Washington University Dispensary in St. Louis found that physicians and midwives had "an equal share in the nefarious practice" of illegal abortion. Of fifty-one women who had had induced abortions, physicians and midwives each had induced 24 percent of them.[78] A New York study of the patient histories of 10,000 working-class women found that physicians had induced almost four times as many abortions as had midwives,[79] while a study of III convictions for illegal abortion in New York between 1925 and 1950 found that the abortionists were midwives in 22.5 percent of the cases and doctors in 27.9 percent.[80] Investigators of midwives in Chicago, New York, Boston, and Baltimore suspected that 5 percent to more than 50 percent of midwives practiced illegal abortion.[81] Though studies conducted at the time estimated the proportion of midwives involved in abortion, they never asked the same question of the medical profession, an omission that reveals the investigators' automatic respect for the medical profession and automatic suspicion of midwives. There is no way to determine what proportion of either group performed abortions, but patient histories and mortality data indicate that both midwives and doctors did.

Emily Projahn was thirty-three years old and had given birth to four children, two of whom survived. In August of 1916 her period did not come. It did not show up in September. After having missed her period for two months, she and her husband visited a doctor whom her husband had seen previously, Dr. C. W. Mercereau at 4954 Milwaukee Avenue. It was a Friday evening and they spoke to him of their trouble. Dr. Mercereau agreed to do the operation and told them the fee would be $10 and $2 for calling on her afterwards. They paid half the fee that night. Mr. Projahn later explained that the doctor "asked me to be quiet and not say anything more about it. I said I would." The doctor then shut the door and prepared to perform the operation. He had his patient lie in a surgical chair and used an instrument. Mrs. Projahn called the instrument a "womb opener." Her husband described it as "nickel-plated, silver-like" and "ten or twelve inches long." The doctor told her to "stay on her feet until she got sick enough to go to bed." When they got home that evening, Mrs. Projahn was bleeding. A week later she called Dr. Mercereau, who came to their home and prescribed medicine. He visited her at home twice. After three weeks of chills and fever, she called in a second doctor, who hospitalized her.[82]

Emily Projahn's abortion was not atypical. The operation was performed in the physician's office, and the doctor followed up by visiting her at home and prescribing medications. Apparently, most physicians performed abortions in their offices.[83] A number of physicians saw their patients one or more times after the operation. Both the patients and their abortionists expected doctors to provide continuing care, as they would with any other health problem. Repeated visits, as in the case of one woman whose doctor saw her five additional times, indicated the procedure had gone badly.[84]

Some physician-abortionists managed their own hospitals. The existence of these hospitals emphasizes the ubiquity of abortion and suggests that some practiced rather openly without fear of trouble. In the 1920s in Chicago, Dr. Amante Rongetti, a regularly licensed physician and surgeon, performed abortions in his own Ashland Boulevard Hospital with beds for twenty-five patients. Dr. Justin L. Mitchell was the medical head of the Michigan Boulevard Sanitarium, where he performed illegal abortions.[85]

Physician fees for abortion varied widely in this period, ranging from $10 to $175. On average, physicians received $48; the most frequently paid amount was $50.[86] Dr. Mercereau charged the Projahns a low fee. Several doctors received less than they asked for. One doctor demanded $150 for the abortion he performed on Ester Reed. When her mother objected, he cruelly told her to sell her furniture and clothing to get the money. Reed's mother gave him $50, and, though he complained, he began the procedure and two days later finished it at their home.[87]

Doctors induced abortions by methods described in medical texts. There were three ways to induce an abortion: by ingesting drugs, a method generally viewed as dangerous or ineffective by the medical profession; by introducing something, such as a rubber catheter, a gauze tampon, or other object, into the cervix to irritate it, bring on contractions, and cause the woman to miscarry; or by dilating the cervix with metal dilators or gauze tampons and then using a curette, a spoon-shaped instrument, to scrape fetal and placental tissue out of the uterus (preferably with the woman under anesthesia). The latter was known as a dilation and curettage, or "D & C."[88] Probably most physicians used instruments to induce abortions.[89] Dr. Mercereau may have induced Mrs. Projahn's miscarriage by introducing through the cervix a uterine sound, a slender, pointed instrument for measuring the depth of the uterus. Three Chicago physicians introduced catheters to bring about abortions. Four sold drugs. Pills were cheaper than an operation, which made them a popular first attempt. If they failed, however, the woman faced a later (more risky, and possibly more expensive) abortion. At least one doctor used chloroform during the operation, and two used gauze. According to Edna Lamb's statement in 1917, Dr. Charles Kline-top packed her cervix with gauze in order to induce an abortion.[90] In the words of one nurse, she and the doctor made it look "just like a woman just having a miscarriage."[91]

The majority of the Chicago physician-abortionists I have identified were Regulars, and a third belonged to the AMA. Over a third belonged to the Chicago Medical Society or the Illinois State Medical Society. Five of the physician-abortionists were Homeopaths, one an

Eclectic. Of this group of thirty-eight physician-abortionists, most were men, seven were women. Although these findings cannot be extended to the universe of physician-abortionists, they establish the involvement of regular, mainstream physicians in abortion.[92]

The women who went to midwives for abortions were mostly of a different class than the women who found physician-abortionists. Native-born, middle-class women were most likely to see physicians; immigrant and working-class women were more likely to go to immigrant midwives. Most of Chicago's midwives and their clients in delivery or abortion cases were white, European immigrants. Over 97 percent of the city's midwives were foreign-born. The few native-born white or black midwives practicing in Chicago may have performed abortions as well, but they have not appeared in the sources.[93] Immigrant women probably preferred immigrant midwives when they needed abortions for the same reasons they preferred them during childbirth—midwives were female, foreign-born, and cheap.

In 1916, Rosie Kawera of Chicago asked a friend to go with her to visit Mrs. Wilhelmina Benn, a licensed midwife. Kawera explained to her friend that "she had a little baby; she wanted to get some medicine to get it out." Kawera was twenty-nine years old, Russian-born, married to a "moulder," mother of an eleven-month-old baby, and two months pregnant. She borrowed $10 from her brother and went to Mrs. Benn's. While her friend waited in the kitchen, Kawera went into the bedroom, where Mrs. Benn inserted what Kawera called "a little pipe." Mrs. Benn told Kawera to keep it in overnight and to phone whenever she got "sick."[94]

Midwives sympathized with women who faced unwanted pregnancies. When the male reporter for the *Times* approached Mme. Schoenian, she told him, "I feel so sorry for the poor things and do all I can for them." The reporter concluded that Schoenian expressed the feelings of most of Chicago's midwives: they felt "sympathy for the 'poor girl'" and considered performing abortions "a benevolent undertaking." The reporter seemed to suggest that midwives had a feminist analysis of abortion, believing that "the necessity for secrecy came from 'man's inhumanity to man'—or woman rather."[95] It is unlikely that immigrant women who refused to be attended by male doctors during childbirth considered going to men for abortions.[96]

Not only did midwives identify with their patients as women, they shared their culture and language. Rosie Kawera and her midwife, Mrs. Benn, were both Russian-born. Frauciszka Gawlik, Austrian-born and married to a Polish man, went to a Polish- and German-speaking mid-wife for her abortion.[97] Though the majority of native-born, white women had physicians attend them during childbirth, some, knowing of midwives' reputation for being abortionists, may have looked for midwives when they needed abortions.

Finally, midwives charged about half as much as doctors, whether for performing an abortion or delivering a baby. Both midwives and doctors, however, charged twice as much for abortions as they did for deliveries. Midwives charged about $10 for attending a birth; doctors charged $20 to $25. A 1910 investigation found midwives' average fee for an abortion was almost $28.[98] My sample of Chicago midwives and physicians who performed abortions at the turn of the century indicates that midwives charged, on the average, $20 for an abortion.[99]

Once a woman found a midwife willing to perform an abortion and they agreed upon a price, they had to decide when and where the pro-cedure would be performed. Midwives provided abortions and after-care in several different locations: in the homes of their patients, in their own offices or homes, or in the homes of other women who acted as nurses. The different places in which midwives worked reflected the va-riety in the location of medical care in the early twentieth century. Some midwives performed abortions at their own homes. Mrs. Kawera went to Mrs. Benn's home for her abortion. Mrs. Jennie Carantzalis, a licensed midwife and nurse, had an office with a receptionist in her own home. Other midwives induced abortions at their patients' homes, as did Mrs. Babetta Newmayer. Midwives visited their abortion patients at home to check on their recovery just as midwives checked up on pa-tients following a delivery.[100]

Some midwives had their abortion patients stay with them or at an-other woman's home for a few days so that they could oversee their re-covery. For some patients, particularly single women who wanted to keep their pregnancies secret, being able to abort and recover for a few days somewhere other than their own homes was a distinct advantage. One 1910 investigation reported that half of the midwives who agreed to perform an abortion (six of twelve midwives) wanted to keep the pa-tient in their homes for a few days after the procedure. One midwife, who used drugs to induce abortions, reportedly "said the patient could stay with her so she could watch the case." When Esther Stark went to midwife Mary Groh for an abortion, Groh arranged to have her board with Mrs. Scholtes for a few days after her "treatment." Midwives could not practice in hospitals, but, in a sense, some midwives created their own informal "hospitals" when they arranged for other women to nurse abortion patients in a setting that was neither the patient's home nor the practitioner's office.[101]

A few midwives had busy abortion practices and seemed to work almost exclusively as abortionists. The Chicago Vice Commission found four women waiting for abortions in one midwife's basement apartment. Another midwife, the commission reported, "said she had a patient in the house and another one who had just had an operation was in the next room."[102] For the women having abortions, it may have been reassuring to recover surrounded by other women sharing the same experience.

Midwives used drugs and instruments to induce abortions. Studies of Chicago midwives in 1908 and 1913 found both in their possession. One investigator commented, "A midwife who has in her equipment a speculum, uterine sounds, dilators, curettes and wired gum catheters, is beyond all question or doubt carrying on a criminal practice." Some midwives, like Hattie Chlevinski and Mrs. Veronica Ripczynski, gave their abortion patients special teas. Midwife Sophie Mann advised her patient to take hot baths, to use a hot water bottle on her stomach, and to use some other remedy "concerning vinegar" (perhaps a douche?).[103]

Midwives Cecilia Styskal, Catherine Haisler, and Jennie Carantzalis all used rubber catheters to induce abortions for their patients. Mrs. Wilhelmina Benn, who inserted "a little pipe" in her patient, may have been using a catheter too. Inducing abortions by inserting a catheter into the cervix to irritate the uterus and induce labor was a common method—used both by physicians and by women at home. At a 1931 trial for criminal abortion, a sixteen-year-old woman described in detail the abortion induced for her by Jennie Carantzalis. She recalled that the midwife had her lie down on a table and inserted "an instrument that opens up" into her vagina (perhaps a dilator?). "She started turning it around there, and it hurt me. . . . I started bleeding and then she took a long instrument that looked like a scissors and she put cotton in them." The woman explained that the midwife "dipped [the cotton] in some liquid and put it in my vagina and was cleaning it out. . . . Then she put a long rubber tube un [sic] me." The midwife inserted more cotton and then, the woman recalled, "she gave me something to put around me, because I was flowing real fast. . . . She said, sit down on the chair a few minutes, and you will be all right." Carantzalis prescribed quinine pills to be taken every three hours, told her to walk around, and instructed that the tube "was supposed to be taken out within

24 hours, the next day at 4:00 o'clock." The next day the young woman was feverish, had "terrific pains," and aborted the fetus.[104]

The Chicago case study shows that midwives and doctors practiced abortion in similar ways. Both prescribed drugs and used catheters to induce miscarriages. Physicians used instruments most frequently, though a few midwives carried curettes in their bags. Some physicians and midwives, as the 1888 exposé made evident, worked together. However, doctors charged twice as much as midwives for abortion services, a pricing structure that matched the class of the practitioners and their patients.

As a general rule, midwives and physicians cared for different patient populations. Midwives primarily served poor, immigrant women, while doctors primarily attended native-born and more affluent women. Both shared class, ethnicity, and culture with their patients; shared backgrounds probably eased women's anxieties. Some women may have crossed these boundaries of background and neighborhood in order to find strangers, whom they believed likelier to perform an abortion or found easier to consult because they did not personally know them.

Midwives shared the experiences of womanhood with their patients, which male physicians could not. Though women who wanted abortions often tried to get them from female physicians, expecting that gender identity would produce aid, many female doctors refused. Some women physicians did perform abortions, and they may have understood this in terms of gender, but there is no way to discover whether, in terms of their relative numbers, more male or more female physicians provided abortions. Contrary to the expectations of women then and some feminists now, the evidence does not allow us to assume that female physicians were more likely to respond to women's demands and perform abortions. The evidence for the turn of the century suggests the opposite, since feminists abhorred abortion and many, many male physicians provided abortions. As midwives disappeared from northern cities by the 1930s,[105] poor women lost a group of practitioners who identified with their gender, culture, and class and provided a range of reproductive services.

This chapter has emphasized the availability of abortion and its ongoing, successful practice, yet the safety of illegal abortions needs to be considered. Even though most women survived their abortions, many died. In 1910, for example, the Cook County coroner recorded the deaths of fifty-two women due to abortion. Seventeen, or 33 percent, had been caused by self-induced abortions, suggesting the dangers of self-reliance. Eight, or 15 percent, followed criminal abortions. In twenty-seven deaths, the cause was unknown—some may have been miscarriages, some illegal abortions. The proportion of deaths known to be caused by criminal abortions was typical.[106] No doubt additional abortion-related deaths were ascribed to other causes.[107] Some abortionists were truly terrible. Dr. Lucy Hagenow, for example, provided abortions in her offices on the north side of Chicago and caused the deaths of (at least) six women due to abortion in 1896, 1899, 1905, 1906, and 1907 and, after being imprisoned for a number of years, operated on another woman who died in 1926.[108] This list of deaths caused by one person is stunning. It is important to remember abortionists such as this one while keeping in mind that the available records overemphasize abortion deaths. Hagenow's imprisonment protected women who sought abortions for several years.

The mortality associated with abortion must be assessed within the context of overall maternal mortality. Childbearing was dangerous, and pregnant women feared dying during childbirth. In the 1920s, observers believed that at least 20,000 women died each year in the United States due to puerperal causes. In 1930, the United States still had one of the highest maternal mortality rates in the world, and this rate did not fall until the late 1930s.[109] The U.S. Children's Bureau's scrupulous study of maternal mortality in fifteen states found that induced abortions were responsible for at least 14 percent of the maternal deaths, and the rate was higher in urban areas.[110] It is impossible to determine the risk associated with the abortion procedure itself since we do not know the total number of abortions induced or the number of abortion-related deaths. Most likely abortion was more dangerous than childbirth since it always required intervention with instruments and hands that could introduce infections, whereas some women delivered without interference. Nor can we ascertain the relative responsibility of different practitioners without knowing who performed abortions and with what results.

Nonetheless, I suspect that midwives and doctors had comparable safety records for abortions. I do not think we should assume, as most contemporary observers did, that midwives were necessarily more dangerous than physicians. Medical studies of maternal mortality from the 1910s, 1920s, and 1930s repeatedly showed that midwives had lower mortality rates than physicians.[111] Of course, skill at delivering babies does not automatically translate into skill in performing abortions. Other evidence shows that midwives and physicians were responsible

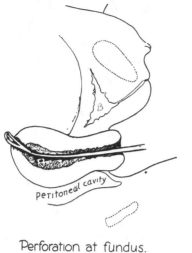

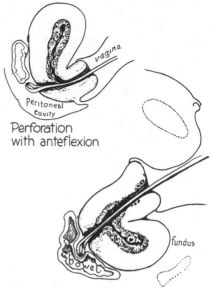

Perforation
with anteflexion

Perforation at fundus.

Perforation with retroflexion

Plate 2. Perforation of the uterus with the curette was one of the hazards of abortion: it could occur during an induced abortion or as a result of a physician's attempt to treat an abortion. Illustration by Robert Latou Dickinson in Frederick J. Taussig, *Abortion, Spontaneous and Induced: Medical and Social Aspects* (St. Louis: C.V. Mosby, 1936), 231. Courtesy C.V. Mosby Co.

for similar numbers of abortion-related deaths. Cook County coroner's records of women's deaths resulting from abortion between 1905 and 1915 showed that out of over one hundred cases where women had died because of criminal abortions, midwives were responsible in fifty-four cases; physicians, in forty-nine. In Milwaukee between 1903 and 1908, of thirty-two abortion-related fatalities, seven of the abortions were performed by doctors, three by midwives, and four were self-induced; in the remaining eighteen cases, who performed the abortions was unknown. A Minneapolis study of abortion-related deaths between 1927 and 1936 found physicians responsible for more than twice as many deaths as midwives.[112]

Finally, physicians' growing use of the curette in abortion cases contributed to the number of abortion-related deaths. (See plate 2.) One expert in obstetrics and abortion, Frederick J. Taussig, observed that as physicians increasingly performed abortions and attended miscarriages, where they did emergency curettements as recommended by most specialists, the rate of uterine perforations and deaths as a result of perforation rose steadily. "The agent most frequently responsible for this injury, it must be confessed, is the physician," Taussig concluded. "The midwife and lay abortionist are relatively less responsible."[113]

As the problem of perforation makes clear, operations performed by physicians at the turn of the century could be quite risky for the woman patient. And though skilled physicians could perform therapeutic abortions safely,[114] not all physicians were competent. Surgery expanded steadily after 1880 with the development of antiseptic and aseptic technique, and the growing number of operations performed by general practitioners, rather than specialists in surgery, became an issue of concern to specialists and the public.[115] As physicians increasingly intervened in pregnancy, whether to deliver a baby, induce an abortion, or curette an incomplete abortion (spontaneous or induced), they sometimes introduced infections and injured their patients.

Answering the question "Who was better, doctors or midwives?" is less important than recognizing that the great variation in education and skill of medical practitioners and the lack of oversight over their practices at the turn of the century meant that the safety of obstetrical procedures varied a great deal. The risk associated with an abortion depended on the technical expertise of the individual practitioner— whether midwife or doctor.[116] Some of the midwives and physicians who induced abortions were quite talented at the operation; others were incompetent and injured or killed their patients. The privacy and autonomy of medical practice that allowed doctors to perform abortions for their patients in this period also allowed every general practitioner, regardless of skill or training, to perform surgical operations such as curettages. The very conditions that permitted the widespread practice of abortion added to the risks of abortion.

CHAPTER 3

Antiabortion Campaigns, Private and Public

"A generation ago," Dr. Joseph Taber Johnson recalled, the AMA had crusaded against abortion and succeeded in winning new laws against it, but that campaign had failed to convince women of the immorality of abortion. Dr. Johnson encouraged his colleagues at the June 7, 1895, meeting of the Washington, D.C., Obstetrical and Gynecological Society to join a new crusade against abortion. "Abortion is now fully as frequent as it ever was in this country," Johnson reported. Furthermore, he told them, "it is alarmingly on the increase; not only is this believed to be true of the cities, but the remotest country districts seem to be infected also." Worse, women still believed early abortions before quickening to be harmless. The blame for this "dense ignorance," Johnson argued, lay with the medical profession, as did the responsibility for enlightening the populace; "[it is] the moral and Christian duty of our profession to correct" the "popular belief" about the life of the fetus. He urged a renewed effort by the nation's doctors, particularly the specialists in obstetrics and gynecology to whom he spoke, to reeducate the public and suppress abortion.[1]

At the turn of the century a second antiabortion campaign, led by physicians such as Dr. Johnson, developed in reaction to the obvious availability and popular acceptance of abortion. These new opponents of abortion faced a difficult task. They could not lobby state legislators to pass laws, since abortion had already been criminalized. Instead, their fight took new cultural and political forms. They had to convince both the general population and the medical profession that abortion was wrong. As we have seen, the public still accepted abortion, many physicians sympathized with women who sought abortions, and some physicians performed abortions. Furthermore, this project did not have a clear victory in sight the way that campaigns for new laws did. This generation of abortion opponents hoped to change Americans' thinking and secure the ongoing enforcement of the criminal abortion laws.

The new antiabortion crusade pursued a three-pronged strategy. Medical efforts focused, first, on reeducating American women and the public about the immorality and dangers of abortion. This cultural campaign took place in physicians' offices and patients' homes during individual encounters as well as in public group forums. Second, antiabortion physicians worked internally within medical societies to eliminate abortionists from the medical profession. Third, the antiabortion campaign moved its focus from state legislatures to the local level, where the new laws were enforced. The new activists sought an alliance with state officials in enforcing the law. Antiabortionists identified an entire group of practitioners they believed responsible for illegal abortion: immigrant midwives. The attempt by specialists in obstetrics to restrict their competitors was the most visible and public aspect of the new campaign. The purging of the profession was treated as a private problem.

One scholar has called the era of illegal abortion "the century of silence."[2] Abortion was not a political issue in the sense that it has become today; it neither played a role in national presidential elections nor reached the U.S. Supreme Court. Yet during the Progressive Era, abortion became a contested issue of interest to politicians and the target of new legislation at both the local and state levels. As the campaign against midwives became intertwined with the campaign against abortion, abortion was repoliticized. In a broader sense, abortion became politicized as physicians and others challenged traditional thinking and behavior and promoted new meanings of pregnancy and abortion. By 1920, the medical campaign against abortion had faded as physicians turned their attention to more pressing questions concerning public policy and reproduction that social movements had brought to the national stage: birth control and the Sheppard-Towner Act for improving maternal and infant health.

The antiabortion campaign points to the important role played by nongovernmental agencies in policing abortion. As voluntary medical societies and reform groups took up enforcing the criminal abortion laws, they essentially acted as part of the state. Indeed, official government agencies and the police relied upon private individuals and agencies to assist in enforcing the laws; in the abortion case, state officials expected the medical profession to act as a leader to repress the practice, particularly within the profession's own ranks. Physicians who spoke vehemently against abortion represented the official view of medicine that the profession presented to the public, but, as we have seen, the public image projected by the leaders of medicine did not accurately represent the attitudes and actions of all physicians. Although many doctors participated in abortion in contradiction of their profession's norms, few openly challenged the official attitude.

As in the earlier antiabortion campaign, specialists in obstetrics took the lead. Just as nineteenth-century Regulars had fought abortion as part of a larger campaign to wrest control over medical practice from competing sects, specialists in obstetrics and gynecology aspired to achieve greater authority over pregnancy and childbirth and to raise their specialty's status.[3] And, as in the past, physicians asserted their sense of moral superiority through this antiabortion campaign. Some, such as Dr. Johnson, who referred to the doctor's "Christian duty," saw the battle against abortion as a missionary effort. Specialists in obstetrics and gynecology claimed the moral authority of religious leaders and the right and duty to make reproductive decisions.

Leadership for a revived antiabortion campaign came out of the national meetings of the AMA's Section on Obstetrics and Gynecology.[4] In 1893, 1906, 1908, and 1911, the chairmen of the section, Doctors J. Milton Duff, Charles Bacon, Walter B. Dorsett, and H. G. Wetherhill, addressed the need for the suppression of abortion in their annual speeches to the section.[5] These men carried on a tradition begun in the mid–nineteenth century by Dr. Humphreys Storer and continued by his son, Dr. Horatio Storer, of articulating opposition to abortion and pressing for its control.[6] J. Milton Duff, chairman of the AMA Section on Obstetrics in 1893, called abortion "a pernicious crime against God and society." The medical profession, he argued, needed to "educate the public up to a thorough appreciation of the pernicious results of this evil."[7] The Chicago Medical Society's antiabortion activities provide an example of obstetricians' investment in the subject.[8] When the society formed a new Committee on Criminal Abortion in 1904, all of the new members, Doctors Rudolph Holmes, Charles Sumner Bacon, and Charles B. Reed, were specialists in obstetrics who became national leaders of their specialty.[9]

Although African American physicians worried about abortion, they never organized an antiabortion campaign as did white physicians in the AMA. Individuals might sometimes try to discourage abortion among African Americans, but the National Medical Association's *Journal* did not regularly report on abortion as did *JAMA*. Instead, it focused on fighting discrimination against African American doctors and patients.[10]

The new medical campaign against abortion aimed to disabuse women of their traditional belief that life did not begin until after quickening. Many women "ignorantly maintained" the belief that abortion prior to quickening was permissible, commented Charles B. Reed, a member of the Chicago Medical Society's abortion committee. Americans needed to be taught, he maintained, that "the fertilized egg contains all the hopes and possibilities of a mature foetus" and that quickening was irrelevant.[11]

Physicians boasted of their success in reversing women's plans to abort. Dr. Mary A. Dixon-Jones of New York told of spending hours talking of the "evil" of abortion to women who sought abortions from her. She sometimes wrote personal letters to dissuade women from having abortions. "Many beautiful little children," she wrote with pride, "are now walking the streets that I have saved." One Chicago physician reported refusing the requests of two "young married women who were both frantic when they found themselves pregnant shortly after marriage. By talking to them kindly and by showing them the terrible results following abortion," he prevented the abortions.[12] These doctors congratulated themselves for restoring the usual gender norms and producing babies.

At a 1904 Kentucky medical meeting, Dr. E. E. Hume told a detailed story that shows how some doctors acted as moral ministers to their patients. His report allows us to listen in on a conversation between a doctor and his patients and to hear what some doctors said to deter abortions. A husband and wife had visited Hume's office, both "anxious to have her relieved." He spoke of "the crime of abortion, and murder." When he discovered they both belonged to the church, he "began to preach to them." Hume recalled his sermon for the assembled doctors: "This is a life, as soon as impregnation occurs. . . . I told them that it would be murder to cause an abortion and asked them how they would like to appear before the great King, and find that child in front of them, and its blood dripping from their fingers. . . . I told them they ought to ask God to forgive the very thought which they had in their hearts." His preaching succeeded. "The woman told me," he recalled, "that she would never try to abort again."[13]

Women's responses to these moral denunciations of abortion varied from terror to hilarity. Though this ideological "information" devastated some and persuaded them to give up their original intentions, others were not convinced. As one Colorado doctor admitted, "Some people . . . will laugh at the doctor for telling them that it is murder to kill an unborn infant." Despite the ridicule the physician might have to endure, the doctor urged "every physician to try to educate the people up to a higher standard."[14]

Other physicians emphasized the mortal, rather than the moral, dangers of abortion in their effort to persuade women to cease the practice. These doctors were consciously constructing the idea that abortion was deadly. Chicago's Dr. Holmes suggested that if doctors downplayed moral arguments and instead stressed the physical risks to women of abortion, they would be more successful in discouraging abortion. "Well-directed arguments concerning the dangers of having the operation done are," Holmes argued, "more effective than too strong presentations of the moral aspect." He warned that when a doctor told a woman that she was committing a crime and "breaking a moral law, he arouses her enmity from the suggestion implied that she is immoral or criminal."[15] His comments highlight the challenge physicians faced when they tried to teach women to adopt the official medical attitude toward abortion.

When an unmarried woman sought an abortion, many physicians pressed her to marry instead. Physicians intervened in these crises in the way that a minister or father figure might. As a result of one Tennessee doctor's efforts, several couples had "quietly married." He advised the unwed women to "take a revolver with them, and if the young man refuses to marry, to kill him on the spot." In a nice twist on tradition, she, rather than her father, would force the "shotgun marriage."[16]

Antiabortion physicians took their ideological campaign to the public. The Chicago Medical Society expected its Criminal Abortion Committee "to exercise an influence toward restraining the evil and checking the debauchment of the minds of the profession and the community." In 1904, the society's Criminal Abortion Committee presented a public forum on abortion at Chicago's public library.[17] A St. Louis settlement house sponsored "a series of medical lectures for women" organized by Dr. Frederick J. Taussig. One lecture focused on abortion. Anticipating the tactics of recent antiabortionists, Taussig "instructed the nurse who gave the lecture to show an enlarged picture of an embryo of six weeks." He remarked, "I think pictures like that of the six weeks' embryo will keep many women from having an abortion done."[18] The scientific image was used to convince women that the fetus was alive even before quickening, contrary to popular belief. Unfortunately, we do not know how audiences reacted to these exaggerated representations of the embryo in early pregnancy. Doctors alone did not create the discourse of abortion as dangerous. Popular media helped to create a cultural image that equated abortion with death,[19] and women seeking birth control at clinics encountered antiabortion messages from staff and posters on the wall.[20]

A concern about practicing medicine for financial gain threaded its way through medical and popular discussions of abortion. When turn-of-the-century physicians talked about abortion, some used prostitution as their metaphor. They railed against the physician who "prostitutes his profession."[21] Their words expressed the fragility of medical reputations. One Philadelphia doctor described the physician who performed abortions as "an unscrupulous, unprincipled member of the medical profession who prostitutes his skill for gain, and subsists like a vampire upon the blood of an unborn generation." Furthermore, he charged, "graduates of the best medical schools have proved false to their noble vocation and have brought dishonor upon themselves and, to a certain degree, discredit upon the grand profession of medicine."[22]

The language of prostitution is an interesting one for a mostly male profession to adopt. It underlines the character of the antiabortion campaign as a purity campaign and the importance to the profession of maintaining its reputation as highly moral. It also points to an underlying fear of association with illicit sexuality. Prostitution as a rule referred to the sexual and economic exploitation of women by men. Men, without risk of shame or social rejection, bought sexual services, whereas women sold the one thing money should not buy, their virtue. But in the abortion transaction, male physicians accepted money from women; women symbolically exploited medical men. The male physician who did abortions risked his reputation and his medical license. Moreover, in the thinking of antiabortionists, the physician-abortionist not only degraded himself, but, just as prostitutes embarrassed all of womanhood, degraded the medical profession as a whole.

This language betrayed doctors' anxieties about medicine as a business. Physicians' economic concerns were evident in the medical ethical standards of the day. Professional ethics focused, on the one hand, on eliminating competition between doctors by banning advertising and establishing uniform fees and, on the other hand, on making sure that

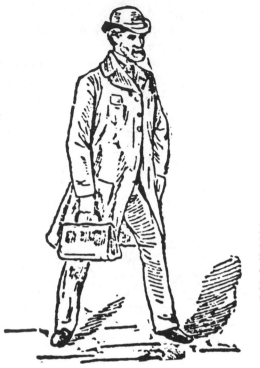

Plate 3. "One of the Reputable Physicians." Note the difference in clothing and demeanor in the depiction of the two types of physicians. *Chicago Times,* December 23, 1888, p. 9.

patients who could pay for medical care did not receive charitable services. In attacking physicians who accepted money for doing abortions, physicians attempted to deny and separate themselves from the ways in which money colored the practice of medicine for all practitioners. The 1888 *Times* exposé represented the difference between the good doctors who did not perform abortions and the bad doctors who did by depicting the "reputable" physician as distinguished but not opulent and the physician-abortionist as a man decked out in furs and top hat. (See plates 3 and 4.)

Anxiety about the damage done by physician-abortionists to the reputation of the medical profession as a whole fueled medical efforts to remove abortionists from their own associations. Physician-abortionists "blacken . . . our profession," the president of the AMA's Section on Obstetrics told his colleagues at the 1893 meeting; they should be "stamped as villains" and prosecuted.[23] "We must purge our ranks of the men who are daily disgracing it" by performing abortions, declared a Maine physician. "We comfort ourselves with the thought

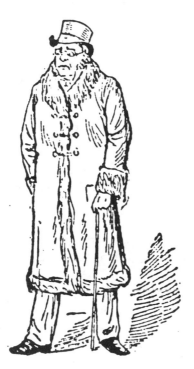

Plate 4. "One of the Abortionists." *Chicago Times,* December 23, 1888, p. 9.

that midwives and renegade physicians are the ones that are doing the most of this work," but, he charged, members of the state and local medical societies practiced abortion. He "beg[ged]" the profession to "begin at once an earnest warfare against the abortionist wherever he may be found."[24]

The response of medical societies to abortion was mixed, however, for they both policed and protected their own members. The Massachusetts Medical Society ousted several members for performing abortions; the Chicago Medical Society expelled Dr. George Lotz in 1912 after he testified at a coroner's inquest and admitted performing an abortion that caused a woman's death.[25] Yet the society exonerated some and ignored others, as it had in 1888. Dr. Carey Culbertson described the committee in 1911 "as a sort of bureau to which the general practitioner can come for information and to bring his data when he is caught in a case of criminal abortion." Physicians who had attempted to repair the results of an illegal abortion, or had attended a woman who miscarried, might find themselves facing criminal charges. The committee promised to help them.[26]

In addition to conducting internal purges of the medical profession, antiabortion activists helped state authorities enforce the law. The Chicago Medical Society's abortion committee forged cooperative relationships with state officials in the investigation of abortionists. "The time has come for this society to take an active part in aiding the prosecution of notorious abortionists," declared Dr. Holmes, the committee's chairman, in 1904. He suggested working with the Cook County coroner and the Chicago and State of Illinois Boards of Health. The committee developed close ties with the coroner's office; the coroner notified the committee of criminal abortion cases and usually one of the committee's members went to the inquest. "In the past year, the chairman of the committee," Dr. Holmes reported in 1906, "secured the arrest of two operators: one, a midwife, was indicted for murder and awaits trial; the other is a physicians, [*sic*] reputed to be an abortionist." [27]

Local medical society representatives (all specialists) acted in the capacity of the coroner. At inquests they questioned witnesses and suspects and collected evidence for future prosecution. Although they were not elected to or employed by the coroner's office, the coroner deferred to their medical knowledge and expected physicians to participate in these cases. State prosecutors spoke to the medical society and taught physicians how to collect evidence to be used against abortionists. [28] Physicians in other cities made similar alliances with state officials. The Philadelphia County Medical Society, for example, formed a committee in 1904 "to aid the legally constituted county officials in securing evidence for the conviction of the criminal abortionist." As a result of this cooperative crusade, the society could boast of having helped imprison at least twelve abortionists and scaring the rest away. [29]

By privately funding and conducting investigations into abortion with undercover detectives, organized medicine voluntarily joined the state in enforcing the criminal abortion laws. Local medical societies around the country supported post office investigations and prosecutions for abortion under the Comstock Law as a way to stop abortion advertising. In October 1906, Dr. Holmes reported to the Chicago Medical Society on the abortion committee's great success in getting Chicago newspapers to cease accepting abortion advertisements. A priest helped visit Chicago's daily papers. After these visits, four daily papers "agreed to refuse all advertisements which concerned the treatment of female complaints." The committee's attorney helped further by threatening to prosecute. Two months later the medical society's board of trustees granted the committee $100 to "to suppress illegal advertising in the lay press."[30] A San Francisco physician, who copied Holmes's methods to remove abortion advertising from local newspapers, reported that the society hired "female detectives" to "visit the various advertising abortionists and get them to consent to perform an abortion." The society sent affidavits from their detectives "to the post office inspector who then sends a stop order to each of the newspapers in which the 'ad' appeared, informing them that the papers would be refused the mails if the objectionable ads were not removed." This worked, but their success was short-lived because the abortionists "soon . . . circumvent this order, and in a few weeks we found that Dr. G. W. O'Donnell became Dr. G. W. Olcot."[31]

The AMA similarly assisted the state in the suppression of the abortifacient trade and the prosecution of abortionists. The AMA created its own Bureau of Investigation in 1906 to investigate and collect information on quackery and patent medicines. The bureau became a semiofficial agency relied upon by government authorities. Individual doctors notified it of abortionists and abortifacients, often including flyers or advertisements in their letters.[32] In addition, the bureau collected information and advertisements on its own and gave this evidence to post office authorities for investigation and prosecution. Government agencies as well as private charities, business organizations, and individuals consulted with the AMA. In 1938 the AMA reported advising the U.S. Post Office, the Food and Drug Administration, the Federal Trade Commission, the Federal Bureau of Investigation, and state and city boards of health. "Frequently," the AMA official reported, authorities asked the bureau to "open its files to them and spend hours . . . discussing . . . the medical viewpoint on the subjects of their investigations." Federal prosecutors asked the AMA to provide expert witnesses in trials against sellers of abortifacients.[33]

Although organized medicine won the respect of state agents and achieved a measure of success in combating abortion, antiabortion leaders ruefully admitted that the profession at large only reluctantly supported antiabortion campaigns. The first chairman of the Chicago Medical Society's Criminal Abortion Committee, Rudolph Holmes, revealed the impotence of the medical regulation of abortion. "I have come to the conclusion," he remarked in 1908, "that the public does not want, the profession does not want, the women in particular do not want, any aggressive campaign against the crime of abortion." For several years he had gathered evidence and gained promises from doctors that they would testify against abortionists, but time and again they disappeared on the day of trial, whereas Medical Society members testified for "notorious abortionist[s]."[34] The situation did not change. The committee had "pushed" branch medical societies to put the topic of abortion on their agendas, "but some societies do not seem at all anxious to have the matter brought up."[35] In 1912 Dr. C. H. Parkes admitted that the coroner and prosecutors, with whom the committee worked, "are firmly convinced that the profession of Chicago and the Chicago Medical Society is apathetic in the extreme, in matters relating to criminal abortion."[36]

At the national level, obstetricians within the AMA found the same indifference to criminal abortion. At the 1908 meeting of the AMA, the chairman of the Section on Obstetrics, Walter B. Dorsett, proposed the creation of a standing "National Committee on Criminal Abortion" and Chicago's Charles Bacon presented the proposal to the AMA's House of Delegates. They proposed forming a national committee to investigate the criminal abortion laws and urged state medical societies to form similar committees, which would meet annually to report their "progress . . . toward the suppression of criminal abortion." Other AMA members did not share the obstetricians' enthusiasm for controlling abortion: the resolution disappeared in committee.[37]

The Anti-midwife Antiabortion Campaign

The antiabortion campaign had its greatest success when it focused its attention not on physicians or on the women who had abortions, but on midwives. Between 1890 and 1920, physicians, public-health workers, and reformers across the United States debated "the midwife problem."[38] Part of the "problem," as many observers defined it, was the practice of abortion by midwives. F. Elisabeth Crowell, a nurse and an investigator of midwives, reported in 1907 that New York City officials and physicians agreed that midwives were primarily responsible for abortion. "Indeed," she concluded, "some go so far as to say that the two terms 'midwife' and 'abortionist' are synonymous."[39] As obstetricians tried to establish their specialty, they focused on midwives as the source of their field's low status and led a campaign to control their competitors.[40] Identifying midwives as abortionists proved to be an effective weapon in the battle to bring midwives under medical scrutiny, and state control. The anti-midwife and antiabortion campaigns became intertwined into one. This campaign arose out of the interests of a small group of specialists, but it won public attention and legislative action as it spoke to larger social concerns about the welfare of immigrant motherhood and the sexuality of young women in the modern American city.

Physicians downplayed the medical side of the abortion story and stressed the role played by midwives, suggesting that all midwives were dangerous. Specialists in obstetrics led this campaign, but condemning midwives for abortion implicitly made all physicians appear morally upright in contrast and shifted attention away from the abortion practices of physicians. Attributing abortion to midwives matched obstetricians' custom of proclaiming their own superiority over midwives (and, later, general practitioners), whom they blamed for overall maternal mortality.[41]

Although scholars have studied the turn-of-the-century medical opposition to midwives, they have not analyzed the role of abortion in the movement to restrict midwifery. Earlier feminist historians of midwifery concentrated on analyzing the medical battle to gain control of obstetrics and comparing physician and midwife safety in childbirth. Most recently, historians have uncovered the details of midwives' birthing practices and have paid greater attention to the history of rural and African American midwives.[42] Abortion was a crucial element of the turn-of-the-century campaign to control urban midwives and one that historians have overlooked.

Tracing the anti-midwife antiabortion campaign as it developed in Chicago provides an opportunity to observe how a debate that began within the medical profession became part of popular discourse and political action. As the medical story of midwives and abortion caught the attention of different groups, each gave the story its own emphasis. Nonetheless, all advanced the obstetricians' program to restrict midwives' practices. The combined campaign to control abortion and midwifery took the form of a classic Progressive Era reform movement: a coalition of private interest groups—doctors, female reformers, nurses, and journalists—of the native-born, white middle-class, identified a problem, investigated and documented its extent in "objective" reports, and mobilized to promote a state-sponsored solution.[43] Also typical of Progressives, the "problem" of midwives and abortion was located in the neighborhoods of the "other," among the city's immigrant masses. Neither the perception that immigrant midwives posed a "problem" nor the tendency to link midwives with abortion was unique to Chicago physicians and reformers.[44] The leaders of medicine and reform in Chicago not only advocated midwife regulations in their own city, they influenced the shape of national health policy.[45]

As the campaign against midwives and abortion moved out of the medical arena and reform circles and into the newspapers, it was strengthened by and became part of the many urban sex reform movements that marked the period. Like other sex reform drives at the turn of the century, the anti-midwife antiabortion campaign identified female sexual behavior and sexual commerce as alarming, and related, urban problems. Americans identified cities as sites where innocents, especially women, were seduced and endangered. Chicago had a notorious reputation as a city of pleasure and vice. The investigations, newspaper exposés, and reform campaigns around prostitution, statutory rape, "women adrift," "birth control," and "race suicide" all attest to the profound upheaval in gender and sexuality that urban industrialization encouraged and made visible. In cities like Chicago it was becoming apparent that newly independent working women were breaking old rules governing sexual behavior and charting new sexual territories that allowed, even celebrated, sexual pleasure separated from procreation and marriage. The era's urban sex reform movements reveal contradictory anxieties about women's newfound sexual freedom and the sexual danger they faced in the city. Sex reformers treated women as both victims of male lust and independent pleasure seekers themselves.[46] Abortion highlighted women's new sexual liberty; women's deaths as a result of abortion emphasized the dangers of sex. The obstetricians' campaign to restrict midwives succeeded, in part, because the antiabortion campaign channeled anxiety about female sexuality into support for the medical program of midwife control.

One of Chicago's specialists in obstetrics helped launch the national medical campaign to control midwives at an international meeting held in Washington, D.C., in September 1893. Dr. Eliza H. Root presented a paper to the section on obstetrics at the Pan-American Medical Congress in which she analyzed the problem of inadequate medical training in obstetrics as well as the results of the unregulated practice of untrained midwives. Root charged midwives with causing infections and inducing abortions, but remarked that untrained physicians posed even greater dangers to their patients. She suggested instituting "the outdoor plan," which would give medical students needed clinical experience by having them attend births in the homes of poor patients.[47]

Although Root's talk focused more on the need to improve the obstetrical education of doctors than on midwives' practices, the specialists at the meeting set an important precedent by focusing their discussion on what they regarded as the crimes and inadequacies of midwives. In so doing, they relegated to the background the problems of poor obstetrical practices by physicians and poor obstetrical training in medical education. As a result of Root's paper and the ensuing discussion, the congress's section on obstetrics took what may have been the first collective international and national action against midwives. The section appointed a committee, headed by Root, which drafted a resolution that "protest[ed] . . . the irregular practice of obstetrics by midwives" and called upon the states to require training and testing of midwives before licensing them. The section voted unanimously in support of the resolution and planned to deliver a copy of its resolution to the board of health or medical licensing of each state.[48] These specialists in obstetrics expected state officials to carry out policies written in the interest of the medical profession and without consultation with midwives, birthing women, or elected officials. Over the next two decades specialists continued to follow the pattern set at the 1893 medical congress.

It is notable that the specialist whose paper inspired this early action in the medical campaign against midwives was a female physician. Many women physicians shared Root's interest in controlling midwifery. Chicago's Dr. Sarah Hackett Stevenson, one of the most prominent female physicians of the nineteenth century, corroborated Root's comments at the meeting and "spoke at length upon the incompetency of foreign midwives in Chicago."[49] The *Woman's Medical Journal* proudly reported on Root's presentation at the Congress, describing it as a "strong and powerful paper on the evils of midwifery, and the desirability of a national law for the extermination of this class."[50]

Root's interest in midwives grew out of her dual identities as a specialist in obstetrics and as a female physician; both groups saw midwives as their rivals. Female physicians had fought to differentiate themselves from less educated and less honored midwives. Women had often based their claims to join the medical profession on their sex and what they could offer women patients during childbirth or gynecological procedures: special feminine sympathy, modesty, and safety in a feminine atmosphere free of the fear of sexual impropriety.[51] Midwives, however, also offered sympathy based on their shared womanhood and on shared class and cultural backgrounds as well. Dr. Stevenson had made the

competition between female health practitioners explicit a few years earlier. She wrote of the need for "stringent laws against midwives. There
is no longer necessity for this class," she argued, because "women
physicians and trained nurses more than fill the demand." Dr. Elizabeth
Jarrett of New York labeled midwives "ignorant, unskillful, [and] dirty"
and looked forward to their replacement by superior female physicians.
"The woman doctor and the midwife," she declared, "have nothing in
common." [52]

The events of the anti-midwife antiabortion campaign highlight the
ways in which class and education could divide women. The campaign
against midwives was more than simply a battle between male physicians and female midwives; the dynamics of class, ethnicity, and professional interests complicate the picture. [53] Female physicians and reformers joined the turn-of-the-century campaign to control the intertwined
"problems" of midwives and abortion. Their involvement in an antiabortion campaign was unprecedented. The earlier medical crusade
had attacked feminists, female physicians, and middle-class women in
general as well as abortion. [54]

Attention to the abortion practices of some midwives enabled specialists in obstetrics and health officials to impose greater control over
all midwives. In 1896 the Chicago City Health Department enacted pio-
neering regulations for midwives on the theory that controlling midwives would control abortion. Dr. Charles S. Bacon, the president
of the health department's obstetric staff, declared that "the practice of
abortion has become a very great evil, largely as a result of a lack of
midwife control." Bacon credited the state board of health with initiating "the movement" for midwife regulation by publishing the details of
thirty-four abortion-related deaths caused by midwives. "These cases in
Chicago," he explained, "were the immediate cause of the movement
which led to the establishment of the system of midwife regulation that
now prevails." The Chicago Health Department wrote twelve rules for
midwives, which the state board of health approved in 1896. One rule
forbade "any midwife hav[ing] in her possession . . . any drug or instrument or other article which may be used to procure an abortion." [55]

In securing the twelve rules for midwives in 1896, Chicago obstetricians won the power to oversee midwives a decade before New York
City doctors and succeeded in defining childbirth as a medical event
long before the national midwife debates reached their peak in the
1910s. [56] Bacon and the other obstetricians in the health department
were concerned about more than midwives' abortion practices—they

resented midwives' obstetric practices in general. As Bacon explained, doctors "objec[t] to midwives" because they "usurp the functions of physicians." Midwives took business that, physicians believed, rightfully belonged to them. In addition, he blamed midwives for raising maternal mortality.[57]

The rules for midwives were written from the perspective of the newly specializing field of obstetrics, which viewed childbearing as a pathological event requiring special medical expertise. The regulations narrowly defined the role of midwives in the birthing process and put midwives directly under the supervision of the city's leading obstetricians. The rules required midwives to register with the Chicago medical inspector of midwives and to keep casebooks and allowed them to attend only "cases of natural labor." In cases of "unnatural" or "abnormal" labor, the rules obliged midwives to call in a physician. To enforce these regulations, the health department organized its own voluntary obstetric staff of "the most eminent men in the city." The staff, of fifty-one obstetricians and ten other doctors, was expected to "attend cases when called on by the midwives, to inspect her [case]book and outfit and in general to help in carrying out the regulations." Department obstetricians also investigated maternal deaths and, when necessary, "impress[ed] the offending midwife with new ideas of their [*sic*] responsibility."[58] Yet, despite the new rules, as later events showed, the health department and its obstetricians had by no means gained complete control over Chicago midwives. Nor had the practice of abortion disappeared.

As the Chicago Medical Society's Criminal Abortion Committee reached the unhappy conclusion that physicians did not support their efforts to bring physician-abortionists to law, they turned their attention to another group. The committee had discovered the "relatively great frequency of the crime of abortion among midwives" and, in 1907, proposed that the society form a new Committee on Midwives to investigate midwives, which it did. The society supported the close scrutiny of their competitors, not their colleagues.[59]

Obstetricians within the medical society joined hands with female reformers to investigate midwifery in Chicago. Hull-House, the settlement house started by Jane Addams, agreed to finance the investigation and the Visiting Nurse Association assisted. Reformers and nurses, like physicians, assumed that high maternal and infant mortality rates, particularly among poor and immigrant populations, could be attributed to midwives. Investigations of midwives were part of a number of activities—such as clean milk drives and classes to teach women about good nutrition and prenatal and infant care—pursued by female urban reformers who hoped to improve the health of poor immigrant women and their families.[60] Gender awareness informed the analysis of the female physicians, nurses, and reformers who joined the effort to regulate midwives. They saw themselves as protectors of other classes of women. Reformers focused on improving the maternal health of poor and immigrant (married) women and protecting young (unmarried) working women from sexual seduction and exploitation.

Rudolph Holmes, head of the medical society's abortion committee and an obstetrician, chaired the new Committee on Midwives. The new committee included Dr. Bacon; Dr. Herbert M. Stowe, another obstetrician; and two female physicians involved in reform, Doctors Alice Hamilton and Caroline Hedger, who shared an interest in maternal and infant health and were associated with Hull-House and the University of Chicago Settlement House respectively.[61] The committee hired Miss F. Elisabeth Crowell to investigate Chicago's midwives. Crowell, a registered nurse and charity worker, had investigated New York midwives two years before and had published an influential and critical report on her investigation. Of the 500 New York midwives she investigated, she suspected that 35 percent practiced abortion.[62] The Chicago committee modeled their investigation of midwives on the New York study, as did Baltimore reformers.[63]

The Chicago Medical Society's Committee on Midwives found, as expected, that the practice of abortion thrived among Chicago's midwives. More than two hundred of the five or six hundred midwives in Chicago were investigated. The committee's "special detective" found that a full third of Chicago's midwives "should be classified as criminal." She found forty-nine midwives willing to operate, four who offered to sell drugs, five who had been indicted for criminal abortion deaths, and twenty-two whom she marked as "suspicious." Nineteen took patients into their homes and ran what the report labeled "abortion shops."[64]

The "detective" uncovered alliances between physicians and midwives in the illegal abortion trade. She visited one physician who ran a midwifery school and who, for an added fee, instructed students in the "*modus operandi* of successful abortion work." The committee also found physicians and midwives who split an abortion practice and the fees. "In the case of a disastrous finale," the committee reported, "the cloak of an honorable calling is wide enough to cover and hide from suspicion both the criminal physician and the criminal midwife." If the midwife had any trouble, she called her physician collaborator, who, if necessary, signed a false death certificate, assigning death to perhaps "pneumonia" or "cardiac failure." [65]

In spite of the evidence of the medical practice of abortion, the 1908 report on "The Midwives of Chicago" blamed midwives alone for illegal abortion and pressed for increased state control over them. "It is generally conceded," wrote Crowell in the committee's report, published in *JAMA,* "that midwives are the chief agents in procuring . . . abortions." [66] The committee compared the state regulation of medicine and midwifery and found that "the laws governing . . . midwifery are utterly absurd and inadequate" compared to those regulating obstetrics. The state required medical students to attend three obstetrical cases, but made no similar requirements of midwives. [67] The committee favored raising the standards for midwives and educating them. No matter how midwives' training improved, however, Crowell argued for the "regulation and inspection of the midwife's practice after she has been turned loose . . . on an ignorant and credulous community." Ideally, the investigators suggested, the state board of health would employ inspectors to supervise Chicago's midwives and "immediately suspen[d]" the licenses of those responsible for infected or mismanaged cases. [68]

As the committee condemned midwives for abortion, it glossed over the involvement of doctors in this criminal practice. It did not recommend that the state inspect the medical practices of physicians and immediately suspend their licenses for abortion or mismanagement. The medical profession preferred to conduct its own, quiet, internal investigations of physicians and expel physician-abortionists itself rather than inviting state agents to oversee medical practices. Physicians could lose their licenses for performing abortions, but in Illinois, only after having been convicted of abortion and having had a hearing before the state board of health. However, since it was extremely difficult for the state to win convictions for criminal abortion, few doctors stood the chance of losing their licenses for illegal abortion. [69] Furthermore, the committee assumed that physicians had better obstetrical training than midwives, but, because of the patterns of social childbirth, some midwives, had, in fact, observed more deliveries than had young doctors. [70]

As a result of the 1908 investigation, Chicago midwives faced increased surveillance and new municipal rules. Again, an investigation initiated because some midwives practiced abortion resulted in restrictions on the birthing practices of all midwives. Although the president of the Illinois Board of Health doubted a new state licensing law for midwives could be won, local officials acted on the report. The Chicago City Council amended the hospital ordinance to prevent midwives and others from treating confinement cases in their own homes. The revised ordinance made anything resembling an "abortion shop" illegal. At the same time, the ordinance preserved hospitals as institutions under medical control. It had not been unusual at the turn of the century for business women to set up private hospitals in their homes, which served the needs of both patients and physicians. The new ordinance prohibited midwives from bringing patients into their own homes or anywhere else unless licensed by the city, but permitted only physicians to obtain licenses for hospitals or maternity centers.[71]

In September 1910, the much talked about Chicago midwives talked back through the legal system and a local paper. Chicago midwives, normally the objects of discussion among middle-class professionals, officials, and reformers, inserted themselves into the debate and told their own, very different story. In the midwives' version, the midwife "problem" was not abortion, but the blackmailing of midwives by state officials. Chicago midwives began investigating the investigators and documenting official corruption and abuse of midwives. They presented to the state's attorney's office twelve affidavits complaining of mistreatment by Illinois health officials. The midwives accused Charles G. Hoffman, an assistant attorney for the state board of health, of threatening midwives with prosecution and extorting them. A meeting of seventy midwives resolved to call on "every midwife in Chicago" and collect additional affidavits from any who had been victimized. A committee was appointed and began work immediately. By the time the city's midwives assembled at a "mass meeting" two weeks later, they had organized themselves into two organizations, the Chicago Midwives' Association and the Midwives' Anti-Graft Association. The midwives demanded that the governor fire Hoffman. They presented additional affidavits telling of abuse, planned a petition, and listened to speeches protesting the state's treatment of midwives.[72]

Mrs. Marie Rolick told the crowd of a visit by a state board of health "spy," who had asked for an abortion. Mrs. Rolick warned other midwives of a male " 'hobble-skirted' spy with curly, wavy, blond hair," who would try to trick them. The male spy, "masquerading as a girl," came with another man and knocked on Rolick's door. Rolick reported that "the man offered me $35 to perform an operation and I only laughed.

He persisted and," she said, "I got angry, grabbed a revolver and threatened to shoot. The 'girl' grabbed her dresses around her and she had a pair of trousers on. . . . my suspicions were well founded." [73]

Mrs. Rolick's "thrilling tale," as the local newspaper billed it, turned the tables on local officials.[74] As investigators and state officials warned midwives to beware of practicing abortion, this midwife warned investigators to beware of midwives armed and willing to fire. Whether or not male investigators really cross-dressed in order to catch midwives, Rolick refashioned the story told by investigators like Miss Crowell and cast herself as a heroine in the drama. In Rolick's narrative there were "spies" (a more malicious term than *investigator*) who hoped to catch midwives performing abortions. The midwife herself appears to be smart and strong—she knew a spy when she saw one and fearlessly threatened "her" with a gun. Unfortunately, the outcome of Chicago midwives' protests and organizing in 1910 remains unclear.

Chicago's midwives showed themselves to be neither passive in the face of attacks nor ignorant about how to defend themselves. These press reports are rare documents in the history of midwifery for they record an episode when midwives united to articulate their opposition to mistreatment by state health officials.[75] The 1910 incident suggests that historians need to revise their assumptions about midwives' inability to organize and defend themselves.[76] Chicago midwives were less isolated both from each other and from American political culture than is usually assumed. And yet midwife organization and resistance was sporadic and ultimately ineffective in preserving midwifery as a craft. Chicago midwives tried to shift attention to abuse by state officers, but they lacked the political and social power to gain control of local debates.

Within weeks of the midwives' public complaints about spies, they were again the subject of secret investigations. The 1910 state-sponsored study of vice in Chicago suggests that reformers imagined abortion, midwives, and prostitution to be linked in the same sexual underground. Investigators for the Chicago vice commission "visited" Chicago's midwives in order to discover whether they performed abortions. Although the vice commission noted that there was "some doubt as to whether or not there is any connection between the practice of abortion and the social evil," they argued for one. "Incidents are on record," the commission informed city officials, "where girls who have had abortions performed have become reckless and discouraged, and have actually entered upon a life of prostitution." Reformers understood both abortion and prostitution as part of the same exploitative commerce in female sexuality. Both were sexually deviant and both symbolized the dangers the city posed to virtuous women.[77]

The vice commission investigated twenty midwives who had raised the commission's suspicions by advertising. The report showed that midwives knew they were often under surveillance: three told the secret investigators that "people at the City Hall watched them." Six refused to perform abortions, the commission agents reported, two referred them to someone else, and, "the *remaining twelve* agreed to perform the supposed abortion for different sums of money" (emphasis in original). Although the commission suspected certain physicians and pharmacists of being in the abortion business, it did not look into their practices. The commission excused its partial inquiry with the explanation that "time has been too limited."[78] Reformers expected to investigate midwives; they were the usual target of investigation, and even when evidence indicated that others participated in illegal activities, reformers did not feel compelled to inspect them. In short, probing the practices of midwives had become a habit.

Neither the rules for midwives enacted by the health department in 1896 nor the 1908 ordinance forbidding the institution of hospitals by midwives (let alone the laws forbidding abortion) put a stop to midwives' obstetric and abortion practices. One influential reformer, Grace Abbott, a Hull-House resident and founder of the Immigrants' Protective League, concluded in a March 1915 report that the recommendations made by the 1908 Committee on Midwives had come to naught.[79]

Abbott urged a new strategy: recognizing midwives and training them. Even though her colleagues at Hull-House had participated in the investigation of midwives with the Chicago Medical Society seven years earlier, "laymen and doctors," Abbott now reported, "ha[d] divided . . . into two opposing camps." The policy of Hull-House reformers to listen to their neighbors, particularly immigrant women, had given them a fresh perspective on midwives. Abbott dismissed the fixation on the abortion practices of some midwives as irrelevant to the question of their safety as birthing attendants. Abbott recognized that poor immigrant women relied on midwives to attend them during childbirth and that improving midwives' skills could improve the maternal and infant health of the foreign-born community. Though Abbott criticized physicians and suggested a policy many would dislike, she reassured them that physicians well-trained in obstetrics were

preferable to midwives and that supporters of midwife training and licensing did not intend to "make a doctor out of a midwife." Immigrants, however, she pointed out, preferred midwives because they
were women and often refused to be seen by male physicians. The "traditions and prejudices" of immigrant women and men made midwives
inevitable and their training a necessity.[80]

Abbott made a concrete proposal for carrying out the public policy
she favored: Cook County Hospital should open a school for midwives.
A 1913 investigation, she reported, found seventy-one midwives who
welcomed the idea. Abbott had surveyed the training opportunities
available to midwives and concluded that what little Chicago had to offer was terrible. Several physicians ran their own officially unrecognized
proprietary schools for midwives, but Abbott questioned their quali-
fications and judged the training worthless because midwives merely
listened to lectures without observing actual deliveries. (This had been
the tradition in medical education as well. In fact, one of the nation's
leading obstetricians reported that most medical students observed
only one delivery.) Abbott again reassured the medical community that
training midwives would not hurt physicians; since medical students
did not work in the maternity ward at the county hospital, her proposal
"would not mean the sacrifice of medical students to the training of
midwives."[81]

Abortion in Chicago exploded into public view just two months after the publication of Abbott's report, when the bizarre abortion-
related death of Miss Anna Johnson appeared on the front pages of the
city's newspapers. On May 26, 1915, Anna Johnson was found dead
with a bullet hole in her head in the home of Dr. Eva Shaver, a graduate of a "notorious" medical school shut down by the state board of
health. Newspapers told a confusing and ever-changing story of Johnson's death. Dr. Shaver claimed that she had recently hired Johnson as
a maid and the girl had committed suicide. Police speculated that
Shaver had killed Johnson in an attempt to cover up a badly performed
abortion and looked for dead babies buried under the floors of the
doctor's home. Johnson's "sweetheart," Marshall Hostetler, told the
coroner that the couple had met at a dancehall over a year before and
had planned to marry. When she discovered her pregnancy, he bought
abortifacient pills from Dr. Shaver's son for Johnson, and when those
failed to work, he arranged for her to go to Dr. Shaver's home for an illegal operation. Johnson had tried "to hide her shame" by having an
abortion and ended up murdered.[82]

Although the accused abortionist in this case was a physician, this incident revived the campaign against midwives and abortion and infused it with a new vitality. Journalists and officials still assumed that female practitioners were midwives, and midwives, abortionists.[83] The Johnson case illuminates the Progressive Era's understanding of abortion as sexually dangerous and as symbolic of heterosexual relations. Press coverage of the story followed well-worn paths in the newspaper trade and in sexual discourse. The story titillated Chicago's citizens and sold papers while it reinforced the sense of the city as a place of sexual danger for young unmarried women.[84]

The coverage of Johnson's death sent different messages about abortion than had the 1888 exposé, which had suggested it was easy for women to get an abortion. A new story was being constructed. The story now told by the press warned young women that challenging sexual norms could kill them. Newspaper headlines such as "Unmarried Lead Deaths" and "Health Committee to Take up Baby and Women Killing Inquiry at Once" all emphasized the deaths of unmarried women following abortions. The *Tribune* grandly displayed photos of Shaver's apartment, Anna Johnson, and the pills she had taken. (See plate 5.) The paper emphasized the certainty that death followed on the heels of abortion by listing, in a separate column next to the photos, the names and accounts of twenty-four Chicago women who had died because of abortions in the last five months. "How many girls die in Chicago each year as Anna Johnson died?" the *Tribune* asked. The paper answered that the coroner reported that abortions had caused at least "601 deaths in the last eight years!"[85]

This report, however, exaggerated the number of deaths due to criminal abortions induced by midwives, physicians, and others. No more than 15 percent of these abortion deaths were identified as caused by criminal abortions. Some of the abortion-related deaths recorded by the coroner had followed miscarriages (spontaneous abortions), and many more were the result of self-induced abortions, a dangerous practice rarely mentioned in the press. Furthermore, not all of the women who had abortions or who died from them were young unmarried "girls" like Johnson; most were married and most survived, but newspapers featured the unwed.[86]

At the same time that press coverage emphasized the victimization of unmarried women, it included a strand that blamed married women for "race suicide." The sympathetic tone toward victimized girlhood contained an undertone of fear and anger toward female control of re-

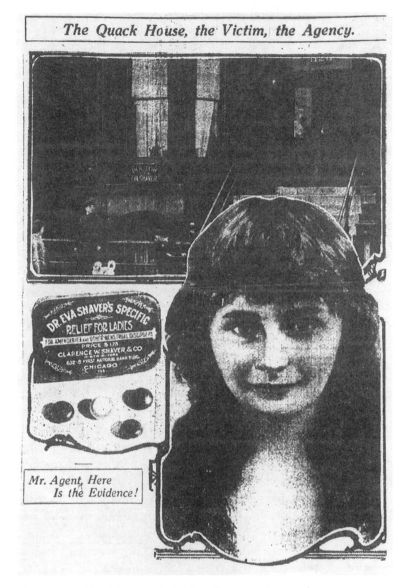

The Quack House, the Victim, the Agency.

Mr. Agent, Here
Is the Evidence!

Plate 5. "The Quack House, the Victim, the Agency." Local newspapers covered abortion as mystery, romance, and crime. In these photos the paper called attention to the pills as "Evidence," luridly labeled Dr. Shaver's office the "House of Murder," and included a portrait of Anna Johnson, the young "victim." The scrollwork was typical of theatrical advertising. Note that the doctor's office and sign faced the street. *Chicago Daily Tribune,* May 29, 1915.

production. Coroner Hoffman, according to one paper, "insisted that retreats wherein 'race suicide' is practiced and preached must be suppressed as a growing menace." His words marked this battle as part of a larger attack on the separation of sex from procreation, the increasing use of contraception by Americans, particularly among the white, native-born elite, and, especially, the feminist movement for birth control. Officials and physicians recognized abortion as one method of birth control and midwives as providers of birth control to the working class. Dr. W. H. Stackable, a member of the Chicago Medical Society's abortion committee, estimated that 60 percent of the women who had abortions were married. Married women had abortions "because they either wish to avoid the responsibility or because they already have large families; neither reason," Stackable remarked, "constitutes a defense." In the midst of this attack on abortion, the circuit court's chief justice refused to grant one woman a divorce because she had had an illegal abortion. Justice John P. McGoorty declared, "A woman who would destroy life in that manner is not fit for decent society. It is the duty of any healthy married woman to bear children. Divorce is refused." To these men of medicine and law, women were obligated to bear children; those who did not deserved to be punished.[87]

The press story of Johnson and Hostetler played on the old theme of male seduction and abandonment of innocent women, but recast the standard gender roles of the tale. In the Johnson melodrama, the woman appeared as the victim, but so too did the man. A second woman performed the lead role of villain. The papers generally presented the lead male in the story, Johnson's "sweetheart," Hostetler, as a victim. Although he was a suspect himself at certain points and had a turbulent (perhaps even violent?) relationship with Johnson, he had lost his beloved sweetheart and "sobbed" and "collapsed" repeatedly at the inquest into her death. He had been duped by the evil Dr. Shaver and her son Clarence into allowing them to induce an abortion and, after Johnson's death, into hiding to avoid the law. Furthermore, it was later reported, as he talked to prosecutors, his life was threatened. The villain in this case became not the young man who had impregnated Johnson and failed to marry her, but the female physician-abortionist, Eva Shaver.[88]

As newspapers reported the Johnson tragedy and highlighted the dangers of abortion, they moved the discussion of abortion and midwifery out of the smaller circles of the medical societies and reform groups and into the public eye. At the same time, the press drew the

public into a medically defined, citywide war on abortion and midwifery. As reporters and officials reworked the abortion story by adding
the exciting angles of sex and murder, they successfully aroused the
curiosity and concern of citizens and politicians. The new story conformed, however, to the analysis of public policy and abortion constructed over the years by specialists in obstetrics. As before, the death
of a woman as a result of abortion prompted an attack on midwives.
This time, however, local press and politicians, not doctors, led the crusade. The new leaders followed doctors in automatically blaming midwives for the problem of abortion in their city and supporting regulation of midwives as the solution even though this meant ignoring that
the Johnson case contradicted their own story because the accused
abortionist was not a midwife at all, but a physician.

Turning Dr. Shaver into a midwife in the discourse reveals the
strength of old prejudices against female physicians. The coroner's declared "war" against abortion immediately turned into a "campaign
against midwives."[89] The *Chicago Herald* cried out, "Midwives under
Fire," and announced that Johnson's death "Turns Searchlight on Maternity Homes and Chicago Midwifery."[90] The "searchlight" never focused on Chicago's medical profession. Coroner Peter Hoffman emphasized the guilt of midwives, though the data collected by his own
office showed midwives and doctors to be almost equally responsible
for women's abortion-related deaths.[91] Dr. Stackable of the Chicago
Medical Society charged that 75 percent of the city's abortionists were
midwives. Although he "admitted" that physicians performed abortions, and called for stricter enforcement of the laws against both midwives and physicians, neither newspapers nor city officials highlighted
the large number of physicians involved in illegal abortion.[92]

Press coverage of Anna Johnson's death inspired local women's organizations to call for the suppression of abortion and regulation of
midwifery. The day after the report of Johnson's death the local press
defended its coverage with the remark that "nothing but publicity and
the arousing of public wrath against the abortionists, say the women's
organizations interested, can check their operations."[93] Dr. Effie L.
Lobdell of the Welfare League of Chicago suggested that physicians
should be able to arrest women who asked them for abortions. The
Woman's City Club favored "more stringent regulation" of midwives,
as did the Chicago Woman's Aid.[94] When Coroner Hoffman vowed to
"exterminat[e] . . . 'wild-cat maternity homes,'" he recognized the
influence of Chicago's club women and asked them to "aid the author-

ities in putting an end to the sale of drugs used in illegal practices."[95] He expected civic and women's organizations to help him eradicate the city's abortionists. The Chicago Medical Society and city ministers soon joined the chorus condemning abortion and endorsed efforts to end its practice in Chicago.[96]

Newspaper readers jumped into the local investigation of "abortion crimes" by writing letters to the "Tribune Quack Department." Several sent names and addresses of abortionists in their neighborhoods. "I would advise," wrote one, "a canvas among the 'lady' physicians and midwives of the west side in the Bohemian settlement," at least two of whom, the writer knew "positively," were abortionists. One woman wrote of her own abortion, but the "crime" in her story was her "former sweetheart's" behavior. He had promised to marry, but then refused. "All that I am living for," she concluded, "is to see the day that they will do justice to men that believe in doing wrong to young girls."[97]

Faced with a public outcry for action, officials at all levels of government quickly enlisted in the battle against abortion by ordering investigations and passing new legislation. Coroner Hoffman led the "war." He suggested that "scores of midwives" used their homes as maternity homes and had their patients pretend to be roomers or servants to cover up their abortion practices. "These wildcat maternity homes and ignorant, lawbreaking midwives must be driven out of Chicago," declared the coroner. The coroner called on other officials to aid him in the fight against abortion. He, the police chief, the city health department, and the state's attorney's office all planned to investigate the maternity centers. The city health department complained that it had no control over midwives and planned, the *Herald* reported, to "seek at once the adoption of an ordinance placing them under its supervision."[98] The Illinois Board of Health's secretary agreed "entirely . . . with the move in the city of Chicago to drive out the abortionists" and promised to "assist in every possible way in the suppression of the evil."[99] Within a few days of Johnson's death, on June 1, 1915, the Chicago City Council unanimously passed a motion ordering its health committee to investigate the underground commerce in abortion as "practiced by midwives and others."[100] U.S. district attorney and post office officials promised inquiries into the abortifacient business.[101]

Local and state health officials invited the local medical society to participate in making public-policy decisions. "Private" and "public" officialdom merged, a characteristic feature of early-twentieth-century

political life. The week after the city council's action, "public and private health officials," the press reported, met at the city health commis-
sioner's office and agreed upon a "co-operative crusade to drive professional abortionists from the city and state." Hoffman had invited the
police chief, the state's attorney, officials from the city and state boards
of health, and members of the Chicago Medical Society to meet, but
not representatives of women's clubs or settlement houses. Although
club women had been important to the coroner for spurring on investigation, they were not included in public-policy discussions. The authorities proposed a state maternity home for "unfortunate girls," a
"higher standard for midwives," and the passage of Illinois House Bill
477, legislation designed to close a loophole in the law that they believed protected abortionists. The bill would allow the state board of
health to revoke the licenses of doctors and midwives who had received
licenses before 1899, many of whom were thought to be abortionists.[102]

There were some exceptions to the common cry. Echoing the proposal made by Abbott a few months earlier, some recommended better
training of midwives. The Chicago Medical Society's president, Dr.
James A. Clark, remarked, "About the most important thing is to raise
the standard of midwives." The county hospitals, he suggested, should
open schools of midwifery. Clark's proposal placed him within the group
of physicians who viewed midwives as a necessity, whose skills could be
improved. Nonetheless, though these physicians held a more sympathetic attitude toward midwives than those who favored an outright
ban on midwives, they shared the belief that midwives should be
brought under greater medical control and, eventually, be replaced by
physicians. Abbott had objected to the obsession with midwives' abortion practices, yet an abortion-related death and an antiabortion antimidwife campaign brought attention to her proposal for midwife education. Despite the support of the medical society's president for a
school for midwives, none opened at Cook County Hospital.[103]

While no advances were made in helping Chicago's midwives improve their skills, the 1915 campaign against abortion strengthened the
state's enforcement of the criminal abortion laws. The Illinois legislature corrected the Medical Practice Act to allow the state to revoke licenses of midwives and physicians licensed before 1899. In Chicago,
police made more arrests for abortion that year than ever before, top-
ping the previous year's high with forty-seven arrests. Dr. Shaver was
held for trial for Anna Johnson's death and in 1916 convicted of
manslaughter for the abortion-related death of another woman.[104]

The events surrounding Anna Johnson's death in 1915 showed how the program to control midwives could advance when it became attached to social anxiety about female sexuality. Specialists who sought increased state control over midwives had political success because, in the public arena, their proposal to control midwives promised not only to control the abortion business, but also to "protect" young, unmarried women from the twin dangers of sex and death. The Johnson case reminded young women that claiming sexual freedom and control over their own fertility could be deadly.

The message was mixed, however; while some took heed of newspaper warnings, others ignored them. Mrs. Cecile Hauptli and Edna Lamb talked about a newspaper story and "what a number of girls did die from abortions." Yet they agreed it was "a very well known fact" that some doctors performed abortions, and they named two. "If you know where to look," Lamb remarked, "you can find doctors all over the city, that will do those things." They had gotten the message that "girls did die" because of abortions, but they discounted the deadly story told by the newspapers. Finding a safe abortionist, Lamb's remarks suggested, was a matter of being savvy.[105]

The newspapers' emphasis on the danger of midwives made at least one Chicago citizen doubt midwives' skills and take his daughter to a doctor instead for an abortion. This man recalled telling the doctor, "The newspaper got it many cases where midwifes [*sic*] kill many young girls and young women." The doctor reassured him: "Don't you be afraid. It is no danger at all." During the procedure, the doctor perforated his patient's uterus, pulled out her intestines, and caused her death. The physician responsible for this disaster was Dr. Charles R. A. Windmueller, a graduate of the University of Illinois College of Medicine in Chicago, a licensed regular physician, and an AMA member.[106]

Neither press nor politicians initiated a war against doctors as a result of this young woman's death. Dr. Windmueller was held to the grand jury for the woman's death, but physicians as a group were not blamed for abortion. In contrast to midwives, who were regularly condemned for abortion as a group, physicians caught doing illegal (and fatal) abortions were treated as disreputable individuals, not as representatives of their entire profession.

The combined campaign to control both midwives and abortion faded in Chicago despite the intense attention given abortion by reporters and politicians in the late spring of 1915. The Chicago City Council neither received a requested report on midwives nor passed any ordinances to regulate them further. In 1916, the number of arrests for abortion fell to little more than half of the previous year's total.[107] Press coverage of abortion still inspired local prosecutors to bring cases to court more quickly, but antiabortion campaigns did not turn into anti-midwife crusades. The *Chicago Examiner,* for instance, ran a series on the deaths of young women due to abortion in 1918. The paper claimed that its "exposé . . . of a ring of unscrupulous doctors who prey upon young girls' misfortunes" had convinced the prosecutor to bring several old abortion cases to trial.[108] The accused abortionists included both physicians and midwives, but this exposé did not target midwives and did not result in new regulations governing their practices.

In turn-of-the-century Chicago, specialists in obstetrics won increased state supervision and restriction of the city's midwives in 1896, 1908, and 1915. In each instance, the identification of midwives as abortionists facilitated the passage of new rules controlling midwives' practices. However, obstetricians did not have the social power to dictate regulation of their competitors: their narrow professional interests had to appeal to other concerns to achieve political success. As their professional rivalry merged with popular discourse about women in the city, the specialists' program to control midwives made headway. Reformers, whether interested in lowering maternal mortality among immigrant women or fighting vice, investigated midwives. When reporters and city officials connected midwives and abortion to contemporary anxieties about the sexual vulnerability and independence of single women, politicians at every level acted to control midwives. Reformers, reporters, and politicians all reworked the midwife story and put their own slant on it, yet they followed the medical line that linked midwives to abortion and urged their regulation as the solution. Controlling midwives seemed to be the answer to an array of perceived social problems. Meanwhile, the role of physicians in performing abortions was overlooked. Stigmatizing midwives as abortionists was only one weapon used by specialists in their political campaign to suppress midwifery. But, as the events in Chicago show, it proved to be a powerful one.

Although antiabortion physicians won their battle for greater control over midwives, one physician's remarks revealed that they lost the war to convince women that abortion was evil. In 1922, a frustrated Dr. Palmer Findley, a specialist from Omaha, observed that "the laity" still believed "that there can be no life until fetal movements are felt." Quickening continued to have real moral meaning for women. "We often find women of unquestioned moral standing bitterly resenting their state of pregnancy, and . . . determined to put an end to the whole affair." But, he reported, "when the date of quickening arrives and they are conscious of sheltering and nourishing a human life, their viewpoint is completely changed."[109] Although this doctor seemed astonished at the persistence of these ideas, his story emphasizes that people took seriously this particular event—the movement of the fetus—as an indication of life. The public, and even much of the medical profession, had not adopted the new thinking that treated conception as the beginning of life and equated it with a child. Although the campaign had not convinced the public that abortion was wrong or stopped its practice, it did create a more hostile environment in which women sought abortions. Women may have felt harassed by physicians who gave them sermons, and some may have felt guilty; others found it harder to obtain abortions when local physicians and politicians cracked down on the abortion trade.

By 1920, the national campaigns against midwives and abortion had come to an end. The Progressive Era's antiabortion campaign had failed to ignite most physicians, to purge physician-abortionists from the profession, or to eradicate abortion. Few doctors talked anymore about the evil of criminal abortion and how to combat it. Palmer Findley was an exception, and he sounded archaic in 1922. The physician who remained committed to the antiabortion campaigns of the past, Findley remarked, "however courageous, will find little encouragement and much embarrassment if he fights alone."[110] The medical discussion of abortion narrowed in the 1920s to the ongoing internal medical debate about whether, when, and how to perform therapeutic abortions.

Changes in the larger context regarding reproduction and public policy help explain the decline of the antimidwife antiabortion campaign. Interest in midwives and abortion as "problems" faded as reformers and activist physicians shifted their attention to other national policy questions, namely maternal and infant health and birth control. Once the women's movement won passage of the Sheppard-Towner Act in 1921, which provided federal matching funds to the states to improve maternal and infant health, the majority of the medical profession turned to battling the act instead of midwives and abortion. Physicians feared government control of medicine and the loss of private-paying patients more than midwives who served the poor.[111]

Leadership for and against Sheppard-Towner came from Chicago. Grace Abbott was appointed head of the federal agency that implemented the Sheppard-Towner Act. Reformers wholeheartedly supported the federal mandate to improve maternal and infant health; the AMA actively fought it. Female reformers and physicians interested in maternal health who had initially supported the investigation and control of midwives adopted a more respectful attitude toward them as they learned more about midwives and the birthing women they served.[112] Although a handful of Chicago physicians, including Doctors Bacon and Hedger, supported the act, the state of Illinois, home of the AMA, was one of only three states that refused to participate in the program.[113]

Not only had a reform movement won the passage of the Sheppard-Towner Act, but another threatening movement, the birth control movement, had arisen during the years of the antiabortion campaign. No group defended abortion, but an increasingly strong and broad-based movement advocated contraceptive use. The birth control movement proclaimed women's right to limit their childbearing and advocated the legalization of contraceptives. For individuals ideologically opposed to female reproductive freedom, birth control was the issue to be fought, not abortion. The birth control movement challenged the law and the medical profession by opening clinics where activists gave women birth control information and devices. Furthermore, birth controllers criticized the medical profession for withholding contraceptives and accused it of being too willing to perform therapeutic abortions.[114] Physicians committed to upholding moral standards, dedicated to stopping women's efforts to limit childbearing, and alarmed at the activities of nonphysicians fought the new birth control movement from the mid-1910s into the 1930s. Their number included some of the physicians active in the antiabortion campaign.[115] Hostile physicians linked the two reform movements by using birth control to attack Sheppard-Towner supporters.[116]

When Congress abolished the Sheppard-Towner Act in 1929 under pressure from the AMA and politically conservative groups, midwives were of little consequence to specialists in obstetrics. By the 1930s, obstetrics was an established specialty and midwives were disappearing from northern cities like Chicago. Obstetricians no longer needed to prop up their own authority by discrediting their competitors or by proclaiming their moral purity. Furthermore, although reformers and doctors had split over Sheppard-Towner, the programs instituted under this act achieved many of the aims of the medical campaign to control midwives. The act encouraged state monitoring of midwives and urged pregnant women to seek physicians as attendants.[117]

The medical fight against abortion, waged in private encounters between female patients and physicians as well as in public political and cultural realms, waned as other issues came to the forefront and the professional concerns that had energized the campaign's leaders subsided. Despite the multifaceted nature of the turn-of-the-century medical campaign against abortion, the practice of abortion continued through the early twentieth century. Antiabortionists had lost the cultural fight to reeducate the public about abortion. They had established, however, important links with the state in making public policy concerning reproduction and in enforcing the criminal abortion laws.

CHAPTER 4

Interrogations and Investigations

In March 1916, Mrs. Carolina Petrovitis, a Lithuanian immigrant to Chicago and mother of two small children, was in terrible pain following her abortion when her friends called in Dr. Kahn.[1] The doctor asked her, "Who did it for you[?]" He "coaxed" her to answer, then told her, "if you won[']t tell me what was done to you I can't handle your case." When Petrovitis finally revealed that a midwife had performed an abortion, Dr. Maurice Kahn called for an ambulance, sent her to a hospital, told the hospital physician of the situation, and suggested he "communicate with the Coroner's office." Three police officers soon arrived to question Carolina Petrovitis. With the permission of the hospital physician, Sgt. William E. O'Connor "instructed" an intern to "tell her she is going to die." The sergeant and another officer accompanied the intern to the woman's bedside, and, as the doctor told Petrovitis of her impending death, she "started to cry—her eyes watered." Sure that Petrovitis realized she was about to die, the police then collected a "dying declaration" from her in which she named the midwife who performed her abortion, told where and when it was done, the price paid, and described the instruments used. Later, the police brought in the midwife and asked Petrovitis "if this was the woman." She nodded "yes." A third police officer drew up another dying statement "covering the facts." As he read the third statement back to Carolina, she lay in bed "in pain, vomiting;" she made her "mark" on the statement. And then she died.

This chapter answers an important question in the history of reproduction: how did the state enforce the criminal abortion laws? From the mid-nineteenth-century criminalization of abortion through the 1930s, the state chiefly prosecuted abortionists after a woman died as a result of an illegal abortion. This account, drawn from the Cook County Coroner's Inquest into Carolina Petrovitis's death in 1916, provides an example of standard medical and investigative procedures used in criminal abortion cases. As is evident from the work of the three police officers in the Petrovitis case, the state had a strong interest in obtaining dying declarations from women who had had illegal abortions. Dying declarations were crucial pieces of evidence for the successful prosecution of criminal abortion cases, and therefore state officials focused on collecting them. For over half a century, state officials in Chicago and across the nation followed the same methods of enforcing the criminal abortion laws. Enforcement was marked by continuity. Not until the end of the Depression, as a result of changes in medicine and abortion practices in the 1930s, did the patterns of controlling abortion change.

Petrovitis's experience illustrates the intimate questioning endured by women during an official investigation into abortion. In abortion cases, the investigative procedures themselves constituted a form of control and punishment. These cases point to the gendered nature of punishment. Recognizing the impact of the criminal abortion laws on women requires looking closely at the details of women's experiences: the interactions between women and their doctors and between women and police and lower-level state officials. Our understanding of what punishment is needs to be refined and redefined, particularly in cases of women who violate sexual norms, to include more subtle methods of disciplining individuals. Gender informed the nature of punishment. The penalties imposed upon women for having illegal abortions were not fines or jail sentences, but humiliating interrogation about sexual matters by male officials—often while women were on their death beds—and public exposure of their abortions. Police, coroner's officers, and prosecutors followed standard procedures during investigations of abortion in order to achieve the larger end of putting abortionists out of business. No evidence suggests that officials consciously created or carried out these investigative procedures in order to harass women, yet the procedures were, nonetheless, punitive. For government officials, the procedures were routine. For the women subjected to these routine investigative procedures, they were frightening and shameful once-in-a-lifetime events. Moreover, media attention to abortion deaths was a crucial component of the enforcement system; publicity warned all women that those who strayed from marriage and motherhood would suffer death and shameful publicity. Because of the singular importance of sexual purity to female social reputation and identity, public exposure could effectively punish women for the transgression of abortion.

The criminal abortion laws and their enforcement not only prohibited abortion, but demanded conformity to gender norms, which required men and women to marry, women to bear children, and men to bear the financial responsibility of children. Although most women who had abortions were married, state officials focused special attention on unwed women and their partners. Coroner's inquests into abortion deaths of unwed women reveal a state interest in forcing working-class men to marry the women they made pregnant. Historians of sexuality have given little attention to the regulation of male heterosexuality, concentrating instead on the sexual control of women and "deviants."[2] Yet, as I was surprised to find, in the late nineteenth and early twentieth centuries the state punished unmarried, working-class men whose lovers died after an abortion. The sexual double standard persisted, but the state imposed penalties upon men, in certain unusual situations, when they failed to carry out their paternal obligation to marry their pregnant lovers and head a nuclear family. Unmarried men implicated in abortion deaths, like women, endured embarrassing questions about their sexual behavior, but in general, the state punished men in more conventionally recognized ways: arresting, jailing, and prosecuting them.

State efforts to control abortion were part of a turn-of-the-century trend toward growing state intervention in sexual and family matters. In enforcing marriage when pregnancy resulted from premarital sex, state officials seemed to be willing to take over another traditional responsibility of the male patriarch. The punishment of unmarried men in cases of abortion-related deaths of unmarried women may have at the same time been a response to feminist demands for male sexual responsibility. Much of this promotion of marriage occurred in the newly created juvenile court system, which female reformers had helped create and in which they participated.[3]

The Petrovitis story reveals some of the ways in which physicians and hospitals served the state in collecting evidence in criminal abortion cases. State officials pulled physicians into a partnership in the suppression of abortion by threatening them with prosecution. Although some physicians voluntarily worked to enforce the criminal abortion laws, others would have preferred to have nothing to do with it. To obtain evidence against abortionists, state prosecutors needed physicians to report abortions and collect dying declarations from their patients. Without doctors' cooperation, police and prosecutors could do little to suppress abortion. In illegal abortion cases, doctors found themselves caught in the middle between their responsibilities to their patients and the demands of government officials. The state regulation of doctors in abortion cases coincided with expanding governmental control of medicine through licensing laws and medical practice acts.[4]

In enforcing the criminal abortion laws, prosecutors learned to concentrate on cases where they had a "victim"—a woman who had died at the hands of a criminal abortionist. Popular tolerance of abortion had tempered enforcement of the criminal abortion laws and helped create the focus on fatalities. In 1903, attorney H. H. Hawkins reviewed Colorado's record and concluded, "No one is prosecuted in Colorado for abortion except where death occurs. . . . The law only applies to the man who is so unskilful as to kill his patient."[5] To some extent this emphasis protected women by locking up some of the worst abortionists. Yet the criminalization of abortion contributed to the dangers of abortion because it restricted access to better trained and more careful practitioners. In Illinois, thirty-seven out of forty-three different abortion cases on which the Supreme Court of Illinois ruled between 1870 and 1940 involved a woman's death. Because prosecutors focused on abortionists responsible for abortion-related deaths, they relied upon dying declarations, like those obtained from Petrovitis, and coroner's inquests as sources of evidence. The Illinois Supreme Court commented on dying declarations in almost a third of the cases it heard where a woman died because of an abortion.[6]

Prosecutors won few convictions for abortion, however. But counting convictions for abortion underestimates and obscures the state's serious interest in enforcing the criminal abortion laws. Analysis of the entire investigative process is necessary to bring to light the state's effort to suppress abortion. Police arrests for abortion and inquests into abortion deaths indicate a greater degree of interest in repressing abortion than suggested by the number of convictions. (See figure 1.) Between 1902 and 1934 in Chicago, the state's attorney's office annually prosecuted at most a handful of criminal abortion cases and never won more than one or two convictions a year. In one ten-year period, less than one-quarter of the prosecutions for murder by abortion resulted

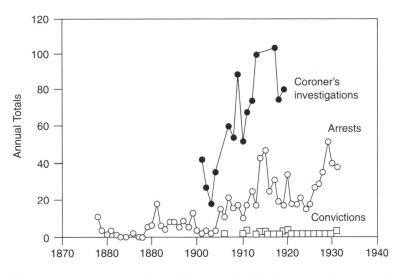

Figure 1. Coroner's investigations of abortion-related deaths compared to arrests and convictions for abortion, Chicago, 1878–1931.

SOURCES: Chicago Department of Police, *Report of General Superintendent of Police of the City of Chicago*, 1878–1912, Municipal Reference Collection, Chicago Public Library, Chicago, Illinois (MRC); Chicago Department of Police, *Annual Report*, 1913–1931, MRC; "Chicago Medical Society. Regular Meeting, Held November 23, 1904, Symposium on Criminal Abortion," *JAMA* 43 (December 17, 1904): 1890.

in a conviction.[7] In contrast, police made at least ten arrests annually for abortion after 1905, averaged twenty-five or twenty-six annual arrests during the 1910s and 1920s, and made almost forty arrests each year in the early 1930s. Police stepped up their arrests under political pressure. The peak years for arrests for abortion coincided with organized efforts against abortion. For example, a peak in 1905 is probably due to the Chicago Medical Society's renewed efforts to eradicate abortion, and the peak in 1912 matches the coordinated, nationwide raids by the U.S. Post Office on people who used the mail to sell contraceptive or abortion instruments or services.[8]

The coroner conducted even more inquests into abortion deaths every year. Between 1901 and 1919, the years for which figures are available, the Cook County coroner investigated an average of over sixty abortion deaths a year, from a low of eighteen in 1903 to a high of 103 in 1917. Not all of these abortion-related deaths followed criminal abortions; some were "accidental," "self-induced," or "spontaneous" abortions, and others were the result of an "undetermined" cause, but, because the coroner had to determine the cause of death, these deaths were investigated like criminal cases.[9] Between 1905 and 1919, the coroner sent an average of twelve suspects a year to the grand jury.[10] The level of legal action against abortion steadily increased over time, but the number of convictions did not change at all. Most of the rise over time in abortion inquests and arrests is probably explained by Chicago's growing population, though the rise may also reflect intensified efforts by state officials to control abortion.

Abortion investigations began, as in the Petrovitis case, when physicians or hospitals noticed a "suspicious" case and reported it to the police or Cook County coroner.[11] In the first stage of an investigation, a woman was questioned by her doctor and might be questioned again by police or special investigators sent by the coroner. Each interrogation was an attempt to obtain a legally valid dying declaration, in which the woman admitted her abortion and named her abortionist. A dying declaration not only led police to suspects, but was itself a crucial piece of evidence that could be introduced at criminal trials. As one lawyer observed, it was almost "impossible" to obtain evidence of criminal abortion any other way.[12]

The dying declaration was an unusual legal instrument that allowed the words of the dead to enter the courtroom. Legally, a dying declaration is an exception to the hearsay rule, which excludes the courtroom use of information that has been received second-hand. Common law allowed the admission of dying declarations as evidence in homicide cases, and states permitted this exception in abortion cases as well.[13] Courts treated dying declarations as though given under oath, based on the common-law assumption that a dying person would not lie because she was, as the coroner put it during the inquest on Petrovitis, "about to leave the worlds—to meet her maker." This exception allowed prosecutors to present, in court, the dying declaration as the dead woman's own accusation of who had killed her.[14]

If the woman died, the abortion investigation proceeded to a second stage: an autopsy performed by coroner's physicians and an official coroner's inquest into the woman's death. During the inquest, the coroner or his deputy questioned a series of witnesses and attempted to collect the facts in the case. Police presented for the first time the dying statements they had collected and any other information or individuals uncovered during their investigation. Family members, lovers, friends, midwives, physicians, and hospital staff all testified at these inquests. A coroner's jury then deliberated and decided the cause of death. Although the legal purpose of an inquest was limited to determining the cause of death, the coroner, in fact, wielded significant power. The coroner's inquest was a highly important stage in the legal process since it generally determined whether anyone would be criminally prosecuted. The jury decided the guilt or innocence of various people involved in a case, and, if the jury determined that the woman's death was the result of "murder by abortion,"[15] it ordered the police to hold the suspected abortionist and accomplices. Suspects remained in jail or out on bail until the case was concluded. After the inquest, prosecutors brought the case before the grand jury, which then indicted the suspects. Both prosecutors and the grand jury tended to follow the findings of the coroner's jury; if the coroner's jury failed to accuse anyone of criminal abortion, then prosecutors generally dropped the case. Abortion cases did not come to trial solely after inquests into abortion-related deaths, but most cases in this period followed the death or injury of a woman.[16]

Most of the women subjected to official investigations into their abortions were, like Carolina Petrovitis, working-class women and either foreign-born themselves or daughters of immigrants. The state's focus on working-class women in abortion cases matched the greater policing of working-class people in general.[17] Working-class women's poverty made it more likely that they, rather than middle-class women, would reach official attention for having abortions. All of the forty-four Cook County coroner's inquests available to me were investigations into the abortions and deaths of white, working-class women. Over half were immigrants or daughters of immigrants.[18] Because of their lack of funds, poor women often used inexpensive, and often dangerous, self-induced measures and delayed calling in doctors if they had complications.[19] By the time these women sought medical attention, they were likely to have reached a critical stage and, as a result, come to official attention. Affluent women may have avoided official investigations into their abortions because they had personal relations with private physicians, many of whom never collected or destroyed dying statements or falsified death certificates. Investigations in New York and Philadelphia found 25 to 30 percent of all abortion deaths were falsely attributed to some other cause such as pneumonia or heart failure. If necessary, wealthier families could pressure or pay physicians and officials to keep quiet about a woman's abortion-related death.[20] I found mention of only one case in which the Cook County coroner investigated the abortion-related death of an African American woman during this period; unfortunately, no record of the case exists.[21] If black women were questioned by officials after their abortions, they may have found it upsetting to be questioned by white authorities. An African American physician prosecuted for abortion complained of racist remarks by the coroner's office; African American women dying as a result of abortions may have suffered similar treatment.[22]

For doctors, like Dr. Kahn, who had been called in to attend an emergency case, caring for patients who had had abortions was both a medical challenge and a legal peril. The appropriate response was unclear; even specialists disagreed on what a doctor should do. In emergencies, physicians performed curettements, repaired uterine tears and wounds, tried to stop hemorrhaging, and, most difficult in an age without antibiotics, fought infections.[23] Once a woman had a widespread, septic infection (characterized by chills and fever), death was very likely. If a woman died despite a doctor's efforts, the doctor became a logical suspect in the criminal abortion case. According to New York attorney Almuth Vandiver, police arrested physicians "simply because they were the last physician attending the patient and they had not made their report to the coroner."[24]

The state needed medical cooperation to investigate abortion cases, and state officials won that cooperation by threatening physicians with arrests and prosecution. Physicians learned that if they failed to report criminal abortion cases, the investigative process could be turned against them. At a 1900 meeting of the Illinois State Medical Society, Dr. O. B. Will of Peoria, Illinois, warned his associates of the "responsibilities and dangers" associated with abortion by relating his own "very annoying experience" when a patient died as a result of an abortion. He was indicted as an accessory to a murder for "keeping the circumstances quiet, by not securing a dying statement from the patient, and in not informing the coroner." Will declared that he was not required to notify the coroner and that the woman had refused to make a statement, but his story implied that cooperation with the authorities might help doctors avoid similar notoriety. One doctor told his colleagues horror stories of Boston physicians who had been arrested, tried, and, though acquitted of abortion charges, ousted by the Massachusetts Medical Society. In addition, doctors associated with illegal abortion risked losing their medical licenses. In Illinois, a physician had to be convicted of abortion to lose his or her license, but other states revoked medical licenses without a trial.[25] Physicians learned from tales like these that if they treated women for complications following abortions, they should report the cases to local officials or collect dying declarations themselves in order to avoid being arrested and prosecuted.

Coroner's inquests into abortion deaths, and the negative publicity the coroner could cause, helped enmesh doctors and hospitals within the enforcement system. At inquests into abortion deaths, the coroner regularly reminded attending physicians of "the rule" to call the police or coroner whenever there was evidence that a woman had been "tampered with" and reprimanded those who failed to follow this policy.[26] The fragile reputations of hospitals and physicians could be damaged simply if they were named and associated with an abortion case in the newspapers. At a 1915 inquest into the death of a woman as a result of abortion, the coroner's jury suggested that Rhodes Avenue Hospital, which had cared for the woman, "be severely censured for lax methods in not complying with the rules required in notifying the proper officials . . . and the seeming indifference on the part of physicians and assistants . . . to ascertain who performed said abortion." The hospital protested the censure and the notoriety resulting from newspaper coverage of the case. The superintendent wrote that the hospital had always cooperated with the coroner's office and that "the hospital was not on trial."[27] This publicized reproof warned hospitals and physicians that if they failed to cooperate with state officials, their institutions and careers could be hurt.

By 1917, if not earlier, state authorities had persuaded Chicago's hospitals to pledge their cooperation in the investigation of abortion cases. The city's hospital superintendents reached an agreement with the coroner, chief of police, and state's attorney's office to notify the coroner's office when they saw patients who had had abortions. Furthermore, if it seemed that the woman would die before an official investigator arrived, hospitals agreed to collect the dying declaration themselves. The coroner even provided hospitals with a "blank form" for dying declarations.[28] The official expectation that doctors would report abortion cases to the coroner was not codified, but in the minds of both doctors and state officials, reporting abortions was, as one doctor described it in court, "compulsory."[29]

A few New York physicians voiced the indignation many may have felt towards coroners. They resented the way that police pursued them when they were the last attending physician in an abortion case and then subjected them to "disagreeable inquest[s]." New York physicians felt harassed by the city's coroners, who, the doctors complained, were far too ready to arrest and investigate physicians in criminal abortion cases.[30]

One way to protect themselves from legal trouble and notoriety in abortion cases, physicians learned, was to secure dying declarations. In 1912, the chairman of the Chicago Medical Society's Criminal Abortion Committee, Dr. Charles H. Parkes, reminded the society that "it is extremely easy for anyone to become criminally involved when connected with these cases, unless properly protected." Parkes presented to the medical society a model dying declaration, drafted by State's Attorney John Wayman, that would "stand the supreme court test." Wayman advised the doctors to ask the dying woman the following questions: "Q: Do you believe that you are about to die? . . . Q: Have you any hope of recovery? . . . Q: Do you understand these questions fully? . . . Q: Are you able to give a clear account of the causes of your illness?"[31]

The state's attorney also provided a standardized format for the dying woman's answer. She should answer, "I am Miss———. Believing that I am about to die, and having no hope of recovery, I make the following statement, while of sound mind and in full possession of my faculties." An important part of the statement was establishing that the woman believed she was near death in order for the statement to be considered valid in court. The woman was then expected to name her abortionist, tell when, where, and how the abortion was done, and name the man "responsible" for her pregnant "condition."[32] Although most women who had abortions were married, the state's prosecutors focused on abortions by unwed women, and this formulaic dying declaration assumed that the dying woman would be unmarried.

Physicians advised each other to deny medical care to a woman who had had an abortion until she made a statement. In 1902, the editors of *JAMA* endorsed this policy of (mis)treating abortion patients. *JAMA* quoted a physician who counseled his colleagues to "refuse all responsibility for the patient unless a confession exonerating him from any connection with the crime is given." Twenty years later, Dr. Palmer Findley gave the same advice to obstetricians and gynecologists. "It is common experience," he reported, "that the patient will tell all she knows when made to realize her danger and a double purpose is attained—the physician in charge is protected and the guilty party is revealed."[33]

If a woman refused to give information, the smart doctor, according to these advisers, would walk out and refuse to attend her. And some physicians, like Dr. Kahn in the Petrovitis case, threatened to do just that. In 1916, one Chicago man called in Dr. G. P. Miller to attend his wife, who had been sick for three weeks following her abortion. Dr. Miller told her, "If I take this case . . . I want you to tell me the truth and who did it, who it was. Under the understanding that I was going to leave the house and have nothing to do with it, she told me the whole story."[34] Physicians' refusal to treat abortion cases seems to have reached female consciousness. In 1930, Mathilde Kleinschmidt, ill from her abortion, rejected her boyfriend's plan to call in a second doctor and insisted that he find the doctor who had performed the abortion instead. When he asked why, she explained, "Another doctor won[']t look at me. He won[']t take the case."[35]

Fear of undeserved prosecution encouraged physicians to distrust their female patients. The illegality of abortion compelled doctors to regard all miscarriages as suspect; a woman who claimed to have miscarried might actually have had an illegal abortion in which the attending physician could be implicated. New York attorney Vandiver warned doctors, "Unscrupulous women and their accomplices have it within their power . . . to successfully blackmail the reputable practitioner, who omits the essential precautions for his protection." Dr. Henry Dawson Furniss told a story that encapsulated doctors' worst fears. He had "absolutely refused" to perform an abortion for a woman who later died from one. Under questioning, she used the opportunity to get even with Furniss for spurning her plea for help by blaming him for her abortion.[36]

This case was unusual, however. Few women falsely accused physicians, but many, probably the majority, protected their abortionists by refusing to name them to doctors or police officers. Abortionists, of course, encouraged their patients not to reveal their names.[37] The prosecuting attorney for St. Louis, Ernest F. Oakley, marveled at the loyalty of women who refused to reveal their abortionists' names. Dying declarations, he thought, were obtained in only "four out of ten cases." One New York woman, who was hospitalized following her abortion, told the doctors who pressed her to name her abortionist, "She was the only one who would help me, and I won't tell on her."[38]

As doctors tried to protect themselves from prosecution in abortion cases, women's health care suffered. Because they feared prosecution, many physicians treated their female patients badly—by rudely questioning them in attempts to gain dying declarations or by delaying or refusing to provide needed medical care. For example, during the 1915 "war" on abortion in Chicago, the *Tribune* discovered that "publicity has changed the attitude of hospital authorities in regard to the handling of abortion victims." One hospital superintendent would neither admit an abortion patient, nor allow an operation "until he had received orders from the police." In this case, the hospital allowed police to make medical and legal decisions in an abortion case as a result of a local antiabortion campaign. "It was not until detectives had assured the superintendent that an operation was necessary to save Mrs. Lapinski's life and that there would be no trouble for the hospital," the newspaper reported, "that Dr. G. M. Cushing . . . was permitted to take the sufferer to the operating room." In a less dramatic fashion, doctors regularly avoided caring for abortion patients by sending them to hospitals instead of treating them in their homes. In 1929, when Dr. Julius Auerbach was called in to care for a woman who had had an abortion, he refused to examine her and sent her to the county hospital in order to avoid being "implicated" in the case.[39]

Though some frightened doctors threatened to deny medical care to women who had abortions and insisted they make statements, others refused "to act as a policeman" for the state.[40] Dr. Parkes reported that Chicago officials "believe that the best hospitals now smother these cases and hinder in every way the work of investigation." Dr. William Robinson, a political radical who advocated legalized abortion, scorned physicians who "badger[ed]" sick women to make dying statements. "The business of the doctor is to relieve pain, cure disease and save life," he declared, "not to act as a bloodhound [for] the state."[41]

Other doctors found a middle ground between compliance with and rejection of the state's rules. Dr. Henry Kruse asked Edna Lamb about her abortion, but did not inform her that she was about to die, which a valid dying declaration needed. He explained, "We don't do that to patients because sometimes it is ver[y] discouraging and the result is bad." Other doctors questioned their patients about their abortions, but only reported cases to authorities when women died. When women survived, the doctors destroyed their statements and kept the abortions confidential. In fact, the Cook County coroner accepted this practice as one that protected the interests of women who survived their abortions, shielded physicians from possible prosecution, and provided information to authorities in cases of death.[42]

Making a patient's medical history public undermined the private and personal relationships physicians had with their patients. Some physicians expressed their allegiance to maintaining patient confidentiality, regardless of the wishes of authorities. Dr. Louis Frank of Louisville, Kentucky, commented in 1904, "If I was called in I would not give testimony compromising a young lady, and I would not put it on record, no matter what the facts were, and I would not 'give away' a

girl, but would attempt to protect her." Two Philadelphia doctors believed medical ethics barred them from testifying against an abortionist
if it violated a patient's confidentiality.[43]

The names of women who had illegal abortions and the intimate details of their lives periodically hit the newspapers. Press coverage of
abortion-related deaths warned all women of the dangers of abortion:
death and publicity. Sometimes newspapers covered abortion stories
on the front page and included photos; more often, abortion-related
deaths and arrests of abortionists appeared in small announcements.
The story of an unwed woman's seduction and abortion-related death
made exciting copy and could dominate local newspapers for days.
Anna Johnson was the center of attention in 1915; a year later Chicago
and Denver newspapers published Ruth Merriweather's love letters
to a Chicago medical student on trial for his involvement in her abortion-related death.[44] In 1918, the *Chicago Examiner* ran a series of
"*tragedies,*" excerpted from coroner's inquests, which told the stories
of unwed women "*who were killed through illegal operations.*" The articles in this series warned young women of the dangers of seduction and
abortion and also warned rural fathers of the need to protect their
daughters from the dangers of city life.[45] The names and addresses of
married women who had abortions often appeared in the press, but not
as seduction tales.[46] Newspapers sometimes highlighted the fact that
police had found thousands of women's names in an abortionist's
records.[47] In doing so, they threatened women who had abortions that
they too could be named and exposed to the public in the newspaper.

Public exposure of a woman's abortion—through the press or gos-
sip—served to punish women who had abortions, as well as their family members. A Chicago police officer recalled that when he questioned
Mary Shelley, she "remark[ed] that she didn't want the statement in
the newspapers." A few women whose abortions had been reported in
the local press lived to face the shame of public exposure. Doctors observed that even when a woman died after an abortion, families did not
want authorities to investigate because they wanted "to shield her reputation."[48] Some families invited state investigation of abortions and
pursued prosecution, yet they may have resented publicity about the
case. One mother, whose daughter had died because of an illegal abortion, cried at a public hearing that her whole family had "keenly felt the
disgrace" of the crime.[49] When Frances Collins died, police visited "all
houses on both sides" of her home as well as "some ladies" in her old
neighborhood and questioned them in hopes of finding a "woman

confidant." The police failed to locate the friend, but they informed the woman's entire community of her death by abortion and displayed the state's interest in controlling abortion.[50]

For the women whose abortions came to the attention of medical and legal authorities, the demands for dying statements by physicians and police felt punitive. One woman described her hospital experience after an abortion as "very humiliating. The doctors put me through a regular jail examination."[51] In their efforts to obtain dying declarations, police and physicians, usually male, repeatedly questioned women about their private lives, their sexuality, and their abortions; they asked women when they last menstruated, when they went to the abortionist, and what he or she did. Were instruments introduced into "their privates"? If so, what did the instruments look like and how were they used? If the woman was unmarried, she was asked with whom she had been sexually intimate and when, precisely the information that she may have hoped to keep secret by having an abortion. Furthermore, as in the Petrovitis case, it was routine for police to bring the suspected abortionist to the bedside of the dying woman in order for her to identify and accuse her abortionist.[52] Hundreds of women who had abortions may have been questioned annually by physicians, police, or coroner's officers without ever entering official records because they survived their abortions.

To the women, being questioned by police officers about their abortions could seem cruel; to the police officers, the questions, however intrusive, seemed necessary. In the Petrovitis case, Sgt. O'Connor mentioned his own fear of getting in trouble if he failed to question the dying woman. The case was out of his precinct, but he took a statement anyhow, as he testified, "to protect ourselves." He "took no chance" and investigated the case in order "to protect the police department."[53] The sergeant did not explain himself further, but his remarks suggested that in 1916 the police felt under pressure, no doubt from many quarters after the Johnson case the year before, to investigate abortion cases carefully. He did not want to be blamed for ruining the investigation and making prosecution impossible. When presented with an abortion case, this police officer, like the doctor, felt the need for self-protection.

Investigations into a woman's abortion-related death were shameful events for the woman's relatives and friends because state officials required that they speak publicly about sexual matters that they ordinarily kept private and rarely discussed. At the Petrovitis inquest, police officer John A. Gallagher recalled that Petrovitis's sister had translated his questions, but when he reached the questions "about using instruments on her privates . . . the sister could not interpret anymore, didn't want to."[54] In order to document a pregnancy and abortion, the coroner asked questions about menstruation, sexual histories, and women's bodies. Family and friends often evaded such questions, but the coroner simply repeated his questions until he received an answer. Female witnesses, who may have discussed sexual topics only with other women, sometimes hesitated to speak before male officials, attorneys, and a jury of six men. At a 1917 inquest into an abortion death, the dead woman's sister perjured herself during questioning. At a later trial, she explained, "I knew everything but I could not answer all of them on account of all the men around. . . . Because there was so many men around I hated to talk about my poor sister more than I had to." The question she could not answer was, she explained, "about her body. . . . He asked me if the doctor had used any instrument, and I said no at that time."[55] One immigrant woman commented during questioning by the coroner about her friend's abortion, "I am ashamed to tell." Despite her shame, she was forced to tell and to repeat her testimony at the midwife-abortionist's trial.[56]

The coroner's office understood that female family members often shared intimate knowledge about women's bodies and sexual behavior and tried to crack that female network to obtain information. The questioning of nineteen-year-old Julia McElroy at the 1928 inquest into the death of her sister, Eunice McElroy, is a vivid example of how the coroner's staff expected sisters to have specific information, asked personal, shaming questions, and threatened those they suspected of not cooperating.[57] The deputy coroner questioned Julia intensively about the sisters' dating practices and Eunice's sexual behavior. He began with an offer to proceed in "a private chamber" because his questions might embarrass Julia, but he immediately denied the validity of those feelings in the legal arena. As he explained to Julia, "I may put some questions to you that you may think is embarrassing [sic], but it is not. I am just merely questioning you because I am an officer of the law, the coroner." Julia denied knowing anything. The coroner established that the sisters shared a bed. "When was the last time your sister had her last menstrual period? You tell the truth," he ordered. Julia told him that her sister had menstruated over three months earlier, and she denied knowing of a pregnancy. "Q: Well, you know they are supposed to come around and flow once a month unless a person is flowing irregularly? . . . You would know when your sister is unwell. She wears a napkin and you probably wear a napkin when you are not well on account of the odor, isn[']t that a fact?" Julia responded only with silence. The coroner continued to press her for information about Eunice's periods and sexual history. When Julia still maintained her ignorance a few days later, the deputy warned her, "If you don't tell a true story, you are going to get into a jam for a year." On the final day of the inquest, the deputy coroner told Julia that he knew that she had shielded the abortionist. With that, Julia revealed her knowledge and explained that she had been repeating the false story begun by her sister to protect her abortionist. The coroner concluded, "You are lucky you are telling the truth. I would sure send you to jail." The coroner eventually obtained from Julia McElroy evidence helpful for the prosecution of Eunice McElroy's abortionist, but he had put Julia through a grueling experience, asked her graphic, sexual questions, questioned her closely about her sister's and her own dating behavior, and threatened her with jail.

Criminal abortion investigations reveal the importance of marriage—and especially the lack of it—to state officials. When police collected dying statements, they routinely asked about the woman's marital status, and at inquests into the deaths of unmarried women, many of the coroner's questions focused on marital status. The coroner probed to discover whether the man involved had offered marriage. To a man, all claimed to have "promised to marry her." Perhaps men understood that this was the only way they could redeem themselves in the eyes of the law and the community. Yet there is evidence of genuine intention to marry. One man had bought a wedding ring. In some cases, the woman wanted to delay marriage; in others, couples found marriage and children financially impossible. As one man testified, "He went to Dr. Rongetti to get rid of the baby because he could not afford it." [58]

Just as dying women endured intrusive questioning about their abortions, their unmarried lovers endured similar interrogations at inquests. For unmarried women and men alike, the official prying into their private sexual lives, and their own mortification, served as a form of punishment for their illicit sexual behavior. The coroner's questions to Marshall Hostetler about his sexual relationship with his sweetheart, Anna Johnson, were not unusual. The coroner asked Hostetler, "When did you become intimate with her? . . . Have any relations with her? . . . When did that occur? . . . Had you been intimate with her before? . . . How many times? . . . Where did that occur?" [59]

Men, too, tried to avoid answering questions related to sex during public investigations into abortion. Charles Morehouse readily answered numerous questions about his girlfriend's abortion, how they borrowed money, and how the family had tried to avoid an investigation. He explained that the doctor had used "a spray." But when the coroner asked "Where?" Morehouse was silent. "A: No response. Q: What portion of the body? A: Well, the privated [*sic*] parts." [60]

The "sweetheart of the dead girl" could be punished severely for having transgressed sexual norms. [61] When an unwed woman died because of an abortion, her lover was automatically arrested, jailed, interrogated by the police and coroner, and sometimes prosecuted as an accessory to the crime as well. Bob Berry's experience in 1931 was typical. When Alma Bromps died, police officers arrived at Berry's door and arrested and jailed him. The next morning he identified the body of his girlfriend and was questioned at the inquest into her death. He remained in jail for at least a week and ultimately became a witness for the state against the accused abortionist. [62] Unmarried men involved in abortion deaths often spent at least one night in jail before the inquests and, if they had no money to bail themselves out, might spend several days or weeks depending on the length of the inquest. [63] Some spent months in jail while they waited for their cases to come to trial. In 1917 Charles Morehouse spent four months in jail after the death of his girlfriend. The state prosecuted Patrick O'Connell, a laborer, along with Dr. Adolph Buettner for the abortion that led to Nellie Walsh's death. Although O'Connell was acquitted, it appears that he spent the nine months between Walsh's death and his criminal trial in the Cook County jail. Other men were convicted and sentenced to prison for their part in an abortion. [64]

The actions of state officials toward unmarried men in criminal abortion deaths reveal the state's interest in enforcing marriage in cases where an unwed woman got pregnant. The state punished young men for the moral offense of engaging in premarital intercourse and then failing to fulfill the implicit engagement by marrying the women whom they impregnated. Police routinely arrested and incarcerated unmarried men as accomplices in the crime of abortion, and the state's attorney sometimes prosecuted them. In contrast, husbands, some of whom had been just as involved as unmarried men in obtaining abortions, were not automatically arrested or prosecuted as accomplices when their wives died. It was rare for a husband to be arrested or prosecuted. [65]

Bastardy cases heard in Chicago similarly demonstrate the state's desire to see couples marry when pregnancy occurred. In bastardy cases, the unwed woman brought the father to court to register paternity and gain minimal financial support for the child. If the couple did not marry, the man could be fined up to $550 or sentenced to six months in jail. Of 163 bastardy cases studied by a Hull-House investigator, a third ended in marriage. Fourteen couples "settled out of court" by marrying, while forty "married in court." Men who reconsidered their situation once in jail could gain their freedom if they decided to marry the woman and legitimate the child.[66]

The official response to unmarried men in abortion cases, as in bastardy cases, served as a warning to other young men of the dangerous consequences of avoiding marriage and children when pregnancy occurred. Newspaper stories of abortion deaths told of the arrest, imprisonment, and interrogation of the "sweetheart of the dead girl," and young men probably traded detailed information about the events that transpired during abortion investigations.[67] Newspaper coverage of abortions warned women that they could die and men that they could be thrown in jail. Some may have concluded that it was better to marry.

Jilted women could exploit the state's readiness to hold unmarried men accountable in illegal abortions as a weapon to strike back at their lovers. These victimized women, as the law regarded them, could consciously use the law to their own advantage. Alice Grimes of southern Illinois actively encouraged official investigation into her abortion for this reason. Prior to her death in 1896, Grimes told her mother that her boyfriend, James Dunn, "ought to suffer some," as she had. When Grimes learned that her uncle had had Dunn arrested, she told her brother she was "glad of it."[68]

The patterns of investigation were so standardized that when a patient died, abortionists alerted family members and explained to them how to suppress evidence and evade the law.[69] With the silence of family members and fake death certificates,[70] abortionists avoided prosecution, women avoided police interrogation, and their relatives avoided the shame of being publicly associated with illegal abortion.

From the late nineteenth century through the 1930s, the state concentrated on collecting dying declarations and prosecuting abortionists when a woman died. The state's control of abortion was by no means entirely successful, but neither was it insignificant. Thousands of women regularly defied the law and had the abortions they needed. When questioned by doctors or police about their abortions, many defied their interrogators and refused to provide the information needed to prosecute abortionists. Yet the state successfully punished women for having abortions, damaged the relationships between women and their doctors, and undermined women's health care. Officials focused on regulating the sexual behavior of working-class women and men, especially the unmarried. Investigations and inquests into abortion forcefully reminded all involved not only of the illegality of abortion, but also of the power of the state to intervene in the private lives of ordinary people in order to prevent and punish violations of sexual codes that demanded marriage and maternity.

Medicine played a complicated role in the enforcement of the criminal abortion laws. Organized medicine acted as part of the state in policing the practice of abortion by women and by physicians. While some physicians actively sought an alliance with the state in enforcing the criminal abortion laws, most physicians who cooperated with the state's investigations did so out of their fear of being arrested as a suspect in an abortion case. By arming themselves with a dying declaration naming someone else as the abortionist, doctors could avoid prosecution and help the state at the same time. The agreement in Chicago to notify the coroner of abortions became a "law" in a sense. Physicians who did not comply with the informal regulations were treated with suspicion by both their colleagues and state officials.[71]

At inquests into abortion deaths, the state reinforced the norms requiring men to marry the women whom they impregnated. Through arrests, incarceration, interrogation, and prosecution, unmarried women's lovers were punished for illegal abortions as well as for their illicit sexual behavior. The treatment of unmarried men in these cases reveals the implicit assumption of state authorities that unwed women who had had abortions had been forced to do so because their "sweethearts" had refused to marry. This underlying assumption ignored the evident agency of many women who sought abortions and delayed marriage. The punishment of unmarried men maintained age-old patriarchal standards.

Analysis of the investigation of abortion in Chicago illuminates the social punishment inherent in the state's routine processes of investigation and the ways in which punishment has been gendered. The state did not prosecute women for having abortions, but it did punish women through persistent questioning by doctors and police and through public exposure of their abortions. The harassment of sick or dying women in the name of criminal investigation continued until the decriminalization of abortion.

CHAPTER 5

Expansion and Specialization

"My husband has been out of work for over six months and no help is in sight," wrote one mother to Margaret Sanger and the American Birth Control League; "I can't afford more children." Every year she performed two abortions upon herself, and she reported, "I have just now gotten up from an abortion and I don't want to repeat it again."[1] The disaster of the Great Depression touched all aspects of women's lives, including the most intimate ones, and brought about a new high in the incidence of abortion. As jobs evaporated and wages fell, families found themselves living on insecure and scanty funds. Many working people lost their homes; tenants had their belongings put out on the street.[2] Married couples gave up children to orphanages because they could not support them.[3]

As women pressured doctors for help, the medical practice of abortion, legal and illegal, expanded during the 1930s. Physicians granted, for the first time, that social conditions were an essential component of medical judgment in therapeutic abortion cases. Medical recognition of social indications reveals the ways in which political and social forces shaped medical thinking and practice. A handful of radical physicians, who looked to Europe as a model, raised the possibility of liberalizing the abortion law. During these years, abortion became more concentrated in the hands of physicians in both hospitals and private offices as a result of structural changes in medicine.

If we move away from the dramatic narratives about abortion produced at inquests or in newspapers, which tell of the deaths and dangers of abortion, and step into the offices of physician-abortionists, a different story can be discerned. Abortion was not extraordinary, but ordinary. The proverbial "back-alley butcher" story of abortion over-emphasizes fatalities and limits our understanding of the history of illegal abortion.[4] Case studies of the "professional abortionists" and their practices in the 1930s provide a unique opportunity to analyze the experiences of the tens of thousands of women who went to physician-abortionists. Many women had abortions in a setting nearly identical to the doctors' offices where they received other medical care. These doctors specialized in a single procedure, abortion. They used standard medical procedures to perform safe abortions routinely and ran what may be called abortion clinics. Furthermore, abortion specialists were an integral part of regular medicine, as the network of physicians who referred patients to these physician-abortionists demonstrates. The physician-abortionists represent the expansion of abortion during the Depression decade.

The Depression years make vivid the relationship between economics and reproduction. Women had abortions on a massive scale. Married women with children found it impossible to bear the expense of another, and unmarried women could not afford to marry. As young working-class women and men put off marriage during the Depression to support their families or to save money for a wedding, marriage rates fell drastically. Yet while they waited to wed, couples engaged in sexual relations, and women became pregnant. Many had abortions.[5]

During the Depression, married women were routinely fired on the assumption that jobs belonged to men and that women had husbands who supported them. Discrimination against married women forced single women to delay marriage and have abortions in order to keep their jobs. One such woman was a young teacher whose fiancé was unemployed. As her daughter recalled fifty years later, "She got pregnant. What were her choices? Marry, lose her job, and bring a child into a family with no means of support? Not marry, lose her job and reputation, and put the baby up for adoption or keep it?" As this scenario makes clear, she had no "choice." Furthermore, it points to the limitations of the rhetoric of "choice" in reproduction; social forces condition women's reproductive options. The teacher's boyfriend found a local physician who helped her in his office; then she went to a hotel to miscarry. Two years later she married a different man, who had a job, and eventually bore seven children.[6]

That almost a thousand New Jersey women purchased a type of

abortion "insurance" in 1936 demonstrates that abortion was a recurring and common need for many. New Jersey police uncovered a "Birth Control Club" of eight hundred dues-paying and card-carrying members. Membership in the club "entitled them to regular examinations and to illegal operations, when they needed them, at a further fee of $75 and upward." Most of the members were "girl clerks" who worked in Newark's downtown offices. Just as working people made small regular payments for life insurance and funeral coverage, these working women bought a form of health insurance through dues paid to this "club." These women *expected* to have abortions in the future. The club provided a means of blunting the expense of abortions and other gynecological care.[7] When the *New York Times* covered this incident, birth control leaders immediately attacked the headline dubbing this a "birth control" club. The medical director of the American Birth Control League explained that the birth control movement "opposed" abortion and that the two were not the same.[8]

The Depression helped legitimate contraceptives. American society increasingly accepted birth control during the 1930s. Condoms sold briskly in drug stores and gas stations. In 1930, the American Birth Control League had fifty-five birth control clinics in fifteen states; by 1938 there were over five hundred clinics. Hostility toward welfare payments and "relief babies" helped win support for providing birth control to the poor. The federal government quietly sponsored, for the first time, provision of birth control services in the late 1930s. As courts began to overturn the Comstock Laws on contraceptives, they allowed the medical profession to prescribe birth control devices. One 1937 poll found that nearly 80 percent of American women approved of birth control use. That year the AMA finally abandoned its official opposition to birth control. The medical profession had been pushed by the birth control movement into accepting responsibility for contraception.[9] Contraceptives were not foolproof, however.

Greater availability of contraceptives could not alone meet the increased need for control over childbearing. The recognized expert on abortion, Frederick J. Taussig, reported that the number of abortions had grown "throughout the world." He believed it was "due less to [a] laxity of morals than to underlying economic conditions." A New Orleans physician who studied the septic abortion cases at the Charity Hospital found that the number of criminal abortions among poor, white patients rose 166 percent between 1930 and 1931. This surge reflected, he suggested, "the financial pressure . . . on this type of charity patient." Studies of Cincinnati, Minneapolis, New York, and Philadelphia showed that the use of abortion swelled in the early 1930s.[10]

Medical studies and sex surveys demonstrated that women of every social strata turned to abortion in greater numbers during the Depression. Comparative studies by class and race appeared for the first time in the 1930s. Induced abortion rates among white, middle- and upper-class, married women rose during the Depression years. The Kinsey Institute for Sex Research, led by Paul H. Gebhard, analyzed data from over five thousand married, white, mostly highly educated, urban women.[11] The researchers found that "the depression of the 1930's resulted in a larger proportion of pregnancies that were artificially aborted." For every age group of women, born between 1890 and 1919, the highest induced abortion rate occurred during "the depth of the depression." White, married women were determined to avoid bearing children during the Depression: they reduced their rate of conception as well.[12]

In the early years of the Depression, married women aborted more of their first pregnancies than had women of earlier generations. Dr. Regine K. Stix discovered this pattern after interviewing almost a thousand women at a New York City birth control clinic in 1931 and 1932, all of whose incomes were severely reduced by the Depression. The young married woman who had an abortion did so "because she was the bread-winner in the family and could not afford to lose her job, much less produce another mouth to feed. A year or two later," Stix explained, "if her husband was working, she gave up her job and planned a baby or two." The findings of Kinsey researchers suggest that aborting first pregnancies early in marriage might have been a growing trend, particularly among more educated, urban white women.[13]

Married black women, like their white counterparts, used abortion more during the Depression. Since African American women lost their jobs in disproportionate numbers, their need may have been greater than that of white women.[14] Unfortunately, Kinsey researchers did not collect data from black women before 1950, but others documented black women's resort to abortion during the 1930s. Dr. Charles H. Garvin, an esteemed black surgeon from Cleveland, commented in 1932 "that there has been a very definite increase in the numbers of abortions, criminally performed, among the married." The African American press reported on black women's use of abortion.[15] In 1935, Harlem Hospital, which cared for mostly poor black patients, opened a separate ward, "The Abortion Service," to treat the women who came for emergency care following illegal abortions.[16]

A number of studies showed that white and black married women of the same class had abortions at the same rate. A study of reproductive histories collected from forty-five hundred women at a New York clinic between 1930 and 1938 suggested that when class was controlled, working-class women, black and white alike, induced abortions at the same rate. The researchers found that "the incidence of pregnancies and spontaneous and induced abortion [among black women] was identical with that obtained for the entire group."[17] A Houston study found that approximately equal proportions of Mexican, African American, and white women had abortions.[18] Studies like these of women of the same class suggest that any racial differences in overall abortion rates may be explained best by class differences.

The evidence on the practice of abortion by class is somewhat contradictory, but it seems that affluent women had higher abortion *rates* than did working-class women, but working-class and poor women actually had a greater *number* of abortions because they were pregnant more often. The Kinsey group of upper- and middle-class white women aborted 24.3 percent of their pregnancies in 1930 and 18.3 percent in 1935. In contrast, the working-class black and white women in the New York clinic study aborted at about half that rate, or 11.5 percent.[19]

The key difference between black and white women was in their response to pregnancy outside of marriage, not their use of abortion. Unmarried white women who became pregnant were more likely to abort their pregnancies than were African American women in the same situation. Instead, more black women bore children out of wedlock and did so without being ostracized by their families and community. Dr. Virginia Clay Hamilton discovered important differences in abortion behavior between white and black single women during interviews with over five hundred low-income women who entered New York's Bellevue Hospital in 1938 and 1939 following the interruption of pregnancy, whether by miscarriage or induced abortion. Hamilton promised confidentiality and found that "the group showed surprisingly little reluctance to discuss the intimate questions which were put to them." Both white and black unmarried women had higher rates of induced abortion than did married women, but 64 percent of the unmarried white women told of having deliberately induced their abortions compared to only 40 percent of the unmarried black women. "Still more striking," commented Hamilton, was the racial difference in abortion behavior among the previously married. Divorced and widowed black women, "behav[ed] essentially like those still married," while divorced and widowed white women returned to the behavior of unmarried women when faced with illegitimate pregnancies. The level of induced abortions among previously married white women approached the high level of abortions among single white women. The Kinsey report found the same racial differences in the behavior of unmarried women.[20]

The tolerance of illegitimacy among African Americans was tempered by class. As African Americans advanced economically, they held their unwed daughters and sons to more rigid standards of chastity. Similarly, by the time the Kinsey Institute interviewed black women in the 1950s, there were clear class differences in the use of abortion by unmarried black women: those with more education (and presumably more affluence) aborted at a higher rate than those with less education.[21]

Women's religious background made little difference in their abortion rates, though religiosity did make a difference. A study of working-class women in New York in the 1930s found almost identical abortion rates among Catholic, Jewish, and Protestant women.[22] However, researchers found striking differences in the reproductive patterns followed by women of different religious groups, a finding that seems to reflect class differences. Catholic and Jewish women tended to have their children earlier in their lives and began aborting unwanted pregnancies as they got older; Protestant women tended to abort earlier pregnancies and bear children later.[23] The Kinsey Report found for both married and unmarried white women, the more devout the woman, the less likely she was to have an abortion; the more religiously "inactive" a woman, the more likely she was to have an abortion.[24]

Access to physician-induced abortions and reliance upon self-induced methods for abortion varied greatly by class and race. Most affluent white women went to physicians for abortions, while poor women and black women self-induced them. Physicians performed 84 percent of the abortions reported by the white, urban women to Kinsey researchers. Fewer than 10 percent of the affluent white women self-induced their abortions, though black women and poor white women, because of poverty or discrimination in access to medical care, often did so. According to the Kinsey study on abortion, 30 percent of the lower-income and black women reported self-inducing their abortions.[25] Sara Brooks, a black Alabama midwife, recalled her own attempt at abortion in the 1930s. A friend told her to go visit "Annie" to get herself out of "trouble." Annie gave Brooks a mixture of camphor gum and nutmeg. When Brooks took it, she recalled, "It made me *so* sick." The doctor who was called gave her warm baking soda to force her to vomit. She believed she would have otherwise died, as her own mother had after taking turpentine to induce an abortion.[26]

Low-income women's and black women's greater reliance upon self-induced methods of abortion meant that the safety of illegal abortion varied by race and class. Self-induced abortions caused more complications and hospitalization than did those induced by physicians or midwives. Since poor women and black women were more likely to try to self-induce abortions and less likely to go to doctors or midwives, they suffered more complications. Dr. Regine K. Stix learned from interviewing almost a thousand women in 1931 and 1932 that self-induced abortions, as compared to midwife- or physician-induced abortions, had the highest rates of infection and hemorrhage. Women reported having no complications after their abortions in 91 percent of the abortions performed by doctors and 86 percent of those performed by midwives. In contrast, only 24 percent of the self-induced abortions were without complications. Of the women who entered the county hospital in Portland, Oregon, after illegal abortions, more than two-thirds had induced their abortions themselves. It is worth noting that although the majority of complications occurred in self-induced abortions, physicians performed the majority of abortions.[27]

As more women had abortions during the Depression, and perhaps more turned to self-induced measures because of their new poverty, growing numbers of women entered the nation's hospitals for care following their illegal abortions. The Depression deepened an earlier trend toward the hospitalization of women who had abortion-related complications in public hospitals. As childbirth gradually moved into the hospital, so too did abortion.[28] Hospitals separated their abortion cases from other obstetrical cases because of the danger of spreading infection and devoted entire wards to caring for emergency abortion cases. At Cook County Hospital, physicians sent all patients with septic abortions or other obstetrical infections to Ward 41.[29] One intern at Cook County Hospital recalled that in 1928 she saw at least thirty or forty abortion cases in the month and a half she worked there; or, one woman a day and several hundred women a year entered the hospital because of postabortion complications. In 1934, the County Hospital admitted 1,159 abortion cases, and reported twenty-two abortion-related deaths that year. Both black and white patients entered the nation's hospitals for care following illegal abortions.[30]

Doctors and public health reformers began to realize the importance of illegal abortion as a contributor to maternal mortality. The maternal mortality study conducted by the Children's Bureau, first reported on in 1931, spotlighted the magnitude of maternal mortality due to illegal abortion. This study, of over seven thousand maternal deaths in fifteen states in 1927 and 1928, found that illegal abortion was responsible for at least 14 percent of the nation's maternal mortality.[31] Another major study of maternal mortality in New York City by the New York Academy of Medicine found that 12.8 percent of maternal deaths were the result of septic abortion. The New York study also showed that abortion had increased as a cause of death both in absolute numbers and in proportion to other causes of maternal mortality. Taussig estimated that approximately fifteen thousand women died every year in the United States because of abortion.[32]

A few physicians began to talk of reform, and even repeal, of the abortion laws. In 1933, two radical physicians published books favoring the decriminalization of abortion in the United States.[33] Both of the physician-authors, Dr. William J. Robinson and Dr. A. J. Rongy, were Jewish immigrants from Russia who were active in politically radical circles as well as members of mainstream medical organizations. Both belonged to the AMA and the New York State and County Medical Societies. For over thirty years Robinson tried to persuade physicians to provide contraceptives. In 1911, he advocated the legalization of abortion, along with a few others, but the rest of the medical profession quickly dismissed such ideas.[34] When Robinson published his book, he considered the time "ripe" for change. In *The Law against Abortion: Its Perniciousness Demonstrated and Its Repeal Demanded*, Robinson contrasted the poisonings, injuries, and deaths of women who had illegal abortions in the United States with the safety record of more than a decade of legal abortions performed by physicians in the Soviet Union.[35]

Rongy offered a different tactic in his book, *Abortion: Legal or Illegal?* He advocated an expansion of the legitimate reasons for therapeutic abortions, which would come close to legalizing abortion. The American public, Rongy argued, already accepted abortion as a "social necessity." "No matter how callous the average physician appears to be," Rongy contended, "he is not left unaffected by the pathetic and often pitiful pleadings of the woman to whom a new pregnancy is a genuine cause of distress." Because of such experiences, most doctors, Rongy declared, privately supported liberalizing the abortion laws. Yet physicians feared to voice publicly their support for legal change. Rongy argued that the legal exception for therapeutic abortions set a precedent that could be used. The indications for abortions should be expanded.[36]

Although Rongy's book "evoked a controversy," a serious public debate on the merits of liberalizing the abortion laws did not develop.[37] One reason it did not was that it was censored. Rongy complained that "the august New York *Times* refused to allow the publisher to advertise" his book.[38] Open discussion of abortion frightened publishers, some of whom opted for silence on the subject. One magazine had its staff of fourteen discuss whether an article on abortion should be published, then protected itself further by giving the article to "several hundred women" who were asked whether it was objectionable. None of the women objected, but before publishing the article, the editors deleted certain graphic paragraphs as a result of reader comments. Though the author of the article referred to Rongy's book, she did not say a word about his proposal to liberalize access to abortion. Instead, she emphasized the dangers of abortion and advised, "Have your baby!"[39] Another reporter discovered that citizens who relied upon libraries for information would have a difficult time learning anything about abortion. The New York Public Library possessed no literature on abortion except the sections included in the Children's Bureau maternal mortality study, and the Academy of Medicine refused to allow nonphysicians to see books on contraception and abortion.[40] American medical publications similarly avoided open debate on the question of reforming the criminal abortion laws. A *JAMA* reviewer described both books as "omens of an expansion in the United States of the demand for sex freedom" and criticized them for ignoring "the evils that may follow . . . repeal or relaxation" of the criminal abortion laws.[41]

The reviewer may have feared that the United States would see, as Europe had, the rise of a feminist and socialist movement for legal abortion. The Soviet Union had legalized abortion in 1920, and socialists and feminists had made the legalization of abortion an issue in Germany, Austria, Switzerland, and England.[42] In England, a movement for the legalization of abortion arose out of the organizing of leftist-feminists active in the birth control movement. In the 1920s these feminists learned that working-class women used abortion as their form of birth control. Furthermore, studies showed that deaths because of illegal abortion contributed greatly to maternal mortality. In 1936, a group of middle-class feminists committed to the interests of the working class and socialism formed an organization, the Abortion Law Reform Association (ALRA), to demand that abortion be made legal and accessible. The ALRA found support among working-class women in England and helped bring them to speak on their own behalf at parliamentary hearings on abortion.[43]

A widespread and vocal political movement for the legalization of abortion never developed in the United States, as it did in England and in Europe. Nonetheless, the challenge to the status quo by a small group of radicals in the 1930s and earlier should not be overlooked. The movements to legalize abortion in the 1960s and 1970s had their roots in earlier efforts during the Depression era. Birth controllers, reformers, physicians, and a small segment of the general public were aware of the possibility of decriminalizing abortion. The birth control movement reported on the Soviet Union and on European efforts to legalize abortion, as did medical journals and some popular magazines,[44] and a handful of leftist women authors addressed the topic of abortion in their fiction.[45]

Though a few M.D.s advocated greater access to abortion in the Depression years, birth controllers continued to treat abortion as taboo. Occasionally birth control clinic staff quietly helped women find abortions,[46] but publicly birth controllers adamantly rejected abortion. The birth controllers were no more brave than mainstream physicians when it came to abortion. A surprising legislative attempt to legalize abortion proves the point. In 1939 a Colorado physician-legislator, Senator George A. Glenn, introduced a bill that would have legalized abortion in his state. How much support he had is unknown. He may have been inspired by radicals within his profession or by a recent case in England that allowed therapeutic abortions to be performed for a greater number of reasons. Margaret Sanger's secretary wrote privately that she believed Sanger would agree with Glenn "that women should be free to terminate pregnancies where it is not desired—but . . . she believes that abortion always represents a physical risk and that contraception is infinitely preferable." When Glenn publicly referred to abortion as "birth control" in his bill, however, Sanger's secretary frantically sent a telegram and letters urging him to change the wording of his bill because they did not want contraception equated with abortion.[47] Birth controllers' fear of abortion underlines the radicalism of women's claim to reproductive rights.

Popular abortion reform movements developed in Europe in the 1920s and 1930s; why not in the United States? In the U.S. as in England, working-class women constantly made it clear to birth controllers that they relied upon abortion, but no organization comparable to the ALRA formed to demand the decriminalization of abortion in the United States. The weakness of working class and socialist movements in this country—and the weak links between feminists, birth controllers, and socialists—hampered the development of a similar political movement around abortion. The red scare after World War I devastated the women's movement and the left, which had actively supported the early birth control movement and which, in Europe, nurtured the movement to legalize abortion.[48] As the American birth control movement withdrew from the left and became a movement of middle-class professionals, the association of legal abortion with Soviet socialism surely tainted the notion among American birth control supporters, who were themselves under assault. The U.S. birth control movement maintained an antiabortion stance and argued for the legitimacy of contraceptives by arguing that birth control could eliminate illegal abortion (a position shared with the more mainstream birth control movement in England). The refusal of American birth controllers to engage in a discussion about liberalizing access to abortion ensured that a public discussion of the idea never developed.[49]

In 1936, a third physician published a book on abortion in the U.S., advocating more moderate reform of the nation's abortion laws than that envisioned by radical thinkers. Dr. Frederick J. Taussig, an obstetrician-gynecologist, wrote a treatise on the subject, which the National Committee on Maternal Health published. The detailed scientific and medical content of Taussig's book, together with its moderate political stance, made it the standard authority on abortion for decades.[50] Taussig offered a model law more socially conservative than Rongy's and less radical than the legalization demanded by Robinson. Taussig had criticized Rongy for being too lenient, asserting that a "lowering of moral tone" would result if unmarried women and widows were allowed to obtain legal abortions.[51] Taussig suggested that modifying state abortion laws to allow physicians to perform a few more therapeutic abortions would not arouse much opposition. At the same time, his reform would restrict physicians' practices. Regular physicians would be allowed to perform therapeutic abortions only after consultation with another physician and in a licensed hospital. Taussig's reform law would allow abortions for rape victims, for retarded women, for girls under sixteen years of age, and for poor women with burdensome household responsibilities.[52]

Many who felt they needed abortions would not be covered. Taussig did not design his proposal to serve all the women already obtaining illegal abortions. He excluded women whose reasons for abortion would offend social conservatives—such as married women who wanted to delay childbearing or did not want to give up their jobs. His proposal denied abortions to unwed women over sixteen years old and to divorced or widowed women who hoped to avoid the shame of bearing an illegitimate child. Taussig felt confident that his law would decrease "the number of secret abortions," while the provisions requiring medical consultation and practice in a hospital would prevent "abuse."[53]

Taussig had called on the medical profession to push for reform, but despite his prominence and the support of the National Committee on Maternal Health, the profession as a whole did not seek liberalization of the nation's abortion laws in the 1930s. The prestige of exclusive medical groups could not erase the association of abortion law reform with radicalism and feminism nor overcome physicians' hostility to being allied with these groups. Furthermore, such a limited model law that rejected women's own perceptions of when they needed abortions and that lacked support from the birth control movement had little chance of gaining popular support.

Although few physicians joined the political challenge of the laws, physicians nonetheless liberalized access to "therapeutic" abortion. During the 1930s, individual physicians and the profession as a whole accepted a de facto expansion of the accepted indications for therapeutic abortions along exactly the social lines proposed by Taussig. In fact, Taussig's proposed legal reform encompassed the broadened indications for therapeutic abortions that he believed to be already accepted by "current medical practice and public opinion" and "in agreement with 'mass opinion.'"[54] A 1939 poll of the nation's medical students confirmed the medical acceptance of abortion. The majority of the medical students, 68 percent, were willing to perform abortions if they were legal.[55]

Therapeutic abortion for women who had tuberculosis illustrates how social conditions entered medical judgment. Tuberculosis of the lungs was the most frequent reason for therapeutic abortion, though there was disagreement over this indication. At the turn of the century, physicians observed that the condition of women who had tuberculosis declined with pregnancy. Physicians urged women with tuberculosis to avoid pregnancy and agreed that when a tubercular woman became pregnant, a therapeutic abortion should be performed to prevent her decline and death. Over the course of thirty years, physicians learned the benefits of rest, saw that the effects of pregnancy on tuberculosis depended on whether the woman had active or latent tuberculosis, and began to revise their views. Typically, Taussig reported, physicians believed latent cases of tuberculosis did not justify abortions, but active cases did.[56]

As Taussig noted, the decision whether to abort the pregnant woman with tuberculosis "is intimately bound up with the social-economic status of the patient." Although doctors disagreed on when tuberculosis made an abortion necessary, they agreed each case had to be examined "from all angles, social as well as medical" before a decision could be made. Long-term bed rest and treatment in a sanatorium could bring a woman with active tuberculosis to a safe delivery. Few could pay for sanatorium care, however, and in those cases, Taussig believed that abortion was justified. He explained how the number of children, housework, and poverty entered into the physician's assessment of proper treatment in these cases. His explanation demonstrates how an affluent woman's desire for a baby, or a poor woman's distress at the prospect, could be incorporated into the physician's decision regarding the necessity of therapeutic abortion.[57]

In a poorly nourished woman with a large family, we must regard the saving of fetal life with less concern than in the woman who can and will carry out sanatorium treatment for the required period of time during and after her pregnancy, and for whom the saving of the child is a matter of great concern. In such women with but one or no children we may, even in active cases, refrain from intervention, while in those whose external conditions make the pregnancy and the subsequent care of the child a serious burden, we would incline more readily, even in latent cases, to an interruption.[58]

The desperate poverty and hunger of many Americans during the Depression similarly entered medical diagnosis. Taussig rejected the Soviet policy of providing abortions for women who already had large families, but reached the same conclusion by medicalizing the problems of large, low-income families. A large family, he suggested, could be detrimental to the health of both a woman and her family. On that basis, an abortion could be medically justified. Abortions in cases of asthma, weight loss, and physical depletion were legitimate, according to Taussig, when the woman had "heavy household duties" and children whom she could not care for or feed adequately. Taussig admitted that conservatives would disagree and that American laws did not allow abortions until a woman's health had already declined, but he favored allowing physicians to perform therapeutic abortions in order "to preserve the health of the mother and the integrity and well being of the family."[59]

As medical advances made it increasingly possible for physicians to bring pregnancies to term for patients with threatening diseases, determining whether an abortion should be performed became more complicated. Changes in the treatment of tuberculosis, heart disease, and vomiting made it possible for more women with these conditions to deliver babies. With adequate rest, women with tuberculosis or heart disease could successfully go through labor. In cases of excessive vomiting, glucose and vitamin feedings could remove the threat of death. Cesarean section had replaced abortion as the response to contracted pelvis. All of these were important advances for women who wanted children. For those who did not, they might prefer abortion and to avoid risks to their own health. The ambiguity of medicine and the ambiguity of the social situation made determining the correct decision difficult.[60]

Taussig's acceptance of broadening the medical indications for therapeutic abortions to include social and economic reasons helped legitimate what was already accepted practice among many doctors. Taussig explained that since the world war "there have been two movements running counter to each other" in terms of their medical and political views of therapeutic abortion: on the one hand, some advocated the liberalization of indications for therapeutic abortion to include social indications; on the other hand, socially conservative doctors argued that therapeutic abortion should be done rarely and never for social reasons.[61] The latter group rejected looking to the circumstances of the patient as part of medicine. Taussig's belief in the necessity of considering the pregnant woman's social situation favored and strengthened one stream of medical thought.

The debate was not only about abortion specifically, but about the nature of medical practice and the relationship between the patient's social world and sickness and health. Should medical decisions be made exclusively on the basis of medical facts about the patient's body and scientific knowledge? Or did the physician have to take into account the person and his or her family, work responsibilities, capacities, and interests? Though the discussion was not framed this way, these issues lay at the heart of divergent medical beliefs about therapeutic abortion. The opposing responses are different methods for dealing with ambiguity in medical knowledge and practice. On one side, physicians recognize the ambiguity inherent in medicine, acknowledge that there are choices to be made, and advocate looking at the larger picture in order to help make the appropriate decision. On the other, physicians handle ambiguity by denying it. When there is doubt, they suggest, there is but one answer. They present a rule to be followed in all cases and in-

sist that all other information is irrelevant. Taussig's discussion of tuberculosis showed, however, that although a physician might take the
conservative medical stance that a tubercular woman should get rest in
an institution and carry the pregnancy to term, the social issues were
inescapable. A low-income woman was unable to follow the doctor's
prescription to spend months in an institution.

Even though Taussig believed social conditions, family need, and income should be considered by the doctor, he resisted addressing the
question of what the patient herself wanted. Physicians who debated
the indications for therapeutic abortion all shared the assumption that
doctors would make decisions for patients. Radical physicians like
Robinson and Rongy, in contrast, assumed that women themselves
would determine when an abortion was necessary. Although mainstream medical thinking assumed that abortion decisions were under
physicians' control, plenty of physicians listened to their patients and
helped them obtain abortions. Allowing physicians to treat social reasons as legitimate medical reasons created some space in which women
and their families could make their preferences known and physicians
could listen.

Despite the objections of some, physicians did perform therapeutic
abortions for economic reasons. An editorial comment in *JAMA* confirmed that physicians performed abortions out of sympathy for destitute patients. "Poverty," the editor asserted, "does not constitute an
indication for abortion." Yet, he admitted, "there is no doubt that in
the United States many abortions are performed for borderline cases in
which there is a strong ethical indication plus a more or less minor
medical ailment."[62] The expansion of therapeutic abortions benefited
women who wanted abortions and who found doctors who could, and
would, justify them on combined medical and social grounds.

Because patients with complications from illegal abortions increasingly went to hospitals, the problem of illegal abortion became visible
to doctors in an unprecedented way. The suffering that so many doctors witnessed made many willing to help women seeking abortions. In
previous years many doctors had privately observed the horrible results
of illegal abortion and tried to cope with them individually in patients'
homes or their own offices. In the Depression decade, as interns, residents, staff, and specialists in hospitals, doctors observed, on a larger
scale, the continuous stream of patients needing emergency care as a
result of illegal abortions. From his days as a hospital intern, Dr. Rongy
recalled a young woman who was hospitalized following her abortion

and her mother who stayed by her side for ten days until her daughter died of septicemia. This "tragedy . . . left a profound impression." [63] A physician who interned at Freedmen's Hospital in Washington, D.C., in the 1930s later recalled attending a hemorrhaging woman who "still had the straightened-out coat hanger hanging from her vagina." [64] In hospital wards, doctors saw women with septic infections, perforations of the uterus, hemorrhages, and mutilation of intestines and other organs caused by self-induced abortions or ineptly performed operations.

The hospital atmosphere, one surmises, made more doctors aware of medical participation in underground abortion services and the stretching of indications to perform therapeutic abortions. In past decades, almost every general practitioner or specialist in obstetrics had been approached at least once by a woman seeking an abortion. The demand generated by the disaster of the Depression increased the number of women knocking on doctors' doors for help. Hospitals concentrated abortion and physicians in one place. In the hospital, doctors could observe each other, talk informally, and spread rumors about physicians' involvement in abortion. Such an atmosphere, I suspect, helped forge a liberal consensus within a section of the medical profession about the horrors of self-induced and poorly performed criminal abortions, together with an acceptance of performing abortions for needy patients or referring them to abortionists.

Abortion Specialists and Clinics

"The demand of women to have abortions," Dr. Rongy observed in 1933, "has become so insistent" that physicians had become more tolerant. A few, he reported, were now "specialists in abortion, who devote themselves to that work to the exclusion of any other part of medical activity." As the Depression damaged physicians' finances, more became interested in abortion practice. [65] The disappearance from northern cities of immigrant midwives added to the pressure upon physicians to perform abortions.

Labeling these physician-abortionists "specialists" referred not to postgraduate education or board certification, but to an exclusive practice and expertise. [66] Even in this unrecognized specialty, however, some physicians obtained additional training in abortion procedures in the United States and Europe. Several abortionists, like their counterparts in other specialties, devised their own instruments and techniques.[67] Rongy believed that as physicians made abortion their "specialty," the dangers of illegal abortion diminished because doctors purchased equipment, used anesthesia and antiseptic procedures, and gained skill in performing abortions.[68]

The medical profession unofficially recognized this specialty by referring patients to physician-abortionists. The specialization in abortion benefited not only the women who wanted abortions, but also physicians who did not themselves perform abortions. Patients could go to skilled practitioners, and physicians could send their patients to colleagues whom they trusted. Numerous doctors avoided performing abortions themselves but participated in abortion by sending patients to specialists. These physician-abortionists were not isolated, but often well-connected and highly regarded by their peers.

Most cities had several physicians who "specialized" in abortion, and many small towns had at least one physician-abortionist. New York's medical examiner knew of "75 physicians" who "specialize exclusively in boot-leg abortions."[69] In the mid-1930s one businessman set up a chain of abortion clinics in cities on the West Coast.[70] Doctors Gabler, Keemer, and Timanus, of Chicago, Detroit, and Baltimore respectively, were physician-abortionists who performed abortions for tens of thousands of women during the 1930s. The decades-long existence of these specialty practices points to the tolerance and accessibility of abortion during these years.

Physician-abortionists practiced in a legally and medically gray area. It was not always clear whether they performed illegal abortions or legal, therapeutic abortions. As physicians, the law allowed them to perform therapeutic abortions in order to preserve a woman's life, but abortion was illegal and frowned upon by the profession. What made physician-abortionists different from other doctors was the volume of abortions performed, often to the exclusion of other medical practice. As long as these physicians received referrals from other physicians, practiced safely, and avoided police interference, they might consider the abortions to be therapeutic. Yet any physician who regularly performed abortions also knew that the procedure was criminal and that he or she practiced on a fine line. Most probably realized that they had crossed that line into illegality.

It is difficult for the historian to gain access to patient records, and this is particularly true for an illegal procedure. Yet I have uncovered records of abortion patients and have reconstructed, for the first time, the daily practice of an underground abortion clinic and the characteristics of its clientele. Seventy patient records of women who had abortions at a Chicago clinic owned by Dr. Josephine Gabler have been preserved in legal documents. These records are a rare find. Analysis of these patient records illuminates the inner workings of a health-care institution that provided crucial reproductive services to thousands of women for decades. The Gabler clinic (later run by Ada Martin) serves as a case study of a specialty practice and reveals the abortion experiences of many women who found physician-abortionists.[71]

Dr. Josephine Gabler was a major source of abortions for Chicago women and other Midwesterners in the 1930s. She graduated from an Illinois medical school in 1905 and received her Illinois medical license that year.[72] She established herself as a specialist in abortion by the late 1920s, perhaps earlier. Over eighteen thousand abortions were performed at her State Street office between 1932 and 1941.[73] In other words, the clinic provided approximately two thousand abortions a year—about five a day, if it operated seven days a week.[74] Dr. Gabler, and other doctors who worked at the State Street office, provided needed abortion services to women from the entire region, including patients from Illinois, Indiana, Michigan, and Wisconsin.[75]

The abortion practice at 190 North State Street in the heart of downtown Chicago was busy and well connected to the Chicago medical community. In January 1940, after more than a decade of business, Dr. Gabler sold her abortion practice to her receptionist, Ada Martin. Gabler retired to Florida, and Martin thereafter managed the practice, arranging for physicians like Dr. Henry James Millstone to perform the abortions.[76] Some of the patients discussed here had abortions before 1940, when Dr. Gabler practiced; others had abortions after Martin purchased the practice.

Numerous women found their way to the State Street office through physicians. Although the medical profession officially condemned abortion, this does not mean that physicians did not participate in illegal abortion.[77] In fact, Dr. Gabler's practice and doctors' referrals to her reveal that many women sought help from physicians—and received it. The Gabler-Martin clinic demonstrates that doctors have been more responsive to the demands of their female patients—even demands for an illegal procedure—than previously suspected. Over two hundred doctors, including some of Chicago's most prominent physicians and AMA members, referred patients to Gabler and Martin for abortions.[78] Of the patients where the person who referred the women can be identified, nearly half had been referred by a doctor.[79] When Mrs. Helen B. learned of her pregnancy in 1940, she wanted an abortion. She "finally persuaded" her doctor that she needed an abortion and was given Dr. Josephine Gabler's business card.[80] The use of business cards itself emphasizes the openness of abortion practice in this period. After Gabler's retirement, the business still used her name and doctors still referred to her. Pharmacists, nurses, and beauty shop operators sent patients as well.[81] As the referrals indicate, women who needed abortions appealed to health-care workers at all levels and visited an exclusive female institution, the beauty salon, for information.

Gabler and Martin showed their appreciation for referrals—and encouraged their colleagues and allies to keep referring—by paying commissions to those who sent patients. Investigators reported that the payments were usually fifteen dollars each, which was about a quarter of the average fee for abortion.[82] When other specialists worked out this type of mutually beneficial arrangement, medical leaders called it "fee-splitting" and deplored it as unethical. Nonetheless, fee-splitting was common among early-twentieth-century doctors, partly because specialists earned so much more than general practitioners.[83]

The other major path to an abortionist's office was through women's personal networks. An abortionist's name and address were critical information, which women shared with each other. In this sample, of the cases where the source of the referral is identifiable, almost a third of the patients found their way to the clinic through friends.[84] Two others knew of the clinic through female relatives, a sister and a sister-in-law. Several had been there before. Every woman who went to 190 North State Street for an abortion became a potential source of information for others in the same predicament. The process of finding a connection could take time; and as time slipped away, the abortion became more difficult, dangerous, and costly. Access to Dr. Gabler and other abortionists depended upon a woman's fortune in tapping into a knowledgeable network. Some never found a safe abortionist.[85]

Women fortunate enough to obtain Gabler's name and address went to the sixth floor of 190 North State Street and checked in with a receptionist.[86] The receptionist (who was first Martin, and later Josephine Kuder) collected information from the patient on a medical record, determined how far the pregnancy had progressed by asking when the woman had last menstruated, told the woman the price of the abortion procedure, and arranged an appointment. On the day of the abortion, the woman was told to undress and put on "a white apron." Mrs. Martin then took her into the operating room, where she was laid on a table, her arms strapped down and her legs raised, and her "private part" shaved, the standard medical procedure in childbirth as well. Mrs. Martin covered the woman's eyes with a towel and then gave her gas to put her to sleep during the operation. One woman woke up during the procedure and felt someone "scraping" her womb. After the operation, the patient rested for about forty-five minutes, received printed instructions from Mrs. Martin outlining how she should care for herself following the abortion, and then went home. Another re-called being given "a card with instructions . . . about hot baths and not to take them. It is similar to the things when you are pregnant and you have a baby in the hospital and about not having anything to do with your husband for so many days afterwards." Finally, Martin ad-monished the patients not to call anyone else if they had problems, but to call the office, which had a twenty-four-hour answering service. Pa-tients were scheduled to return for a checkup; some came the next day, others ten days or six weeks later.[87]

In many ways, the experience of getting an abortion at the State Street clinic was like going into any other doctor's office for medical care. Referrals from physicians, note taking by a receptionist, women dressed in white uniforms, instruments and delivery tables, and the in-structions for after-care were all typical in a doctor's office—and famil-iar to women who had previously delivered babies in hospitals. The women received anesthesia and, apparently, a dilation and curettage of the uterus—the same procedure they would have had if they had a le-gal, therapeutic abortion in the hospital.[88]

Nonetheless, the criminality of abortion made its practice clandes-tine. Two safeguards designed to shield the people performing abor-tions made the procedures in Martin's office different from legal, hospi-tal procedures: covering the eyes of patients in order to make identifying the physician-abortionist impossible and warning women not to go to anyone else if they experienced complications. The clinic did not aban-don its clients if problems developed following the abortion, but they did not want them going to physicians or local hospitals who might alert authorities.

The majority of women in the State Street patient records were mar-ried when they had their abortions. The data for the clinic's patients match the findings of studies that suggest that the majority of women who had abortions before World War II were married.[89] Fifty-six of the seventy women, or a full 80 percent, were married when they had their abortions. Only fourteen were unmarried, though the proportion of unmarried women may be understated.[90]

The married women having abortions followed different patterns to control the timing and number of their children. Over half of the married women (thirty-two women, or 57 percent) had children.[91] Over a third of these women had children under two years old. Mothers seemed strongly motivated to avoid having two babies in diapers at once. Some did not expect to have any more children, like Victoria M., who had three adult children aged twenty-six, twenty-four, and eighteen years old.[92] A second, and large, group of the married women (twenty-four, or 43 percent) had no children at all. This is not what we would expect; we have learned that married women used birth control and abortion after they had children, not before. Unfortunately, the records do not reveal what personal, economic, or social reasons induced these particular women to have abortions, but this group of childless, married women who had abortions is an interesting one that suggests differences in reproductive behavior. Some could be lying, as at least one unmarried woman did, but I know that two were indeed married and childless.[93] Could they represent a significant number of married couples who intended to have no children at all? Since the records do not say how long they had been married, it is possible that these were abortions of prebridal pregnancies. Perhaps some worried about extramarital affairs. Some may have been college students or married to students. Perhaps they needed an abortion because they could not risk losing their jobs. Probably most who had abortions in the early years of their marriages had children later. Class could shape reproduction in complicated ways. Working women and more affluent college women found it necessary to delay childbearing for different reasons and at different times.

The age range of the State Street patients reflected the diversity of women's reproductive patterns and needs. The ages of the women having abortions in this sample ranged from eighteen to forty-eight years, but the majority of women were in their twenties. Their average age was twenty-seven years, but over half were under twenty-five.[94] In 1992, for comparison, most of the women who had abortions were unmarried and under twenty-five years old.[95] Women having abortions in the 1930s and early 1940s were about the same age that they are today. The difference is that most of the women in the Martin case records ended their pregnancies within the context of marriage: 80 percent of the Gabler-Martin clinic patients were married; now, 80 percent are unmarried. Today, most of the women who have abortions do so when they are single and finishing high school or college and expect to bear children later. As Rosalind Petchesky argues, this change marks a "rejection of early marriage as the defining objective in women's lives, and . . . an expectation of economic independence."[96]

It is difficult to determine the class of the women who made up the patients at 190 North State Street, but it seems to have been a mixed group. The records of this office show that we cannot assume that working-class women were never able to get safe abortions from physicians. The availability of safe, illegal abortions depended on more factors than one's class background. Information about income or the occupation of the woman's husband, if married, was not included in the patient records, but the records show that at least a third of the women worked for wages. Most of the married women seem to have been homemakers, but one quarter of the married women (fourteen) worked outside of the home. The group of working women included professional women such as teachers and nurses as well as working-class women such as a waitress, a "wrapper" at a baking company, and a sausage maker. Two women who lived in Evanston and Skokie, Chicago suburbs, may have been more affluent. The various referral networks suggest that women of different classes learned of the State Street clinic.

The racial composition of the women who relied upon the abortion services of Dr. Gabler is even more obscure. There is no racial information in the patient records. Newspaper photos, however, show that Martin and Kuder were white, and the lack of racial identification of witnesses and most of the people charged in the case suggest that most were white, since legal opinions and newspapers at the time often identified black individuals. One person in the Martin case was identified as an African American: Mrs. Roberta Powell, a "colored" nurse from the south side of Chicago, was charged along with Martin.[97] If black women sought connections to abortionists through black nurses, which seems likely, some African Americans *may* have found Gabler through Powell. This is the only hint regarding black women in this case, and, unfortunately, Powell never reemerged in the records.

Most of the women who went to the State Street office for an abortion did so early in their pregnancies. The largest number came for help when they had missed two periods and there was no more hope that they were somehow just off one month. Over 80 percent went to the office for an abortion within two months of their last period; in current terminology, 96 percent of the abortions were during the first trimester.

This pattern matches that of the present; today most abortions are performed in the first eight weeks of pregnancy.[98] Women then and now have tended to have very early abortions.

The fees charged for abortion at 190 State Street ranged between $35 and $300. For the sixty-nine cases with fees noted on the patient record, the mean price—the average—was $67 and the modal price—the price most frequently paid—was $50. Remarkably, the Kinsey study on abortion also found that the average fee for an abortion in the 1930s was $67.[99] These charges were considerable: the average working woman's wage was approximately $20 per week.[100] Nonetheless, an abortion cost less than physician and hospital fees for childbirth.[101]

The prosecutor in the trial of Martin and Kuder charged that the prices "for this criminal operation varied with whatever the traffic would bear,"[102] but my analysis of the office's patient records finds that different factors determined price. One was the length of pregnancy—the further along a woman was, the higher the price. Another was bargaining by patients to lower the price. The more expensive abortions generally occurred at a later point in the pregnancy; the cost of the operation reflected the greater difficulty and risk associated with a later abortion. Of the six abortions that cost over one hundred dollars in this sample, five were of advanced pregnancies.[103] Georgina W. paid one of the highest prices for her abortion, $200, but Martin called hers an "unusual case" because her pregnancy was four months along. In addition, the office arranged for nursing care at an apartment on the south side of Chicago, where she rested for several days. Even Georgina W., however, negotiated the original price down fifty dollars.[104] Paula F., who went to Dr. Gabler for an abortion in 1939, recalled in court that when the receptionist (Kuder) asked how long she had been pregnant, she lied and said "three or four weeks at the most" instead of saying it had been two and a half months. She lied, she explained, because "I know they do charge according to the length of period you have missed and your condition, . . . I knew it would make a big difference in the price." Not only did Paula F. try to cut the price by hiding the progress of her pregnancy, she told the receptionist that she could not afford the quoted price and offered $35 instead. When Kuder told her that "they couldn't think of doing it like that," Paula F. started to walk out, but Kuder stopped her and told her "Well, that will be all right."[105] Some of the variation in prices may have been a result of fitting the fee to the customer, as the prosecutor accused, but this was common among doctors. Physicians accepted lower fees from lower-income patients and collected higher fees from wealthier patients.[106]

The successful bargaining indicates that women did not feel as desperate or as ashamed about abortion as we might expect. Many of the women who walked into the abortionist's office had an idea of what a "fair" price for an abortion should be. Women's willingness to bargain suggests that at least some knew of other abortionists and had other options. The evidence suggests that these women believed they had some control over their illegal abortions. This is really quite remarkable given the criminality of abortion at the time. Gabler and Martin negotiated with their patients and accepted partial payments.[107] Of the twenty-four patients who testified at the trial of Martin and Kuder, over a third told of getting the fees lowered.[108] When Helen N. heard the fee was $65, she objected because she had paid $50 on her previous visit. Her fee for the second abortion was lowered to $50. Some women, like Charlotte B., paid a lower price for their abortions because friends had told them what they had paid. Charlotte B. initially agreed to pay $65 for her abortion when she made her appointment, but when she learned that a "lady friend" had paid less, Charlotte complained and paid only $50.[109] The clinic seemed to be trying to raise its prices, but without success.

Gabler and Martin could provide illegal abortions openly because they paid for protection from the law. Bribery of police and prosecutors underpinned the abortion practice. We only know of the corruption of legal authorities in Chicago because police officer Daniel Moriarity tried to kill Martin in order to silence her. Moriarity hoped to keep his own bribe taking a secret by killing Martin; after mistakenly killing Martin's daughter, he confessed to his own role in illegal abortion. He declared that Martin had paid at least two police officers and two assistant state's attorneys to "fix" any investigations into her business.[110] Moriarity met Martin at a tavern each month, where she "slipped him a $100 note." The payments added up to almost half of his annual income, an enticing sum. In return, Moriarity made sure that attempts to prosecute Mrs. Martin or her associates were bungled. Moriarity reflected, "I always managed to keep the heat off her pretty well until this latest investigation."[111] Hired police protection of abortionists may not have been unusual. One woman who traveled from Wisconsin to Chicago for an abortion by a well-known physician saw a policeman near the physician's office. At first, she recalled, "my fears were that he was a spy; later on I realized he was a paid look-out and protector."[112]

The office at 190 North State Street where thousands of women obtained abortions from a skilled practitioner was not a rarity.[113] Few reputable physicians would induce abortions, but, one New York physician observed, few "would refuse to supply the name and address of one of these abortionists to a patient who applied to them in distress."[114] In Detroit, African American physicians might refer patients to Dr. Edgar Bass Keemer Jr. Dr. Keemer's education, professional career, and social circle were within the African American medical profession. He graduated from Meharry Medical College in Nashville, Tennessee, in 1936, interned at Freedmen's Hospital in Washington, D.C., and took over the practice of a deceased black general practitioner in Indiana. When he moved to Detroit, black physicians helped him open his practice. Keemer was not isolated from other black physicians as an abortionist, but relied upon. Throughout his career as an abortionist, which lasted into the 1970s, Keemer served primarily poor women and black women. In thirty-five years, he performed over thirty thousand abortions.[115]

Dr. Keemer performed his first abortion in 1938. As Keemer told the story, he had refused to perform an abortion for an unmarried woman, who then committed suicide. After this tragedy, Keemer resolved to make amends by performing an abortion for someone else. Within months another woman sought help. She explained, he recalled, that she needed an abortion because she had seven children, her husband earned little, "and we can't hardly feed 'em." Keemer agreed to do the abortion and then realized he did not know how. He contacted the physician-abortionist he knew in Washington to learn the techniques he never learned in medical school.[116]

Keemer's wife, also a physician, played a key role in convincing him to perform abortions. She had wanted to help the first woman, who had come to her expecting a female physician to understand, but Keemer overruled his wife. She was furious. She favored performing abortions because she had had an abortion herself while the couple completed their medical internships. She pointed out Keemer's hypocrisy to him. Although she pushed her husband to do abortions, it is not clear whether Keemer's wife joined the abortion practice.[117]

Keemer's new mentor had performed the abortion for Keemer's wife. "Dr. G." was known as "one of the best practitioners of the forbidden art on the East Coast." This doctor showed Keemer how to use Leunbach's Paste to induce abortions. The advantages of the Leunbach method compared to doing a dilation and curettage, according to Keemer, were in its safety and minimal pain. A dilation and curettage took more time, required extreme care during the curettage to avoid perforation of the uterus, and, if done without anesthesia, was "murderously painful." With the new method, the physician filled a bulb syringe with the paste, a potassium soap solution, and carefully expelled all air in order to avoid introducing an air bubble into the bloodstream, which could kill the patient. Once the air had been removed, the physician introduced the syringe into the cervix, injected the paste into the uterus, and packed the vagina with sterile gauze. The Leunbach method required only "ten minutes on the doctor's table," another advantage of the method, and then the woman could go home. Eighteen hours later, she removed the gauze tampon and a miscarriage occurred with "minimal cramps." Two aspirin, Keemer claimed, usually blunted any pain.[118]

The Leunbach method stimulated the practice of abortion during the 1930s and quickly gained a reputation as dangerous. Keemer had adopted the quintessential abortion method of the decade. A German physician promoted Leunbach's Paste and sold it through the mail to doctors with promises that with it they could safely and easily induce therapeutic abortions instead of performing major operations. A writer for *JAMA* attacked the paste as dangerous, both as a method and because it could easily be used to induce illegal abortions. The chief danger was having a patient die from an air embolism or poisoning; German medical journals had reported twenty-five deaths following the use of this paste. The author warned that abortionists "will turn to such pastes, because of their simplicity." Furthermore, he conceded, "some reputable physicians, now in dire financial straits, may be tempted to use this simple means for inducing abortion."[119] The ease with which Leunbach's paste could be used in the privacy of a doctor's own office helped pull physicians into the abortion trade. When a federal crackdown in the early 1940s dried up Keemer's supply of Leunbach's paste, his abortion practice almost ended. Keemer approached his father, a pharmacist in Nashville, for help. He sent his father a sample, told him why he needed it, and asked him to manufacture it for him. Keemer soon received the paste along with a "note wishing me good luck."[120]

When women came to Keemer's office in Detroit, he took their medical histories, explained the procedure, then performed the brief operation using the Leunbach method to induce a miscarriage. Keemer sent his patients home with printed instructions on caring for themselves and told them to call at any time if they needed help. Keemer or a nurse visited the women at home the next day and did a checkup two weeks later as well. The fee Keemer charged for his first abortion in the late 1930s was $15; by the 1960s he charged on a sliding scale up to $125. If the procedure failed, Keemer returned the fee. In the unusual case where a dilation and curettage was needed, Keemer sent the woman to the hospital, called in a specialist, and paid all fees as well as any money lost by the patient in missing work.[121] Keemer protected his patients by providing after-care; his sense of financial responsibility protected him from complaints and legal interference.

In Baltimore, reputable physicians referred their patients to Dr. George Loutrell Timanus, one of two well-known physician-abortionists in Baltimore. Dr. Timanus had a close relationship to Baltimore's white medical elite at Johns Hopkins University, where the faculty taught Timanus's techniques to their students and called him a friend. Timanus received his M.D. from the University of Maryland Medical School in 1914. From the mid-1920s to his retirement in 1951, he specialized in abortion and provided abortions for women living on the East Coast.[122]

Dr. Timanus's practice was nearly identical to those of Doctors Gabler and Keemer. At Dr. Timanus's office at 1307 Maryland Avenue, patients were greeted by a receptionist and attended by a nurse. Timanus, however, required them to have a letter of referral from a physician. He charged $400, though a referring physician could ask him to lower the fee for less affluent patients, used anesthesia, and performed dilation and curettages. Like Keemer and Gabler, he provided his patients with after-care and phone numbers to call if they had any problems. Timanus's patients seem to have been mostly affluent, probably mostly white, women.[123]

Like Dr. Keemer, Dr. Timanus heard the distress of women faced with pregnancies they could not bear. As chief physician at public playgrounds in Baltimore, he came into contact with working-class mothers of large families and unmarried, pregnant teens. "Schoolteachers," Timanus later recalled, intervened on behalf of schoolgirls, "pleading pitifully for girls who would be banished from school and home if they produced an illegitimate birth." Timanus empathized with the difficulties of poor married women and unmarried girls and began performing abortions in the mid-1920s.[124]

The experiences that moved Doctors Keemer and Timanus to aid women who sought abortions were not exceptional. Most doctors encountered women patients seeking abortions who told similar stories of poverty, excessive childbearing, and illegitimacy. Numerous individual physicians violated the official medical norms that condemned abortion because they could not ignore the dilemmas described by their patients. Many referred them to someone else; only a few doctors bravely turned their sympathy into practice. It is difficult to trace precisely the motivations of those who became abortionists. Money motivated some, as it motivated some to become physicians. Others acted on the political conviction that women had the right to control their own reproduction.[125]

Doctors Gabler, Keemer, and Timanus represent a larger pattern of medical involvement in illegal abortion and an expansion of the medical provision of abortions during the 1930s. Each of these physicians specialized in abortion and had open, busy practices. Hundreds of physicians in their areas trusted them and relied upon them as a resource for abortion services. Their practices were not temporary, but established; they were not located on back alleys, but on main streets. Dr. Gabler had a business card; Dr. Timanus was listed in the phone book and his office had a sign in front.[126] Gabler, Keemer, and Timanus were three of many doctors who performed abortions and were probably among the best available.

Thousands of women obtained abortions from physicians in conventional medical settings and suffered no complications afterwards. Middle-class women, through their private doctors, may have had the best access to the physicians who specialized in abortion. But these specialty abortion practices were not exclusive. A mixed group of patients—working-class and middle-class women, white and black—reached these trusted physicians. The Depression heightened women's need for abortions. The expansion of abortion featured both the acceptance of a wider array of indications for therapeutic abortion and the rise of abortion as a specialty. Women's increased demand for abortions drew the medical profession into providing abortion services.

CHAPTER 6

Raids and Rules

In August 1940, Chicago police raided the Gabler-Martin abortion clinic on 190 North State Street. Police arrested Mrs. Ada Martin, the clinic's new owner; her receptionist, Josephine Kuder; and, as Capt. Thomas Duffy put it, "four girls who were in the office for surgical attention." That raid failed to close Martin's office. Six months later, eighteen police officers again raided the clinic on the morning of February 7, 1941. As Martin later described the events in court, Capt. Duffy entered the office and demanded of her, "Where is your customers?" Then the police "started moving couches and tables and going through all the cupboards and the cash box." The police seized the clinic's furniture, papers, and patient records and arrested Martin and Kuder. Several days later, police entered a business office of Martin's and drilled open a safe from which they confiscated all patient and financial records. The office, Martin recalled, looked "like . . . a bomb shell had hit it." Two and a half months later, police "ransacked" Martin's home and seized more records.[1] When Martin and Kuder came to trial for conspiracy to commit abortion, the prosecution's case against them featured two dozen former patients, who testified about their abortions at the State Street office.

The raid on the State Street office and the subsequent criminal trial of Martin and Kuder are emblematic of the newly aggressive level of the state's suppression of abortion circa 1940. The repression of abortion during the 1940s and 1950s took new forms. Prosecutors no longer focused their energy on the abortionists responsible for women's deaths, but worked to shut down the trusted and skilled abortionists, many of them physicians, who had operated clinics for years with little or no police interference. Authorities still prosecuted the inept abortionists who killed their patients, but this was neither new nor their primary focus. Instead, prosecutors went after clinics that the medical community had essentially endorsed through its widespread referral system. The attack on these established practices meant the destruction of a system that worked well for both women seeking abortions and for physicians. This system had created a space in which thousands of women obtained safe abortions from skilled physicians in an environment nearly identical to that of any other medical practice.

One of the purposes of raiding abortionists' offices was to catch women patients. From the start of the State Street investigation, police and prosecutors intended to find patients. When police raided Martin's practice the first time, they caught "four girls." When they raided again in 1941, Capt. Duffy asked Martin, "Where is your customers?"[2] During a raid of another abortion office on State Street, police broke down a door and "found one woman under an anesthetic on an operating table, and another on a cot, resting after an operation." Detectives questioned both women.[3] If police failed to catch patients on the spot, they looked for patient records to locate former patients for questioning. In the Martin case, police confiscated thousands of patient records.[4]

The new mode of enforcing the criminal abortion laws brought women into contact with the criminal justice system in unprecedented ways. Like the old mode, the state's methods used interrogation and the humiliation of public exposure to penalize women who had abortions. However, rather than relying on dying declarations as the primary evidence against accused abortionists, prosecutors now took the novel approach of looking for healthy female patients to serve as witnesses against their abortionists. Prosecutors showed great persistence in tracking down women who had illegal abortions and routinely brought them into the courtroom and put their abortions on display for judge, jury, and journalist. Women had before felt the force of law during interrogations on their deathbeds; now women were forced to speak of their abortions in the male-dominated spaces of the police station and the courtroom.

Almost simultaneously with the shift in police tactics to control abortion, hospital administrators created new policies to restrict therapeutic abortion. Though the new hospital policies and state efforts to restrict abortion were not part of a coordinated campaign, they were connected. Each reinforced the other. As hospitals constructed barriers to abortion, they acted in conjunction with the state to enforce the criminal abortion laws. The raids and rules together redefined legal and illegal abortion. The definition of legal abortion narrowed in this period, causing that of criminal abortion to broaden. Law and medicine shaped each other.

The new repression of abortion was, in part, a response to the changing circumstances of abortion during the Depression. Abortion became more visible as the practice of therapeutic abortion expanded in hospitals and specialist abortion practices mushroomed. The specialization and institutionalization of abortion during the 1930s facilitated the state's reliance on raiding abortionists' offices. "Professional abortionists," like Dr. Gabler, Dr. Timanus, and Dr. Keemer, had offices, kept regular hours, and had a steady stream of patients coming in.[5] Police officers easily observed their abortion practices.

Medical advances, which improved women's chances of surviving injuries and infections resulting from abortions, contributed to the change in enforcement patterns. The same developments that finally reduced the mortality associated with childbirth reduced the mortality due to abortion. Blood transfusions in the 1930s rescued women hemorrhaging after their abortions; sulfa drugs helped combat infections. Penicillin after World War II, and other antibiotics later, brought about a noticeable decline in overall maternal mortality, including mortality following abortion.[6] State officials quickly adapted their investigative procedures to the new situation—in fact, they took advantage of it. At one trial in which a woman testified against her abortionist, the prosecutor attributed the fact that she was alive and able to appear in court to a recently discovered wonder drug. "Thank God for penicillin," he declared to the jury, "or you might not have had the testimony of Marie L."[7]

But neither medical advances nor structural changes in abortion practice alone can explain the vigorous efforts to suppress abortion. The new repression of abortion was a reaction against the apparent changes in gender and growing female independence. During the Depression women had cut their fertility and appeared to be leaving the home and motherhood for the workplace. World War II accentuated these trends. Furthermore, women's movement into war jobs seemed to contribute to a new "boom" in abortion during the war. Employers' habit of immediately dismissing women upon discovering their pregnancies reinforced the need for abortion.[8] Even though women wore overalls to work in war industries during World War II, Americans were ambivalent about these visible changes. Women's industrial work and high wages might be tolerated "for the duration," but few were prepared to accept these transformations in gender permanently.[9] The renewed repression of abortion reveals a new turn in American society toward pronatalism and "traditional" gender roles often associated with the "feminine mystique" of the 1950s. My work confirms what historians Mary Ryan, Elaine Tyler May, Susan Hartmann, and Linda Gordon have also found: the assault on female independence and the promotion of maternity began in the 1940s, a full decade earlier than generally recognized.[10]

The backlash against abortion reinforced the era's pronatalism. During the 1940s women faced intense social and ideological pressure to bear children. At a 1942 conference on abortion, New York City judge Anna Kross observed, "Today, the pressure is going to be for more and more population." The *Ladies Home Journal* urged women "to correct the mistakes of the 1920s and '30s" by having numerous babies. In the mid-1940s, influential Freudian psychologists equated maternity with female sexual gratification. By the 1950s, the "domestic revival" was in full swing; American women married younger, and the birth rate actually rose for the first time in the twentieth century. Although the push for maternity and domesticity was primarily directed at white women, women of color also felt the pressure to subordinate themselves to men as wives and mothers.[11]

The repression of abortion in this period was new, not normal, and should be incorporated into our understanding of the multifaceted and far-reaching effects of "McCarthyism."[12] The state's surveillance of abortion in this period is another aspect of the political and cultural attack on critical thought and behavior. McCarthyism was devoted not only to eradicating the Communist Party, but to destroying the labor, peace, and interracial movements. As part of the fervent anticommunism of the postwar period, police and government agents investigated and harassed thousands of people for their political views and frightened many more,[13] while the majority learned to conform and keep quiet. Deviation from standard gender and sexual behavior came under attack along with political deviance. State authorities labeled gays and lesbians "perverts and national security risks," and police raided their bars.[14] Abortion symbolized subversiveness, as did these other ideas and activities. In fact, abortion was linked to communism at this time, and red-baiting entered the medical abortion discourse. The attack on abortion and women who sought to control their own reproduction and lives was the dark side of the era's pronatalist ideology.

Raids and Criminal Trials

Raids of abortionists' offices became the national norm during the 1940s and 1950s. Raiding the establishments of criminals—like gambling, prostitution, and bootleg liquor businesses—was not an unknown technique to police, but raids became newly important in the enforcement of the abortion laws. Reflecting on those years, one journalist commented in 1951, "Ten years ago, reform movements and law enforcement drives drove practically all the competent abortionists out of business." [15]

Police and prosecutors around the country duplicated the innovative investigative methods used by Chicago officials in the Martin case. New York police raided several physician-abortionists in the early 1940s.[16] In 1945, police arrested a San Francisco abortionist, who was known as a "careful and clean operator who functioned so openly that a city official described her business as a 'public utility.' " [17] In 1952, after questioning two patients picked up at a bus stop, detectives arrested a Kentucky physician who had been providing abortions since the late 1930s.[18] Police raided the offices of long-time abortionists in Akron, Detroit, Baltimore, Los Angeles, and Portland, Oregon.[19] The Los Angeles police department had a six-member team devoted exclusively to pursuing abortion cases.[20] As police stepped up raids of abortionists' offices during the 1940s and 1950s, corrupt police officers (or their imitators) cashed in by conducting fake raids and extorting abortionists.[21]

The strategy of raiding abortionists' offices not only resulted in the arrest of the abortionist, but also yielded women who had had abortions. The record of the Illinois Supreme Court indicates the importance of women patients to the state's case against abortionists. Of the cases reviewed by the Illinois Supreme Court regarding abortions performed between 1940 and 1960, women testified about their illegal abortions in approximately two-thirds of the cases; only one-third involved a woman's death. In contrast, in the previous seventy years, over 80 percent of the abortion cases heard by the court centered on a woman's death.[22]

After the February 1941 raid of Martin's clinic, police and prosecutors pursued the clinic's patients in order to question them and use them as witnesses.[23] Police entered Martin's offices and home to find the names and addresses of customers. The assistant state's attorney in charge of the investigation, Samuel Papanek, used the thousands of seized records to summon hundreds of former patients. The state's attorney's office sent letters telling women they were expected to attend a scheduled appointment, without saying why. Papanek threatened to subpoena them to the grand jury if they failed to appear. The letters themselves frightened many who received them.[24] Those who obeyed these ominous letters and kept their appointments learned that Martin's office had been raided and saw the records detailing their own abortions. Detectives—both women and men—then questioned the women about their abortions and informed them they might have to testify against Martin and others.

For the women caught in the prosecutor's net, testifying in court had to be traumatic. Prosecutors denied forcing the women to testify against Martin and Kuder, but none had voluntarily complained or offered to testify. Once called to the witness stand, Martin's patients had to speak publicly of pregnancy and abortion in front of a predominantly male audience of judge, attorneys, officials, and newspaper reporters.[25] If they had been unmarried, they had to admit in court their illicit sexuality and sometimes name their lovers. As one woman remarked, testifying at the trial forced her to remember and speak of that which she had "tried to forget." One married woman with three children had never told anyone of her abortion until under questioning she told investigators and again told the court. Evelyn K. felt forced to speak in court against her will. During her testimony she reluctantly named the man who went with her and paid for the abortion, but remarked that "it should be" a secret.[26] Not all women cooperated with the state's attorney; Mary F. refused to testify "for fear her husband w[ould] find out."[27] Others may not have realized they could refuse. Women who believed that the prosecutor was the "court," a "Judge," and "a Sheriff" believed the law had required them to testify.[28]

The state did force women to speak in public courtrooms in order to enforce the criminal abortion laws. In 1942, the New York state legislature passed a statute that compelled women who had gone to abortionists to testify in criminal abortion cases. When a woman who had an abortion refused to testify at a 1949 abortion trial in Chicago, the judge cited her for contempt of court and ordered her to jail for six months. One night in jail convinced the woman to testify the next day. In criminal abortion trials, women often testified under duress.[29]

The prosecutor in the Martin case systematically searched for women who had abortions, but did not pursue the hundreds of physicians who referred patients to Martin's clinic. Martin's business records included the names and addresses of referring physicians, but not a single physician testified about referring patients to the State Street abortion clinic. In this case, the state went after the least powerful people while protecting the more powerful, reputable physicians of Chicago. One woman had to name the man responsible for her pregnancy, but the judge allowed another to withhold the name of the physician who had given her Dr. Gabler's card.[30]

On April 16, 1942, after listening to the testimony of twenty-four of Martin's former patients, the judge hearing the case found both Martin and Kuder guilty of conspiracy to commit abortion and sentenced both to the penitentiary for one to three years.[31] They appealed to the Illinois Supreme Court.

In November 1942, the Illinois Supreme Court overturned Martin and Kuder's convictions because all of the evidence against them had been obtained through the patient records, records that had been illegally seized without a warrant. This ruling was constitutionally significant because the state's highest court confirmed that protections guaranteed in the Bill of Rights against illegal search and seizure applied to state officials. The state court pointed to the Fourth Amendment of the United States Constitution and the corresponding clauses in the Illinois constitution that protected the people "against unreasonable searches and seizures." "It is our duty and the duty of all of the officers of the State," the Illinois Supreme Court sternly reminded the state, "to enforce these constitutional rights preserved to the people." The court condemned the actions of the police and prosecutor in the State Street investigation for their "total disregard of constitutional rights."[32] The U.S. Supreme Court had not found that the restrictions in the U.S. Constitution applied to the behavior of local and state police, but the highest court in the state of Illinois did, forcefully. *State v. Martin* was one of the cases at the state level that recognized and established that the protections against state abuse of power in the U.S. Constitution applied to government authorities at every level. Not until 1961 did the U.S. Supreme Court determine that state authorities could not violate the basic constitutional right against unreasonable search and seizure.[33] The Illinois Supreme Court reversed Martin and Kuder's convictions and remanded them for a new trial.[34]

Newspaper reports of the investigation into Martin's business, which they nicknamed the "loop abortion ring," portrayed abortion as part of the criminal underworld. The investigation exposed corruption in both the police force and the prosecutor's office; Martin's daughter was murdered by a police officer afraid of having his bribe taking discovered.[35] The state charged at least nine people, including two physicians and two nurses. Discovery provoked one physician, who performed abortions for Martin, and his wife, a nurse and his assistant, to commit suicide.[36] The *Chicago Daily Tribune* reported the news on the front page with eye-catching headlines and photos.[37]

These stories enticed readers then and can seduce readers now. There is a danger in getting caught up in the newspaper's story, though; it is easy to recreate the journalists' lurid story line instead of analyzing it.[38] Abortion coverage helped produce the sense that organized crime threatened America. The underworld was a staple of popular news reporting, and, as Lawrence Friedman has noted, the idea of a syndicate provided "a simple and satisfying explanation for at least *some* of the crime that plagued the nation."[39] An illustration for an Oregon newspaper clearly connected abortion to organized crime. The sketch shows a man dressed as a gangster, with a gun in one hand and a cigar in the other; smoke, dollar signs, and a scalpel swirl around his head. In a glance the image conveys the point that the criminal element controlled abortion.[40]

Press coverage of police kicking down doors and raiding abortion offices not only thrilled the public, but also supported the state's efforts to suppress abortion by threatening women, physicians, and others. When the *Chicago Daily Tribune* reported that the police had thousands of Martin's patient records in their hands, they informed everyone involved that they too might be arrested and exposed. "It was the most complete set of records I ever saw," Capt. Duffy declared. "It showed all the patients, their payments, the doctors, nurses, druggists or former patients who had sent them." The paper even printed a sample of a patient record.[41] The policeman's triumph was the patient's and physician's warning. Newspapers further penalized the women in abortion cases by exposing them in their pages. Sometimes papers threatened to but refrained from printing the names of patients or witnesses in abortion cases. At other times, papers named or printed photos of the women—a practice that publicized their illegal abortions and raised questions about their sexual activities.[42]

Since the taint of sexual misbehavior dishonored women uniquely in a way that it did not dishonor men, the public identification of women

who had abortions hurt them. In one instance the prosecutor protected a cooperative female witness by withholding her name from the
press while allowing the papers to name and photograph an uncooper-
ative woman.[43] As this ploy demonstrates, prosecutors understood the
dangers of public exposure to women and used it for their own purposes. Women faced more than the possibility of death when they
sought abortions. The exhibition of women in these cases threatened
all women who had abortions in the past or might have them in the future. Exposure in the papers and interrogation in the courtroom did
not need to happen to every woman who had an abortion to make
women in general understand the dangers of illegal abortion. However,
the state resorted to even more intrusive methods.

On the morning of December 8, 1947, police staked out the apartment of Helen Stanko, a midwife, on the north side of Chicago. Every
twenty or thirty minutes police officers picked up women as they left
Stanko's office; by 10:45 they had accosted eight women. As she walked
along the street away from Stanko's apartment that morning, Clara L.
recalled, "I was forced to go with two men, two detectives." She explained that "one of the officers grabbed my arm. . . . They said they
knew where I had been, and I should come along with them." When
she objected, they showed her their badges. "One fellow even swore. . . .
I still did not want to go. They said if you don't want to cause embarrassment you better go with us or we will call a paddy wagon. So I did
not have any choice." Once the police brought her to the doctor's
office, Clara L. said she was not "forced," but "submitted" to a gynecological exam performed by Dr. Janet Towne in the presence of a po-
licewoman. Dr. Towne examined Clara L., determined she was pregnant, and then removed a rubber catheter placed in the cervix by
Stanko. Clara L. was "too upset and nervous" at the time to remember
what Dr. Towne said to her. When Towne finished, an assistant state's
attorney, Nate Kinnally, and "other men" questioned her in the presence of a court reporter. Then, police drove her to a police station
where she was briefly questioned and where she waited until the police
brought all of the other patients to the station.[44]

Dr. Towne performed an internal pelvic exam on each woman
brought to her by the police, confirmed pregnancy, and removed a rubber catheter from each of them. She found one woman bleeding pro-
fusely and one woman whose cervix had been lacerated. Once Lt.
James P. Hackett received this information, he had Stanko arrested.
Without a warrant, several police entered Stanko's apartment where,

Hackett recounted, they found her "working on an operating table on a patient." Police arrested Stanko, took her patient, and seized Stanko's notebook of patients' names, her instruments, and her medical table.[45] When the police brought Helen Stanko to the station, her patients identified her as their abortionist.

State officials captured women and invaded their bodies as part of their investigation into illegal abortion. The police officers in this case claimed they neither arrested the women patients caught in this raid nor forced them to be medically examined. In the prosecutor's words, they "escorted" the women in unmarked cars to Dr. Towne. Yet anyone picked up by the police or threatened with a paddy wagon, as Clara L. was, would find it difficult to distinguish between her experience and being arrested and hard to resist the ride and medical exam. Although not formally arrested, all of these women were under the control of the police and were implicitly, if not explicitly, threatened with trouble and prosecution themselves. The state argued that Clara L. "consented" to medical examination, but the state's claim was deceptive.[46] Regardless of the language used by officials in court, the police had coerced the women into going with them and into submitting to gynecological exams.

The capture and examination of Stanko's patients had been planned in advance in order to obtain solid evidence for a later criminal trial of Stanko. The state used women's bodies as evidence. Women apprehended in abortion raids in other states were also forced to endure gynecological exams.[47] Police planned the raid on Stanko after one of her patients was hospitalized,[48] but the official response was at least as punitive as protective toward women. Perhaps realizing that forcing an exam by a male physician would provoke resistance, the prosecutor arranged for Dr. Towne's assistance before the raid.[49] Towne's description during the Stanko trial of her pelvic examinations of the women, as well as the introduction into evidence of each catheter she had removed from them, provided crucial evidence for the state's prosecution of Stanko for "attempting to procure an abortion on one Clara L."[50]

Several women caught that December morning testified at Stanko's trial, and some expressed embarrassment at being questioned about their sexual lives in a public forum. Not only had they undergone the fright of being caught, questioned, and examined, the state required them to appear in court. Clara L. was named in the indictment against Helen Stanko and was the first patient to be called to the stand at the February 1948 trial. She told the court that she was a thirty-eight-year-old factory worker and explained how the police caught her on December 8. As she described lying on a table at Stanko's office and how Stanko had inserted a "rubber tube," Clara's voice seems to have grown faint, for the court advised her, "Raise your voice a little, so that the last jurors can hear you." The prosecutor next asked,

Q: Now when you say she inserted some sort of rubber tube in you, will you tell us where she inserted that rubber tube, into what part of your body?
A: Well, I don't know, I would not know what to say.
Q: Was it between your fingers?
A: No.
Q: Tell us what part of your body the tube was inserted in?
A: In between my legs.
Q: At the knees?
A: No.
Q: Well, where? This jury I thinkwill [*sic*] understand.
A: It was inserted in my privates.[51]

Clara L.'s reticence makes it evident that she found it difficult and shameful to discuss her body, her sexual organs, and the abortion procedure in a public courtroom. The prosecutor asked her to name and discuss the treatment of the sexual parts of her body, something never discussed in public—and for many women never in private either. His sarcastic questions were designed to shame. The jury convicted Stanko of attempting to procure an abortion, and the judge sentenced her to five to ten years in prison. She appealed her case to the Illinois Supreme Court, which overturned the conviction. When Stanko was retried, Clara L. and other patients had to testify again. Stanko was convicted a second time.[52]

Only Stanko's defense attorney protested the treatment of the women who had sought abortions from Stanko. At the beginning of Stanko's first trial, her lawyer submitted affidavits arguing that each of her patients had been "illegally arrested and detained, was coerced and forced to submit to physical examination against her will and questioned and forced to make statements against this defendant against her will." The defense argued that since the evidence had been illegally obtained, the witnesses should not be allowed to testify. Throughout the trial and in appeals to the Illinois Supreme Court, the defense attorney suggested that Stanko's patients had been forced to testify against their will, not voluntarily as the state claimed.[53]

The personal violation of each of these eight women during a criminal investigation evoked no judicial concern, even at the highest levels of the judiciary. The treatment of women in the Stanko case suggests that the state did not respect the bodily integrity of its citizens. And, at least in abortion cases, women did not have any rights against involuntary invasion of their bodies. When Stanko appealed to the Illinois Supreme Court twice for her convictions resulting from the 1947 raid, the court expressed no objection to the capturing of women by the police or to the forced gynecological examinations. The Illinois Supreme Court reviewed the two trials of Stanko and overturned her convictions in both cases, once for prejudicial comments by the prosecutor, an erroneous instruction to the jury, and "total disregard of the rights" of the defendant, and once because she had been convicted for a crime other than the one she committed. In both opinions, the court avoided scrutinizing the treatment of the women whose testimony was coerced by the state.[54]

The methods of obtaining evidence and the use of women as witnesses against abortionists punished women by frightening, shaming, and exposing them. In some cases police arrested and fingerprinted women who had abortions; in others prosecutors threatened to prosecute them if they refused to talk.[55] Women were physically captured and endured gynecological exams under duress. As the prosecutor remarked in the *Martin* case, these women had their abortions and then "went about their daily walk of life."[56] When government authorities intervened in abortion, they transformed this part of daily life, this resolution of a personal crisis in a doctor's office, into a public shame.

As women were being caught and dragged into police stations and courtrooms during this crackdown on abortion, physicians began to realize the personal dangers of being involved, however indirectly, in abortion. Physicians had been protected during the Martin and Kuder trial, but state authorities began to threaten doctors who referred patients to abortionists. If referring physicians could be silenced, women's access to professional abortionists might be cut off. In 1942, New York's governor signed an act aimed at the medical community's practice of referring patients to abortionists. The act made the doctor who gave women information about abortion "equally guilty" to those who performed abortions, and New York police arrested physicians who referred patients to abortionists.[57] During a 1954 Chicago investigation, the prosecutor planned to question scores of doctors connected to a local physician-abortionist. "A large percentage of the medical profession," he charged, "is winking at the violation of abortion laws." Furthermore, "he warns," the newspaper reported, "that doctors can be charged as accessories to criminal violations if they steer such patients." Note the language used: what physicians might call referring and women might have seen as helping, the prosecutor labeled "steering"—a word suggesting organized crime. Despite the fact that the prosecutor used reporters to send messages to physicians, he admonished them not to photograph the physicians and simultaneously promised doctors protection from publicity if they cooperated and hounding by the press if they did not.[58] No doubt some doctors stopped telling patients of abortionists.

At the same time, abortion was being linked to communism ideologically. Critics invariably stigmatized radicals and their movements by associating them with sexual license and deviance. This was part of a long history of attacking feminists and radical women by smearing their sexual reputations. One child of communist parents remembers people jeering about "free love" at her mother.[59] *Time* magazine remarked in an article about a convicted abortionist that, in the 1920s, "abortion was *de rigeur* among far left Communists all over the world, as no good female revolutionary was supposed to be hampered by children." *Time's* analysis denied the maternalism of female communists and implied that all leftist women had abortions as a matter of course.[60] Other popular coverage of abortion reported on the legalization of abortion in the Soviet Union, thus connecting a crime in America to communism.[61] Conservative organizations and politicians suppressed discussion of abortion at one college campus.[62]

Furthermore, the national political climate taught Americans to beware of nonconformity. As federal, state, and local agencies went on anticommunist crusades in the 1940s and 1950s, physicians, like everyone else, learned, often unconsciously, that those with unconventional views could be targeted and forced out of their jobs. The pursuit of college professors, scientists, and other professionals served as examples to all of how prestigious and respected professions could suddenly come under state scrutiny and attack. When prosecutors threatened to track down doctors and arrest them, there was every reason to believe them. If professors and state department officials could lose their positions, physicians could imagine the state revoking physicians' medical licenses.[63] The medical profession was traditionally conservative; it had fought off the Sheppard-Towner Act and national health insurance by labeling them "socialized" medicine.[64] Yet the small section of the profession with radical or liberal leanings had reason to fear being singled out by authorities.

When a New York prosecutor initiated an investigation as a result of a physician's comments at a Planned Parenthood meeting, it matched the methods used by the FBI and Congress when chasing "Communists." A prominent physician had spoken at a function of Planned Parenthood and the Brooklyn chapter of the National Council of Jewish Women. Every year, Dr. Louis M. Hellman remarked, about six hundred women came to the county hospital following induced abortions. The prosecutor immediately opened an investigation and called Dr. Hellman to the grand jury because, as he explained, the state required hospitals to report all suspected illegal abortions for investigation, but the hospital had reported only thirty cases, not six hundred. Though the inquiry did not result in any indictments or prosecution, the medical community learned that it was under official surveillance. One suspects that pro–birth control and Jewish organizations were of particular interest to local authorities.[65]

Hospital Rules

In this political climate, medicine turned away from the liberalizing trends of the Depression era and adopted a more conservative stance toward abortion. Medical policy toward and practice of therapeutic abortions changed significantly during the 1940s and 1950s as hospitals invented new rules to regulate therapeutic abortion. Physicians and their institutions patrolled the borders dividing legal and illegal abortion in new ways as obstetric departments created therapeutic abortion committees to control and reduce the practice of abortion. In the past, in the privacy of the physician's office, physicians performed therapeutic abortions without interference. Although the profession urged physicians to consult with other doctors before inducing abortions, nothing required physicians to justify their intentions to anyone. Therapeutic abortion committees grew out of the structural changes of the 1930s coupled with the political conservatism of the 1940s and 1950s, not out of a breakdown in medical consensus.

As obstetrical departments instituted therapeutic abortion committees in the 1940s and 1950s, hospitals voluntarily took on a new role in enforcing the abortion laws and acted as an arm of the state. Hospital abortion committees defined when an abortion was therapeutic and legal, regulated physicians who performed abortions, and standardized the accepted indications for abortion in each hospital. They served as "gatekeepers," granting or denying women access to safe, legal, therapeutic abortions performed in hospitals. The new structure legitimated some therapeutic abortions by preventing others. As hospitals defined and controlled therapeutic abortions performed inside hospitals, they simultaneously defined all abortions performed outside the hospital as illegal.

A Detroit hospital may have created the first therapeutic abortion committee. A 1939 meeting of obstetricians and gynecologists heard the earliest known report of such a committee. Hospital abortion committees were not first formed in the 1950s, but became nearly universal then; they originated more than a decade earlier than generally thought. Dr. Albert E. Catherwood of Detroit reported that Harper Hospital had set up a "permanent therapeutic abortion committee." "Formerly," Catherwood explained, "it was not difficult for any one who wanted to do a therapeutic abortion to get one or two doctors to agree with him." Some physicians, Catherwood and his colleagues believed, performed abortions too readily and too frequently. Under the new policy, the physician who proposed to do a therapeutic abortion presented the case to the hospital's committee, which deliberated on whether or not an abortion should be performed. The committee also considered whether sterilizations should be performed. Catherwood concluded with pride, "We think it a very satisfactory method, and have noted that since the appointment of this permanent committee, the number of therapeutic abortions in Harper Hospital has been greatly reduced."[66] Other hospitals soon adopted Harper Hospital's innovation in abortion control.

Early discussions of therapeutic abortion committees show that physicians feared prosecution for therapeutic abortion and wanted the legal protection afforded by such a committee. During this first reported discussion, Dr. H. Close Hesseltine of the University of Chicago and the Chicago Lying-In Hospital called the therapeutic abortion committee "a very good idea" and noted the "medico-legal protection" it offered.[67] After hearing about Harper Hospital's committee, physicians at Florence Crittenton Hospital in Detroit became worried about their own legal vulnerability. The doctors investigated Michigan law and learned that therapeutic abortion was legal, but concluded that if prosecuted, "the physician had no legal protection." The obstetricians and gynecologists reviewed the therapeutic abortions in their hospital and judged that some "could have been avoided." Faced with this evidence, the hospital imitated Harper Hospital and formed its own committee of three obstetrician-gynecologists to review therapeutic abortion cases and "to protect the physician from inadvertent lapses, medical or legal."[68]

The founders of therapeutic abortion committees and their legal advisers assumed that the law required great caution and that the exception allowing therapeutic abortions would be narrowly interpreted. Physicians never cited a single American case of a doctor being prosecuted for performing a therapeutic abortion in a hospital—nor have I found any—yet they pointed to the need to protect physicians and hospitals from prosecution as the reason for forming therapeutic abortion committees. It seems likely that their fears grew out of traditional concerns about the legal dangers of abortion and the trial of Dr. Aleck Bourne in England.

The famous trial in 1938 of Dr. Bourne for inducing a therapeutic abortion for a fourteen-year-old rape victim may have been the immediate event that inspired hospitals and physicians to examine their policies toward therapeutic abortion and attempt to control its practice. Although none of the published discussion of therapeutic abortion committees explicitly mentioned the *Bourne* case, the timing of the creation of the first committees suggests a link. Bourne had been arrested for performing a therapeutic abortion, prosecuted, and acquitted during the summer of 1938. It was at a 1939 medical meeting that the idea and formation of a hospital therapeutic abortion committee was first announced. The Bourne trial was no obscure case, but one reported in both popular and medical journals in 1938. *Newsweek, Time,* the *New York Times,* and *JAMA* all covered the case. Bourne's was a test case that grew out of a larger social movement to decriminalize abortion in England. He and his supporters hoped to win legal recognition of a more liberal interpretation of the abortion laws. Through the Bourne case, the American public learned of the existence of British medical support for liberalizing access to abortion and American physicians discovered that a reputable physician could be prosecuted for therapeutic abortion.[69]

The doctors' desire for legal protection need not have resulted in restricting the practice of therapeutic abortion, especially since there had been no case in the United States of a physician arrested for therapeutic abortion. As we have seen, the legal system had historically left the definition of therapeutic abortion to the judgment of the medical profession. During the 1930s, reputable physicians in the United States had supported a broadening of the acceptable indications for therapeutic abortion. Organized medicine could have promoted the liberal interpretation of indications for therapeutic abortion put forward by doctors like Taussig and Bourne. Hospitals and their attorneys could have planned to use the precedent created by the *Bourne* case if American officials ever prosecuted a physician or hospital for the performance of a therapeutic abortion in a hospital. These strategies, however, were not pursued. The political conservatism of the period made it increasingly unlikely that the medical profession would follow such a bold course.

The proponents of abortion committees wanted more than legal protection, however; they wanted moral protection for the therapeutic abortions that were performed. When Dr. Hesseltine of Chicago first heard of the committee idea, he noted that "it would give moral support" to those involved in therapeutic abortion.[70] When Doctors Harry A. Pearse and Harold A. Ott described the abortion committee at Florence Crittenton Hospital, they observed that the committee would "conduct its deliberations on a high ethical plane, thereby avoiding the imputation of immorality to the procedures it approves. Thus," they assured their audience, "the attending physician can be certain that any abortion . . . which he may do with the committee's approval will be legally defensible, medically indicated, and *morally acceptable*" (emphasis added). Chicago's Rudolph Holmes applauded the committee plan for insuring the morality of therapeutic abortions. "It would be a great protection to the operator as well as a deterrent to dangerous aspersions by outsiders," he remarked.[71] The committees could make some abortions morally pure and protect medical reputations from attack. Therapeutic abortion committees not only gave their stamp of approval to a select number of abortions, they gave the procedure and the doctor their blessings.

Therapeutic abortion committees provided a way for some members of the obstetrics and gynecology department to impose their views on their colleagues. The new system institutionalized conservative medical views about abortion. When Pearse and Ott explained why Florence Crittenton had created a therapeutic abortion committee in 1940, they pointed to the difficulty of convincing doctors to "curtai[l]" their practice of abortion for preferred patients. Some physicians performed therapeutic abortions in response to the needs of their patients. "Humanitarian impulses cloud professional vision," Pearse and Ott reported, and "the special pleas of intimately known patients" caused physicians' judgment to "laps[e]." Some hospital staff decided that "kindly counsel" should be given to those physicians they deemed unaware of the ambiguous nature of the law. Moral suasion, however, failed to convince these doctors to cease performing therapeutic abortions without strict medical indications. The doctors soon discovered that their advice was "not cheerfully accepted, [but] more frequently is disregarded" by their colleagues.[72] That physicians ignored unasked-for advice is not surprising. Physicians had long disagreed on the indications for therapeutic abortion, as they disagreed on diagnosis and therapeutics in other areas of medicine, but each practiced according to his (or her) best medical judgment. The formation of therapeutic abortion committees, which subjected doctors to oversight, was a new and conservative reform enacted when "kindly counsel" failed to bring about change.

Pearse and Ott detailed the review process of one of the earliest therapeutic abortion committees. Although designed to bring conformity to medical practice in the hospital, the committee nonetheless ran into controversy. In 1940, Florence Crittenton had created a committee of three obstetrician-gynecologists to decide whether or not to allow therapeutic abortions. A physician who wanted approval for a therapeutic abortion submitted a letter to the committee along with the medical indications for the procedure and the recommendations of consultants. The committee then circulated the request among its members. The chairman reviewed the comments and met with members if there were disagreements. If the committee approved a request, the request and the letter of approval were included in the patient's permanent medical record. In 1946, in response to a rise in the number of sterilization procedures, the committee was given the additional task of approving or vetoing sterilizations, a move suggesting that physicians were again listening to patients who wanted to end their childbearing. The following year the committee had to be reorganized into an anonymous committee in order to put a stop to the pleas and complaints being directed at the head of the department whenever a request was denied.[73]

The new structure regulating therapeutic abortions in the hospital limited their number while preserving a small area in which some specialists could still practice legal abortion. Therapeutic abortion committees helped take legal abortion out of the hands of general practitioners and private, nonhospital-based practice and place it in the control of hospital-based specialists in obstetrics. Hospital abortion committees, generally composed of specialists in obstetrics and chiefs of hospital divisions, regulated the medical practice of their colleagues and were particularly concerned about the practices of general practitioners. As these specialists checked the abortion practices of general practitioners, they protected their own right to do therapeutic abortions. Obstetricians regarded themselves, researchers observed, "vis-à-vis the general practitioner, the guardians of standards of practice in this area."[74] Family doctors, because of their knowledge of an entire family and its problems, may have been more likely to consider the whole situation of a woman, rather than sticking to rigidly defined medical indications.[75] The tradition of listening to a patient's story and taking her whole life situation into consideration when reaching medical decisions was being delegitimated. The requirement that physicians obtain the approval of their peers (or superiors) through the committee system changed the relationship between women and their doctors.

During the 1940s and 1950s, hospitals across the nation instituted their own committees to regulate and reduce the practice of therapeutic abortion. The Committee on Abortion created in the early 1940s at the Monmouth Memorial Hospital in Long Branch, New Jersey, was designed "to eliminate the questionable cases." When the California Hospital in Los Angeles established its committee in 1948, the committee rejected half of the proposed therapeutic abortions, thus drastically cutting the number of therapeutic abortions performed there from approximately fifteen per year to six. In 1950, the University of Virginia Hospital, which had averaged over eleven therapeutic abortions per year, created a board to review all cases recommended for psychiatric reasons; a year later, only one abortion had been performed. After Sloane Hospital in New York instituted a review board in 1955, fewer than half as many therapeutic abortions were performed over the next five years. Chicago's Mt. Sinai Hospital formed an anonymous committee in 1956; the following year the number of therapeutic abortions fell from fifteen per year to three.[76]

Probably more important than refusing to authorize therapeutic abortion in specific cases, committees discouraged physicians from seeking approval for abortions. Requiring physicians to commit their medical judgment regarding pregnancy and abortion to writing and then submit supportive arguments based on strict medical indications to a committee for review eliminated some cases immediately. The surveillance itself indicated distrust of physicians and distaste for the procedure. As Dr. Robert A. MacKenzie of Monmouth Memorial Hospital in New Jersey pointed out, "No physician is going to ask the Committee to consider a case which he has not carefully studied, nor about which he does not feel strongly." Physicians who believed in providing therapeutic abortions on more liberal grounds would be unlikely to submit patients to the committee. As a committee approved and disapproved cases, doctors learned not to submit cases like those vetoed in the past. Dr. Alan F. Guttmacher reported that many requests never reached the abortion committee at Mt. Sinai Hospital in New York because doctors asked committee members in advance how they would react to certain requests. "Many physicians are discouraged by telephone conversation or corridor consultation with a single Committee member," Guttmacher reported.[77]

Moreover, abortion committees discouraged women from seeking therapeutic abortions. MacKenzie's report of his hospital's abortion committee made this aspect of its work explicit: "No woman will consent to be taken to the hospital for possible examination and interrogation unless she desperately feels the need for help."[78] Consciously built into the review process were procedures that could be expected to embarrass women patients. Women might have to endure both physical examinations and verbal questioning from several doctors before receiving a therapeutic abortion. This policy was justified, in the minds of some, because some women tried to "abuse" the law and obtain therapeutic abortions for nonmedical reasons. Yet it treated all women as suspects and forced all of them to endure repeated examinations. The University of Virginia Hospital's abortion board reviewed cases with psychiatric indications by having each of the board's three members interview the woman, compare notes, and then decide her fate.[79] Women whose cases might pass muster might prefer to avoid this trying process.

Not only physicians, but hospitals, came under scrutiny for the number of therapeutic abortions performed. Doctors Samuel A. Cosgrove and Patricia A. Carter of the Margaret Hague Maternity Hospital in New Jersey started a competition between hospitals with a 1944 article. The physicians opposed Taussig's call for a broadening of the indications for therapeutic abortion. The authors called for strictly limiting the practice of therapeutic abortion to the rare cases when "the pregnancy threatens the life of the mother *imminently*." Physicians performed so many abortions in the nation's teaching hospitals, Cosgrove and Carter charged, that they could not teach medical students an "abhorrence of abortion in general." Their article presented a table showing the incidence of therapeutic abortion compared to the number of deliveries at seven hospitals. The Johns Hopkins University topped the list with a therapeutic abortion to delivery ratio of 1:35. Margaret Hague proudly came out with the lowest ratio, 1 abortion to 16,750 deliveries.[80]

The medical monitoring of therapeutic abortions is a manifestation of the rise of both conservative medical attitudes toward therapeutic abortion and McCarthyism within medicine. Although Cosgrove and Carter denied wishing to impose their moral values on others, the article's red-baiting and inflammatory language said otherwise. They connected Taussig's call for abortion law reform to Russia and its "amoral and unethical" society. They stigmatized therapeutic abortion—a legal and legitimate procedure—by renaming it "abortion-murder." Nineteenth-century antiabortion activists used this type of language in their campaign to criminalize abortion; their descendants used it to condemn abortions performed to save a pregnant woman's life, abortions long approved by the profession.[81] The article provided a seemingly objective way to judge a hospital's ethical standards. Though a few objected to the language of "murder" and to the insinuation that a comparatively high therapeutic abortion rate meant that a hospital condoned immoral and illegal medical practices,[82] concern about these rates contributed to the restriction of therapeutic abortion.

Political pressure clearly influenced medical policy and practice. Hospital administrators felt pressed by both colleagues and state officials to keep their level of therapeutic abortions down and in line with that of other hospitals. Guttmacher reported forming the abortion board at Mt. Sinai Hospital in 1952 because "it was rumored around New York . . . that Mt. Sinai was an 'easy' place in which to have an abortion." He did not want his obstetrical service's fame, he said, to derive from "its great leniency toward abortion!" He and the other obstetricians decided, Guttmacher reported, "to substitute a conservative, restrictive policy on therapeutic abortion for the liberal, permissive one then in force." Others told of one psychiatrist's experience: the first time he recommended a therapeutic abortion, the district attorney's office called him and told him that he "better watch his step." Dr. Theodore Lidz, of Yale University School of Medicine, noted there was "a tendency on the part of the hospital not to wish to have its rate higher than the rest of the hospitals in the state, because *there might be pressure from someone in the state government*. Thus there is constant care to keep the rates lower" (emphasis added). And, he thought the rates were "dropping" as a result.[83] Doctors at Yale had to be acutely aware of the danger of being associated with abortion or communism given the political situation in Connecticut, where the Catholic Church organized with state politicians to keep birth control illegal and to silence physicians who opposed them.[84]

A few physicians voiced discontent over the shift to a conservative attitude toward therapeutic abortion. At one meeting, several doctors defended therapeutic abortion on more liberal grounds and agreed upon the necessity of considering social and economic conditions. Dr. George H. Ryder's rhetorical questions showed his commitment to the values that had dominated during the Depression era. "Are we to limit therapeutic abortions to medical indications only?" he demanded. "What about hard-working women in poor health, with little money, who already have five or six children? . . . Shall we force them to go through additional pregnancies simply because we think that they shall not die in childbirth?" Dr. Edward A. Schumann went to the heart of the matter: physicians were "apt to be too hyperconservative and think too greatly about the fetus." If pregnancy threatened "disability or death" to a patient or family member, he would "have a small inconsequential fetus removed without concern." These doctors did not doubt the primacy of the pregnant woman's life or the legitimacy of therapeutic abortion. Their views, however, were out of power.[85]

Legal Challenges to the Abortion Laws

Twelve to fifteen police officers invaded Timanus's office on August 21, 1950, burst into his examining room, where they found a patient on an operating table with her skirt up, grabbed all of the patient records, and brought everyone in the office—Timanus, his employees, and his patients—to the police station for interrogation. Six years later, on August 28, 1956, Detroit police raided Dr. Keemer's office, arrested sixteen of his patients, Keemer, his new partner, and two nurses, and collected his patient records.[86] Both physicians had practiced abortion in their cities undisturbed for years, Timanus for almost twenty-five years and Keemer for over ten. Police and prosecutors in Baltimore and Detroit investigated and prosecuted these doctors and their associates in exactly the same way state authorities had in Chicago. Their trials, however, were distinctly different from most abortion cases.

In 1951 and 1958, Dr. Timanus and Dr. Keemer used their own criminal trials as forums for challenging American law on abortion. Both doctors defended themselves against charges of abortion and conspiring to commit abortion by arguing that the abortions were legal. (Usually defendants simply denied having performed abortions.) State laws on abortion provided exceptions for abortions performed for medical reasons, but when a therapeutic abortion was "indicated" was unclear. The Timanus and Keemer cases centered on the definition of a legal, "therapeutic" abortion versus an illegal, "criminal" abortion. Both could have been important test cases of the abortion law, perhaps comparable to the *Bourne* case in England.

Analysis of the trials of Timanus and Keemer reveals the power of medicine to define the law. The distinction between legal and illegal abortions had always been gray. Law did not impose a line dividing legal and illegal, but looked to medicine to mark that line. These cases clarified and shifted the borderline between legal and illegal abortions; in the end, the definition of a therapeutic abortion narrowed to conform to hospital policy and the space in which physicians could legally perform abortions shrank.

As historical records, criminal trial records are quite different from the inquests that were crucial for uncovering abortion in the early twentieth century. At inquests, witnesses were allowed to talk in their own way. The coroner asked questions, but at inquests the rules of criminal trials did not apply, and lawyers rarely cross-examined witnesses. What is said in the courtroom, in contrast, is more planned and coordinated; it is rarely spontaneous.[87] Legal records contain significant information, and I have extracted much from them for this history, but criminal trial records are partial and constructed.

In the Keemer and Timanus cases, the lawyers for the state and defense each constructed their case to present competing definitions of legal abortion. The jury's decision in a criminal trial is based on a sifting of the evidence, but a trial is more than the objective presentation of facts. Every trial contains two sides and each presents not only "facts," but also an argument for the jury. The rules of the courtroom further constrain the presentation of information; the details revealed in court are thus always incomplete. Crucial information may be kept out. The trial is constructed by the lawyers in order to convince the jury of their argument and win—either a conviction for the prosecution or an acquittal for the defense. Lawyers try to control the picture they create and to ask only questions which yield the desired answers.[88] Yet the stories that lawyers try to create break apart as witnesses inject their own concerns into the proceedings. The Timanus case offers an example of how lawyers attempted to construct particular stories and how other stories nonetheless disrupted the neat narrative that the attorneys tried to tell. We can best see how the prosecution and the defense constructed a story about abortion in Timanus's 1951 trial, for which there is a transcript.[89]

The state built its case around the testimony of ten of Timanus's patients, women arrested during the raid or located through seized patient records. In questioning each woman about her pregnancy and abortion, the prosecutor emphasized that these abortions had not been performed for any physical reason. The prosecutor asked Mrs. Eleanor B. and the others, "Was there anything wrong with you physically, any reason why you could not have your child physically?" Mrs. B. answered, "Physically, no."[90]

The defense argued that Dr. Timanus performed legal abortions. He practiced only in consultation with other physicians and induced abortions for reasons of mental health, an acceptable indication. In contrast to the state's construction of therapeutic abortion, the defense referred to the growing acceptance of psychiatric indications for therapeutic abortion. When the defense attorneys cross-examined the women, they highlighted the mental strain of each patient. The attorney asked Mrs. B.,

Q: Why did you want to have your pregnancy interrupted?
A: Well, I wasn't living with my husband. . . .
Q: And it would have upset you terrifically if you had a child?
A: Yes, sir, it would.
Q: What was your mental and nervous state at the time you found out you were pregnant?
A: I wasn't in a very good mental state of mind.
Q: You mean you were pretty desperate?
A: Yes, sir.[91]

With each witness, the defense confirmed that she had first seen another physician who had referred her to Dr. Timanus and that she had been nervous and under great mental distress at the time that she went to Timanus for an abortion. The defense displayed letters from physicians referring patients to Dr. Timanus for "treatment" to show that he had performed abortions only in consultation with other physicians.[92]

As the two sides built their cases, along the way they unintentionally drew out another story: the story of women's lives and the situations that made them need abortions. This story had no place in the plots being created by the opposing lawyers, but the witnesses defied the story lines being produced and inserted their own voices. The female perspective had no legal relevance, though it was key to Timanus's practice and the importance of distinguishing legal and illegal abortion. In asking questions designed to show whether the abortions were justified or not, attorneys drew out the women's own reasons for seeking abortions. The defense attorney asked Mrs. B. why she went to the doctor who referred her to Timanus.

A: What did I go for? . . . Because I had missed a menstrual period.
Q: Well, why did you want to have your pregnancy interrupted?
A: Well, I wasn't living with my husband.

Here is the answer: the importance of an impending divorce in making reproductive decisions seemed completely obvious to the woman who sought the abortion. The defense attorney, however, wanted to draw out the woman's mental state in order to translate the social situation into acceptable medical terms.

Q: And it would have upset you terrifically if you had a child?
A: Yes, sir, it would.[93]

Naoma G. candidly answered that she had gone to Dr. Timanus in 1950 "to have an abortion performed." The defense attorney clarified her feelings,

Q: You weren't married, were you? . . . And you were really pretty much distressed about it weren't you?
A: That is right, well, anybody would.[94]

The ostracism an unmarried woman could expect for bearing a child made abortion necessary for this woman. "Anybody" would feel the same way and, presumably, do the same thing. Again, the defense attorney had to medicalize the social problem, by emphasizing her mental health, in order to claim that the abortion had been performed for medical reasons.

Miss Anne Adams, Timanus's nurse and codefendant, agreed that all of Timanus's patients were upset.

A: I can almost make a blanket statement that every patient that comes to us is highly emotional, is upset with fears. . . . But the procedure is unknown to them, they need reassurance that they will not—it is just like everything else. You are afraid of the unknown. They don't know what is going to happen. Any procedure is feared by any one who associates pain with it.[95]

The nurse first confirmed that all of Timanus's patients were upset, but then stopped herself midsentence as she described their feelings. I suspect that the women "need[ed] reassurance" that they would not be hurt. All patients feared operations; these patients may have been especially fearful since the popular press consistently portrayed abortion as deadly. Adams could not refer to the dangers associated with abortion, however, because she was testifying to the safety, modernity, and legality of Timanus's practice. The story line that the lawyers were working to create in the courtroom, and that she wanted to see succeed, interfered with her desire to tell the female story.

Nonetheless, Adams inserted a woman's perspective throughout her testimony and openly expressed her belief in the need for abortion for single women. She had known of "a single girl" who had been unable to get an abortion. She "had no way of getting married or taking care of an unwanted child," Adams told the court. "The social stigma attached to it upset her; she had no family to turn to, and she found the only answer was to do away with herself." This terrible event explained the importance of doctors like Timanus, "who understood the circumstances of unmarried women." It also explained her interest in later working with him.[96]

Adams's lawyer asked, "Have you any guilt on your own conscience? Just face the jury and tell them." She declared, "I have no feeling of guilt. I feel that Dr. Timanus is doing a great social need, and I am sure any one who has come in contact with patients and has any feeling for any one who is in duress and stress—" The prosecutor interrupted her: "I object to this." The judge sustained him. The rules of the courtroom cut off and silenced Adams's talk about abortion as a "social need."[97] In the past, juries had been understanding, and prosecutors knew that it was nearly impossible to convict accused abortionists unless a woman had died. This prosecutor did not want Adams to sway the jury toward a sympathetic view of the doctor who provided abortions. This moment starkly shows the constructed and controlled nature of testimony in the courtroom. The nurse was not allowed to speak of a woman's view of pregnancy and abortion nor to suggest the need for compassion.

The testimony of Nurse Adams is exceptional. Nurses played an important role in the abortion trade and were frequently arrested during raids, but we know little about them. This source gives us unique insight into the thinking of nurses. Nurse Adams's remarks suggest a special sensitivity to women's need for abortion and that her work held deep meaning for her because of that gendered awareness. Nurses working in regular medical offices sometimes gave patients the names of abortionists; nurses who worked with abortionists eased women's worries and cared for patients before, during, and after the procedure.[98]

The state brought in physicians who contradicted Timanus's claim that he practiced legally. Most damning was the testimony of Dr. Jerome E. Goodman, a gynecologist who appeared as a medical expert. The doctor explained what he would have done if he believed a pregnancy should be "discontinue[d]."

> *A:* Well, I would first admit her to the hospital, get a consultation on her. And in our hospital, before an abortion, what we call a therapeutic abortion, can be performed you have to get two letters, one from the attendant on the staff, and then the case is brought up before a committee, and they, in turn, must pass upon whether a therapeutic abortion is necessary or not.[99]

Dr. Goodman described what had fast become the norm in hospitals across the country. According to him, a therapeutic abortion had less to do with a diagnosis made by a physician than with hospital policy. Therapeutic abortion committees reviewed physicians' decisions to perform abortions and could veto them. Successfully going through the process of review by committee made an abortion legitimate and, thus, "therapeutic." Implicitly, a doctor who had failed to go through a committee had performed an illegal abortion.

When the defense questioned Goodman about his own referral of patients to Timanus, he denied it. Yet one patient testified that the doctor had arranged her abortion by phone, Timanus's secretary confirmed the call, and his name appeared in Timanus's records. Timanus remembered the doctor's betrayal years later. Being abandoned by colleagues who had relied on him seemed to hurt Timanus more than the raid, the trial, and his imprisonment.[100]

The prosecution presented a second gynecologist to bolster its case that the abortions performed by Timanus could not be considered medically necessary. Dr. John Hermon Long had performed a number of therapeutic abortions during his twenty years of practice and what he described did not match Dr. Timanus's practices. The judge questioned him.

> *Court:* In your experience what has been the reason for them?
> *Witness:* Tuberculosis, advanced kidney disease, severe diabetes. . . .
> *Court:* Where is it done?
> *Witness:* In the hospital.

Mr. Orth, the prosecuting attorney, continued the questioning:

Q: What steps do you take before the operation is performed?
A: Ordinarily patients are referred to me by a medical man because they need it, and I don't determine the reason for it actually. I never do myself, but I am merely the surgeon in the case.
Q: All your therapeutic abortions are performed at a hospital?
A: Right.
Q: What hospital is that?
A: Well, usually at Johns Hopkins.[101]

Dr. Long's testimony emphasized two key points for the prosecution: first, therapeutic abortions were performed for diseases and physical reasons only—he listed three. Second, therapeutic abortions were performed in hospitals. Reputable physicians did not perform abortions in their own offices.

The definition of a therapeutic abortion given by Doctors Long and Goodman suggested that physicians universally agreed on the indications for abortion and the procedures to be followed. The two medical witnesses did not discuss existing disagreements within medicine over the indications for therapeutic abortion and did not admit that some doctors accepted social, economic, and psychiatric indications for therapeutic abortion. Medical experts never voluntarily revealed professional disagreements in the courtroom because it undermined their authority, and the defense attorneys did not ask the questions needed to expose the medical debate.[102] The defense doomed its case by failing to bring in their own expert witnesses to testify to the validity of performing therapeutic abortions for mental health. Indeed, by the time of this trial in 1951, psychiatric indications for therapeutic abortion were increasingly common, but the jury never heard about this trend.[103]

Finally, Timanus helped convict himself by clinging to his own sense of professional ethics: he refused to call to the witness stand the doctors who had referred patients to him. Instead, he protected the physicians who had relied upon him and hoped they would voluntarily testify to the legitimacy of his practice. Timanus wrote personal letters asking for support from 353 doctors who had referred patients. None came forward.[104] No one wanted to risk trouble with the law or the profession by defending an accused abortionist. The appearance of colleagues would have shown Timanus to be a member of a respected medical community and a specialist. That some names appeared in the newspapers probably scared them all.[105]

According to the medical experts at this trial, therapeutic abortions were performed for physical indications only, had gone through a hospital review procedure, and were only performed in hospitals. Hospital policy, in the end, convicted Timanus and his employees of illegal abortion. The Maryland Court of Appeals upheld conviction and specifically pointed out that the defense had presented no evidence showing that the abortions had been performed for physical reasons. Timanus was imprisoned for four and a half months and fined $5,000. Anne Adams, the nurse, and Bessie E. Nelson, the secretary, were each fined $1,000 plus costs.[106]

Keemer's trial followed the lines of Timanus's trial. Against legal advice, Keemer insisted on making the legal exception for therapeutic abortion the center of his defense. He too argued that he performed legal, therapeutic abortions for reasons of mental health. Keemer decided to turn his trial into a test case. Unlike Timanus, Keemer had three physicians who testified to Keemer's competency and, most important, agreed that an unwanted pregnancy could threaten a woman's mental and physical health and, thus, her life. However, two other doctors who had agreed to testify for Keemer failed to show up. No medical experts refuted Keemer's claim that these abortions were medically justified. Only four of Keemer's patients testified for the state against him. "Dozens of enraged women," Keemer recalled, told him of being bothered by the police, but many refused to cooperate. Three black patients testified that the stressful circumstances of their lives at the time made having a child "dangerous."[107]

When the prosecutor questioned a young white patient of Keemer's, however, a racist element entered the proceedings. As the prosecutor emphasized that a black man had touched the white woman's "private parts," Keemer later wrote, he "knew . . . that justice was not to be done." Racist notions about black sexual aggression and the need to protect white womanhood from black men ruined Keemer's attempt to make his trial a test case for abortion. Keemer, his colleague, and his assistants were convicted and sent to prison. Keemer served fourteen months.[108]

Oddly, given his political goal of making his case a test of the abortion laws, Keemer did not appeal to the Michigan State Supreme Court. Keemer and his colleague distributed a statement to the press defending themselves as doctors who did "everything in our knowledge as doctors to alleviate physical and mental suffering," but they took it no further. Keemer's attorney believed it would be futile, and Keemer could not pay for an appeal. But more than that, he refused to allow his community to raise the funds for an appeal. "No, I won't accept any defense fund," Keemer later recalled telling a friend who offered to raise money. "A defense fund is just not me."[109] Like Timanus, Keemer envisioned this test case as an individual effort, not a collective one, and, like Timanus, he clung to his own ideas of respectability. Given Keemer's involvement in the Socialist Workers Party and the civil rights movement, this seems a strangely individualistic political move.[110] His personality and his profession precluded enlarging his fight.

In the absence of a professional movement and a social movement advocating liberalization of the abortion laws, neither Timanus's nor Keemer's cases could become test cases. Instead, they confirmed the new restrictiveness of the era. For a case to test the law, it needs to focus on an issue around which lawyers and activists are working to "educate" the courts and society. To have an impact, the case needs to be publicized. For example, when Margaret Sanger claimed women's right to contraceptives in the *Woman Rebel* in 1914 and when she opened the first birth control clinic, she expected to be arrested and to use her arrest to challenge the laws against contraceptives. *Brown v. Board of Education* (1954), which found segregation in the schools to be unconstitutional, grew out of decades of work by the NAACP and the black civil rights movement. These test cases, which challenged and changed the law, grew out of social movements and had their organized and vocal support.[111] Though local papers covered the trials of both Keemer and Timanus, their cases were not understood as radical challenges to the law or to the new methods of suppressing abortion.[112]

For Timanus or Keemer to have successfully reversed the trend toward greater restriction of abortion, they would have needed a social movement behind them. At the very least, if they had tried to recruit other doctors to their cause or to organize sympathetic patients, they might have begun a public discussion about women's need for abortions. As it was, their refusal to do so ensured that the radical potential of their cases went unnoticed, and their efforts were quickly forgotten.

The English example offers a contrast. In the 1930s, Dr. Aleck Bourne succeeded in expanding the indications for therapeutic abortion as a result of his criminal trial for abortion. This case had been organized; it was not one lone individual hoping for justice on the basis of his singular argument. Bourne had *demanded* that authorities arrest him and hoped, he said, "to establish in the eyes of the law that mental health was just as important as physical health." Bourne's trial and legal victory grew out of professional medical support for reform and feminist organizing for women's reproductive rights.[113] The United States had no such movement, feminist or medical, for reform or repeal of the abortion laws until the mid-1950s and 1960s. When a handful of physicians sought arrests as a way of challenging the criminal abortion laws in the late 1960s and early 1970s, they had a larger social movement supporting them, and criminal abortion cases could become test cases.[114]

During the 1940s and 1950s, a nationwide crackdown ended the relative ease of obtaining abortions. The new repression destroyed the old system in which physicians referred patients to abortion specialists who practiced in private clinics and replaced it with new rules and regulations. Hospitals assisted the state by forming therapeutic abortion committees, which further restricted abortion practice. The state's visible interest in stopping the skilled physician-abortionists who had the trust and respect of the medical community magnified the medical community's sense that it needed to be more strict and that those who performed therapeutic abortions needed better legal protection.

Physicians and historians believe that hospitals gained authority over the decisions and practices of physicians only recently, during the 1970s and 1980s, because of new governmental regulation of health care, malpractice suits, and the entrance of corporations into the medical system.[115] Yet therapeutic abortion committees show that hospitals gained control over physicians and medical practice at a much earlier date. Therapeutic abortion committees brought physicians' practices under hospital scrutiny and control over thirty years earlier than generally assumed. These committees were forerunners of the oversight under which nearly all doctors work today. In the forties and fifties, formal committees reviewed and could overrule a physician's medical judgment regarding therapeutic abortion. The committees represented a new intervention in the relationship between physicians and patients and an erosion of physicians' freedom to make medical decisions.

The initial controls on doctors' practices grew out of a politically charged, pronatalist atmosphere hostile to female autonomy. Hospital review of physicians' decisions began with review of reproductive procedures. Review of obstetrical procedures was designed not only to protect women from unnecessary operations, but also to patrol women's own decision making over reproduction. During the 1930s, hospital administrators became concerned about the need to regulate obstetrical operations, partly in response to public criticism of high maternal mortality rates. They were uniquely anxious about abortion, however. A 1935 study alerted hospital administrators of their "duty" to "prevent . . . illegal operations." By 1940, national hospital standards required physicians to consult with other physicians before performing therapeutic abortions. By 1954, the Joint Commission on Accreditation of Hospitals (JCAH) issued standards that required consultation for only three operations—all of them concerning reproduction. First-time cesarean sections, curettages or any procedure in which a "pregnancy may be interrupted," and sterilization required consultation. No other operations required review. The JCAH explained, "We are dealing here with not only prfessional [*sic*] but also moral and legal considerations."[116]

Though new hospital policies restricted the practice of most physicians, they protected specialists and created a small domain in which specialists could perform legal abortions in hospitals without fear. The review of physicians' decisions to perform therapeutic abortions by committees became the mark of a legal abortion. The fact that physicians such as Keemer and Timanus performed abortions frequently and outside hospital walls made their practices, in the eyes of the profession and the law, illegal. Hospital policy delegitimated the tradition of private, out-of-hospital practice of therapeutic abortion.

Doctors Timanus and Keemer's attempts to liberalize the law through their own criminal trials were extraordinary, but their trials achieved precisely the opposite of what they had hoped for. Instead of easing the practice of abortion, the cases confirmed and strengthened the repression of the era. Their cases show how law and medicine were intertwined and mutually reinforcing. In the 1940s and 1950s, hospitals created a new apparatus for reducing the number of therapeutic abortions. This newly instituted committee system redefined the law. No state laws required hospitals to review doctors' decisions to induce abortions. Nonetheless, the creation of restrictive policies governing therapeutic abortion regulated abortion both inside and outside the hospital and delineated what was "legal" and "illegal." Timanus succinctly expressed medicine's role in the courtroom when he remarked, "The profession . . . convicted me."[117]

Women seeking abortions were subjected to more intrusion and scrutiny by both the state and the medical system. They were examined, verbally and physically, by state officials if caught during a raid, or by medical authorities if a therapeutic abortion had been recommended. The state forced women to speak of their pregnancies, sexual partners, and abortions and to name their abortionists in court. Newspaper coverage of raids and criminal trials further exposed and shamed the women who had abortions and the people who provided them. As hospitals restricted access to therapeutic abortion in order to avoid legal trouble, their rules mirrored the state's methods of interrogating, exposing, and embarrassing women. The political atmosphere inhibited discussion of abortion and women's need for it, along with other ideas that challenged the status quo. Silencing, forced speaking, naming names, and public exposure of subversive behavior and beliefs were all characteristic of the McCarthy Era. They aptly describe the period's repression of abortion as well.

CHAPTER 7

Repercussions

"There is . . . more difficulty in locating abortionists today than there used to be," reported Dr. Alfred Kinsey, director of the
Institute for Sex Research in Indiana. "The laws have made it more
difficult . . . to find a physician who will perform it, and that has raised
the cost of abortions."[1] Abortions became harder to obtain, more expensive, and more dangerous as a result of the new repression as hospitals cut access to legal therapeutic abortion and the state shut down established clinics. Accounts of illegal abortions in the 1950s and 1960s
feature a new level of secrecy. Blindfolding and taking women alone to
unknown places for their abortions became the norm. What had been a
fairly open practice became more clandestine as abortionists devised
ways to avoid police detection.

With the new repression of abortion, a discretionary and discriminatory system developed in which class and racial privilege came to the
forefront. Those few who received safe, legal, therapeutic abortions in
hospitals were almost all white women with private health insurance.
Yet almost every woman who looked for an abortion had a difficult
time obtaining one, and many endured frightening and dangerous procedures. Inequality reached into the world of illegal abortion as well.
Low-income women and African American and Latina women suffered
more of the ill effects of criminal abortion than white and wealthy
women. By the early 1960s, the deadly inequality in access to safe abortions by race and class became glaringly obvious. While observers rec-

ognized and deplored the racism and elitism of the abortion system, awareness of the system's inherent sexism remained buried.

Women continued to abort their pregnancies, despite the state and medical repression of abortion. In fact, demand for abortion may have increased in the fifties and sixties. It certainly intensified. Structural changes in women's lives magnified the demand for abortion at the precise moment that the availability of abortion was being severely limited. As Rosalind Petchesky has demonstrated, when women's opportunities and responsibilities expanded in the 1950s and 1960s, their need to control their reproduction grew. Growing numbers of women entered college and the workplace in this period, and both of these male-defined territories required that women postpone and control childbearing. The number of women attending college rose, but this increased attendance was a distinctly middle-class phenomenon, and twice as many white women as black women completed college. Schools and businesses did not provide day-care services and were not structured flexibly so that women could arrange their work around child rearing; yet gender arrangements continued to require that mothers take the entire responsibility for child rearing. Once a woman was visibly pregnant, her school would expel her and her boss fire her. Women were caught in a double bind—required to control their reproduction and forbidden the means of doing so. Many who sought abortions in the postwar period had no room in which to maneuver. Abortion was the only option.[2]

In the early twentieth century, in contrast, married women who wanted abortions had a bit more flexibility if getting one proved difficult. Their reproductive control could aim for decreasing the number of children rather than require absolute infertility for years at a time. For many, if their contraceptive or abortion attempts failed, they could incorporate another child into the family more easily than could women of the fifties. Early-twentieth-century women who did piecework or took in boarders could watch a child in their workplace—their home. It may not have been desirable or easy, but it was possible to adapt to another child. As married women increasingly entered the workforce outside their homes, they did not have that option. Women in school or in the workplace, married or not, needed to control the timing of their childbearing precisely.[3] Some managed both to bear children and keep jobs. African American women have a long history of combining wage earning and child rearing, but it was hard, and they hoped to avoid having to do both at the same time.[4] The structure of education, the economy, and gender helped generate women's need for abortion.

The requirement that unmarried female students remain childless and maintain at least the image of virginity made sex with men, with its risk of pregnancy, dangerous. For a single woman in high school or college, to bear a child meant the abrupt halt to her education. If she carried the pregnancy to term and bore an "illegitimate" child, she would be stigmatized and kicked out of school.[5] If she legitimated the pregnancy by marrying, she was unlikely to continue her education because she would be required to devote herself to full-time child rearing. The new husband and father might have to drop out of school too in order to find a job to support his family. If these were unattractive options, the student could bear a child and give it up for adoption, although that often meant being closeted in an unwed mothers home. Resolving the problem of illegitimate children by leaving them with adoption agencies soared during this period.[6] The growing importance of unwed mothers homes and adoption can be explained by several factors—cultural pronatalism, the mistreatment of single mothers, and the increased difficulty of obtaining abortions. Yet many women found it heartbreaking to give up infants, for whom they knew they could not provide at that time in their lives.[7] In short, pregnancy threatened to destroy a young woman's life and ambitions.

The ability to control their reproduction through abortion enabled women (and men) to continue their education and fulfill societal, familial, and personal goals. The postwar prohibitions on access to birth control and condemnation of childbearing outside of marriage compelled people to marry grooms and brides they did not want to marry. Yet the ideology of romance urged couples to marry for love. Some women bravely chose the danger of abortion for the possibility of a happier future rather than the certainty of a miserable marriage. Abortion was a positive good for women because it allowed them to make decisions about their own futures, delay marriage, be selective about husbands, and improve their lives through education and independent wage earning. For young men as well, the ability of their girlfriends to obtain abortions meant that they could complete their educations and have greater control over the timing of marriage and choice of partners. The constraints facing young unmarried women remain much the same today: contraception and abortion are essential. What is new is that growing numbers of middle-class, single, white women bear children without facing complete social ostracism, though the problems of finances and child care persist. Meanwhile, the New Right is desperately working to restigmatize women who have sex and bear children outside of marriage.[8]

The near impossibility of obtaining birth control in the fifties and sixties raised the danger of intercourse and the fears felt by single women. Physicians and birth control clinics refused to provide contraceptives to unmarried women. In the late 1960s, the health clinic at the University of Illinois in Chicago insisted upon seeing a marriage license before providing birth control. Though some women managed to circumvent these restrictions, all that was left to most to prevent pregnancy were methods that interrupted the flow of lovemaking and required male cooperation—withdrawal, not one of the most effective methods, or condoms. Nonetheless, fortunate women who managed to obtain contraceptives or had careful and trustworthy boyfriends could still find themselves pregnant and in desperate need of abortion.

Unmarried college women feared having their sex lives discovered by college officials or parents. As one 1945 graduate of the University of Wisconsin in Madison recalled, she and other students "hoped that the university authorities . . . knew nothing including your name. College was then in loco parentis and you were put on probation or expelled should the Dean become blatantly aware of all the hanky-panky going on." If students found themselves pregnant, they needed to keep both the pregnancy and their sexual activity secret. One way to do that was by having an abortion. When Rose S. got pregnant at nineteen despite her use of a diaphragm, she "confirmed the pregnancy by seeing, under a false name and equipped with a Woolworth-bought wedding ring, a gynecologist . . . (chosen at random from the phone book)." She acted under a false name because, she explained, "What seemed of paramount importance to me . . . was the secrecy: I not only didn't want anyone in authority to know, I was also anxious that no word leak out to any of my friends and, certainly, family." Once she had confirmed her pregnancy as a "married" woman, as an unmarried college student she arranged for an abortion with "an expert" doctor in Chicago. She had previously accompanied a friend to Chicago for an abortion; she now traveled by train to Chicago for her own abortion at an office much like the Dr. Gabler-Martin clinic on State Street. She had a 6 A.M. appointment, paid $250, more than twice the cost of her out-of-state tuition, and by 9 A.M. was going home by train. The abortion was successful and no one at the university ever discovered it. In later years she more openly discussed her abortions with friends and, when asked for help in locating an abortionist, she had names and telephone numbers ready in her address book.[9]

College students' need for secrecy could be fatal. One woman, who had gone to a southern women's college, remembered another student who had an illegal abortion. "She was too frightened to tell anyone what she had done," she recalled, "so when she developed complications, [she] tried to take care of herself. She locked herself in the bathroom between 2 dorm rooms and quietly bled to death." College students learned a chilling lesson that year about womanhood and the dangers of sex and pregnancy and, perhaps, of the danger of silence as well.[10]

Many more sought out illegal abortionists, but the police crackdown made them harder to find and more expensive. Medical observers agreed that fewer abortionists practiced in New York City in 1955 than had in 1940. The "sharp crackdown" on abortionists in New York had not only reduced their numbers, but the prices charged by the remaining few had more than tripled. Chicago newspaper reports in the 1950s showed that the average fee for abortion in Chicago had more than quadrupled to $325 compared to the average fee of $68 charged in the early 1940s at the Gabler-Martin clinic. One magazine investigated abortion in nine cities in 1955 and found that prices charged by physician-abortionists ranged from $200 to $500.[11]

Finding the money needed to pay for an abortion was a hardship for most. Abortionists could charge hundreds or thousands of dollars depending on the woman's finances. One Chicago woman reported that a friend of hers dropped out of school in order to earn the $500 needed for an illegal abortion. While she worked, her pregnancy progressed. When she was six months pregnant, she had her abortion "in an apartment . . . with no medical backup services."[12] Others took their furniture to pawn shops to raise money for abortions.[13]

There was a notable shift in illegal abortion practices in this period. It was not until the postwar period, quite late in the history of illegal abortion, that women's descriptions of illegal abortions included meeting intermediaries, being blindfolded, and being driven to a secret and unknown place where an unseen and unknown person performed the abortion. Popular magazines at the time emphasized the newly clandestine nature of abortion. When *Ebony*, an African American magazine, covered illegal abortion in its January 1951 issue, it presented abortion as dark and dangerous. A series of dim photographs showed a woman meeting an unknown "contact-man," a cramped room in which the abortionist operated, and police crowded around a bed where a woman had died as a result of her abortion. The emphasis on death was not new in abortion coverage; the depiction of a woman alone meeting an unknown connection was.[14]

Recent narratives of illegal abortions in this period confirm the covert character of the abortion underground. These oral histories and written accounts have been produced as a result of efforts to excavate and preserve women's experiences of the era of illegal abortion. Many informants have told their stories in the hope that their personal histories will generate understanding among politicians and the public about the necessity of legal abortion. The accounts are individual, but patterns stand out and have helped draw a portrait of abortion during the decades immediately preceding *Roe v. Wade*.[15] When one woman met her connection in Baltimore, he blindfolded her and walked her up the stairs, down the halls, and down the stairs to thoroughly confuse her before taking her into a hotel room where the abortionist introduced a catheter. A woman who went to Tampa for an abortion in 1963 recalled being examined by the doctor, then being put in a van with several other women, the entire group blindfolded, and then driven to an unknown location where the abortions were performed. A nineteen-year-old from Madison, Wisconsin, went to Chicago where she "waited on a street corner, was picked up, blindfolded, and driven to a motel in a Cadillac." She commented later, "I know the person who did the abortion was not a doctor. I went through with it because I was desperate."[16]

The clandestine nature of illegal abortions, even if women survived them, sharpened women's awareness of the danger and illegality of abortion. If the Madison woman had experienced any problems, no friend or relative would have been able to find or help her. One woman recalled her fear when she took a friend to the illegal abortionist whom she had previously visited herself: "As I handed her over to strangers at the outside door of the apartment building where the abortion was to be performed, then met the mysterious contact in the park who carefully counted the money, and then waited, waited and waited, I realized how totally at the mercy of unknowns and unknowables my friend was, and I had been." A Detroit student, who found she was pregnant in the spring of 1968, went with a friend to an abortionist who "was upstairs over a store. We were both scared to *death*. The man did the abortion and said not to call him if I had problems." Almost twenty years later the woman seemed to breathe a sigh of relief as she wrote, "Luckily I was O.K."[17]

These memories of illegal abortion point to another element of danger in these secret, anonymous abortions: concern about the medical credentials of the abortionist. One woman remarked that she knew her abortionist was "not a doctor"; another reported a woman who had an abortion six months into her pregnancy "with no medical backup services." Such observations tell of women's fears at the time, which they forced themselves to ignore in the face of their need to avoid bearing a child. At the same time, they point out that what these women accepted as necessary then is unthinkable to them today. Unlike the working women of early-twentieth-century Chicago, most women in the fifties and sixties trusted only white-coated physicians for medical care and knew nothing of other practitioners and their skills. One set of oral histories suggests, however, that some black women may have been more aware and trusting of the alternative practitioners in their neighborhoods than were white women.[18]

Furthermore, having abortions in nonmedical settings alarmed women, and rude abortionists demeaned them. A Milwaukee woman had an abortion without anesthesia and reported that "the 'doctor' smoked a cigar during the entire time." One Chicago abortionist worked "in a dirty T shirt," treated his patients in twenty minutes, "then pushed them out" of the hotel where he worked into a waiting limousine. Another abortionist reeked of alcohol and performed the abortion in the kitchen.[19] The unprofessional demeanor of these abortionists disconcerted many; dirty rooms and drunk practitioners made women worry about injury and infection.

Some abortionists took advantage of their clients' vulnerability in this increasingly secretive situation to sexually harass and exploit them. These men equated abortion with sexual availability and tried to turn their patients into prostitutes. One woman, who had an illegal abortion in the mid-1950s after being raped, recalled the humiliation she felt when the abortionist remarked, "'You can take your pants down now, but you shoulda'—ha!ha!—kept'em on before.'" When he finished the abortion, for which he charged $1,000, he offered to return $20 if she would give him "a 'quick blow job.'" Other abortionists insisted on a trade: sex for abortion. When one sixteen-year-old was propositioned, she walked out. Because she refused to be sexually exploited in exchange for an abortion, she was compelled to give birth and give her child up for adoption.[20]

Since abortionists provided an illegal service, anyone could enter the trade. The crackdown on abortion coupled with the growing demand inevitably attracted more people to this lucrative business that required no specific training. Some women found respectful and skilled abortionists, including both physicians and nonphysicians. Others went to untrained practitioners, including motorcycle mechanics, bartenders, and real-estate agents, who knew little more than that women needed abortions and that inducing them was profitable.[21] The varying prices and the sexual harassment of patients, the unsafe and unsure conditions, could flourish in the black market. Without regulation to ensure competence, all abortion patients were vulnerable.

Illegal abortionists made women go through more connections, shell out more money, and often submit to blindfolding in order to obtain an abortion. Those who went the legal abortion route experienced a different, but similar, set of trials. The therapeutic abortion committees instituted in most hospitals by the 1950s forced women to see more physicians (which meant paying more), have their cases reviewed by a committee, and perhaps submit to interviews. Either way, women looking for abortions had to get around more barriers to obtain them.

Hospital abortion committees not only reviewed physicians' medical decisions in order to uphold new hospital standards, but in some cases also reviewed women's sexual histories and upheld the old sexual double standard. The review policies allowed doctors so inclined to punish 211 unmarried women for their sexual behavior. One committee, which had initially approved a therapeutic abortion, reversed its decision when it learned the woman was unmarried. Some committee members, another member observed, seemed to regard premarital intercourse as a "crime." "Now that she has had her fun," one committee member complained, "she wants us to launder her dirty underwear. From my standpoint she can sweat this one out." Pregnancy exposed an unmarried woman's sexual activity. This hostile physician acted on the common view that such a woman deserved the shame of pregnancy and childbearing out of wedlock as punishment for her sexual misbehavior (and, perhaps, pleasure). Sex itself, and independent female sexuality in particular, this doctor seemed to feel, were "dirty" and repugnant.[22] As these remarks suggest, discomfort about sex could easily pervade committee proceedings. Yet we know of these mean remarks because another doctor reported them as an example of the abuses that occurred in this system. Medical hostility to women seeking therapeutic abortions has been overdrawn.[23] Nonetheless, no matter how sympathetic some individual physicians were, the committee system lent itself to differential assessments of abortion patients.

Yet medical understanding helped open access to abortion along a new path at the same time that it was being increasingly restricted. Psychiatric indications for therapeutic abortion, dismissed as ludicrous earlier in the century,[24] gained new credibility in the 1940s and 1950s. Analysis of therapeutic abortion trends in New York City between 1943 and 1947 showed that abortions for mental illness had "increased steadily" over the period. By 1947, a fifth of the therapeutic abortions had been induced for psychiatric reasons.[25] A study of sixty of the nation's hospitals found that between 1951 and 1960, psychiatric indications accounted for nearly half of all therapeutic abortions.[26] The growing importance of psychiatric indications arose out of the decline of medical complications requiring therapeutic abortion as well as the growing legitimacy of psychiatry.[27]

Physicians and their private-paying female patients together made psychiatric reasons the primary indication for therapeutic abortion. The ambiguity of psychiatric indications made them flexible and available as a category for justifying abortions needed by women. The most important indication for therapeutic abortion at the turn of the century, pernicious vomiting, had been similarly imprecise. Just as late-nineteenth-century and early-twentieth-century women mimicked the symptoms of this dangerous condition to get abortions, in the 1950s and 1960s some women feigned psychiatric problems.[28] Middle-class women, who knew of therapeutic abortion as a possible solution to unwanted pregnancies, demanded them of their doctors in the way that American women always had, but they now referred to a different set of symptoms.

By the 1960s, it was widely known that a woman might obtain a therapeutic abortion if she found the right psychiatrists and said the right words. Women learned to speak of their emotional distress and suicidal intentions. The abortion committee at Mt. Sinai in New York, for example, accepted psychiatric indications only in cases of threatened suicide. "The law says that one may abort to save the life of the mother," Dr. Alan Guttmacher explained, "therefore we insist that suicidal intent must be present in the psychiatric patient in order to validate abortion."[29] One psychiatrist recalled that when women asked him to recommend therapeutic abortions, he simply did so by writing letters that said they were suicidal. He did not question the women seeking his help and, unlike some psychiatrists who doubled their fees, charged nothing. Believing women should be able to decide for themselves and that denial of abortions caused emotional problems, he helped women obtain legal abortions. As word got through the grapevine, more women came to him. Eventually he found the demand overwhelming and, worried that his colleagues might suspect him of extracting huge fees from the women, he ended his involvement.[30]

The suicide threat by no means guaranteed abortion. So many women threatened to commit suicide, the head of a Baltimore hospital's abortion committee recalled, that the claim was "ignored." She told a tragic story of a pregnant teenager who tried to kill herself after learning that her request for a therapeutic abortion had been rejected. The committee reconsidered her case and decided to hospitalize her through her pregnancy in order to save her life. Physicians were using the hospital to enforce childbearing. In the end, this teenager so disrupted the hospital with her multiple suicide attempts that the abortion committee reconsidered a second time and agreed to a therapeutic abortion. Her abortion was granted less because of her own mental health than because of the needs of the hospital and its staff. This particular case highlights the subjectivity of the entire committee system.[31]

Abortions for psychiatric reasons were particularly important for unmarried women in college. One study of the Affiliated Hospitals of the State University of New York at Buffalo found that growing numbers of young, unmarried women were being aborted. The proportion of unmarried women among therapeutic abortion patients had shot up from 7 percent in the 1940s to 41 percent in the early 1960s. Of the single women, almost every one had a therapeutic abortion for psychiatric reasons, 94 percent compared to 48 percent of the married patients. "Possibly, married people are better adjusted and unmarried teen-agers more unstable," the physicians remarked, "but the more likely explanation is that our culture threatens the unmarried gravida with a social stigma which she desperately wishes to avoid by means of abortion."[32] One might add that unmarried college women found sympathy among physicians at university hospitals, who could identify with them as students as well as with their class and race. Such sympathy led them to suggest, along with other reformers in the mid-1960s, that the laws (not sexual behavior, interestingly) needed to change.

Psychiatric indications for abortion sometimes incorporated social and familial reasons, just as tuberculosis had in the past. For example, some psychiatrists regarded therapeutic abortion as a way to prevent future psychiatric problems among the children of women who did not want to bear them. "Most psychiatrists recognize that the woman who states she does not wish to have a baby is unlikely to be a good mother," remarked one psychiatrist in 1955, "and, in the end, we may have several sick children as a result."[33] However, there was a major difference between the socioeconomic indications accepted in the 1930s and those associated with psychiatric indications in the 1940s and 1950s. The former anticipated helping low-income women already overburdened with a large family and housework; the latter primarily served middle-class patients who knew of the indication and could afford psychiatrists.

The new acceptance of psychiatric indications for therapeutic abortions put psychiatrists at the center of tense decisions about when abortions should be performed. If no other medical indication could be found, physicians treated psychiatrists as a last resort, thus making them the final gatekeeper in access to therapeutic abortion. Psychiatrists found themselves under pressure to approve abortions. While the psychiatrist might sympathize with the patient, the nebulousness of the law, Dr. Theodore Lidz felt, required the psychiatrist to be "conservative in his judgment."[34]

Some psychiatrists objected to psychiatric indications out of animosity toward the independence of women. "We know that woman's main role here on earth is to conceive, deliver, and raise children," stated Dr. Sidney Bolter. "The psychiatrist," he warned, "has become the unwitting accomplice" in abortion, taken advantage of by women and their doctors. He urged his colleagues to reverse the trend and to look for psychiatric reasons to advise against therapeutic abortion.[35] Psychiatrists like Bolter were fighting a losing battle, however. The practice of inducing therapeutic abortions for psychiatric reasons continued to rise,[36] though the number performed for this indication never made up the overall decline in therapeutic abortion.

Rubella, which threatened fetal defects, was another new and important indication for abortion from the mid-1950s through the early 1960s. Research had shown that among women who had German measles, or rubella, a few weeks prior to conception or in early pregnancy, about a third of the children would be born with serious defects. Obstetricians generally agreed that a therapeutic abortion should be performed if the fetus had been exposed to rubella during early pregnancy.[37] The response to the dangers of thalidomide, a tranquilizer that could cause fetal defects that became widely known as a result of the Sherri Finkbine case in 1962, showed that much of the public accepted abortion when damage to the fetus was likely.[38]

The acceptance of maternal rubella as an indication for abortion may be read as eugenic, as a method for "improving" the population, but it was neither mandatory nor part of a government program. A distinction must be made between actions taken because they have been imposed by powerful agencies, such as the government or an employer, and decisions made by concerned potential parents. Perhaps this indication should be understood as implicitly taking family capacities and values into consideration and tacitly recognizing a parental right to determine whether they could care for a child born with congenital defects. As Petchesky comments, how to respond to such a possibility is inherently a moral question, and these questions are *"inevitably hard,"* but there is a tremendous difference between a moral question and the political question of who shall make the decision. Furthermore, the social context is crucial. The availability of services for disabled children and their parents influences future possibilities and the ethical choices that potential parents may make. As Michael Bérubé has shown, the lives of the disabled, specifically those born with Down's syndrome, have radically changed in recent years, as have our ideas about the possible future in store for disabled children.[39] Finally, distinctions must be made between decisions about pregnancy and attitudes toward actual children. The same individual who might decide to abort a pregnancy with evidence of fetal defects could devote themselves to a child born with various problems; parents who love and care for a disabled child might seek abortion in order to avoid another. Individual women and their partners regularly face these difficult questions today when they undergo amniocentesis.[40]

Despite new indications, the number of therapeutic abortions dropped dramatically in the two decades following the creation of hospital abortion committees. Individual hospitals boasted of their success in reducing therapeutic abortions since the institution of review committees. Two studies of abortion trends in New York City, the only region that collected long-term data, confirmed their claims. By the early 1960s the number of therapeutic abortions performed in New York City was less than half the number induced twenty years earlier. In the 1940s, New York City physicians performed an average of 710 therapeutic abortions per year; by the early 1960s, they performed fewer than 300. Standardizing these statistics to one thousand live births, the usual method for analyzing trends in maternal health, the rate of therapeutic abortions dropped at an even faster rate: 65 percent between 1943 and 1962.[41] (See figure 2.)

The new restrictions on abortion hit women of color hardest. Racial and economic discrimination limited their access to medical care in

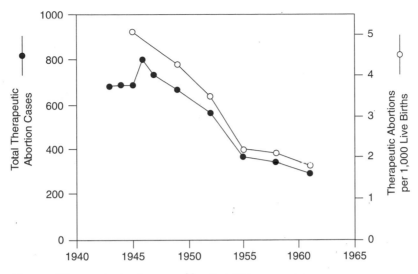

Figure 2. Therapeutic abortion cases, New York City, 1943–1962.
SOURCES: Christopher Tietze, "Therapeutic Abortions in New York City, 1943–1947," *AJOG* 60 (July 1950): 147; Edwin M. Gold et al., "Therapeutic Abortions in New York City: A 20-Year Review," *AJPH* 55 (July 1965): 966, table 2.
NOTE: The average ratio per one thousand live births from 1943 to 1947 is given as 5.1. Data for 1951 to 1962 are reported as totals over three-year intervals. I plot an annual mean at the midpoint year.

general and to safe therapeutic abortions in particular. For the entire period between 1943 and 1962 in New York City, white women had over 91 percent of the therapeutic abortions performed in the city. Furthermore, the decline in the number of therapeutic abortions between 1951 and 1962 was highest among Puerto Ricans and lowest among whites. Public health officials noted that "the disparity . . . between ethnic groups has been widening over the years" and believed it a "medical responsibility . . . to equalize the opportunities for therapeutic abortion."[42] (See figure 3.)

Class inequality in the practice of legal, therapeutic abortions appeared in individual hospitals. Physicians performed the overwhelming majority of therapeutic abortions for private-paying white patients. They performed very few for low-income ward patients. Dr. Robert E. Hall of Columbia University found that at Sloane Hospital in New York, private-paying patients received four times as many therapeutic abortions as did nonpaying ward patients. All but one of the private patients were white. The ward patients were more racially mixed, includ-

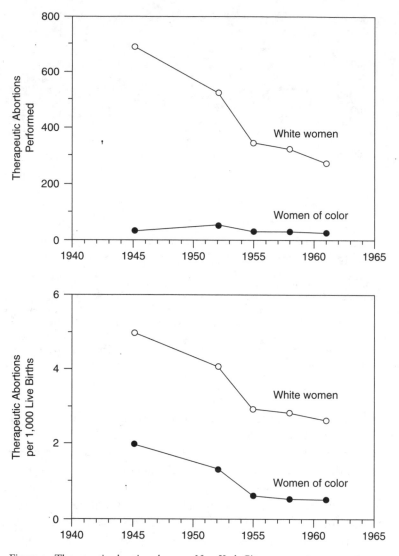

Figure 3. Therapeutic abortion, by race, New York City, 1943–1962.

SOURCES: Christopher Tietze, "Therapeutic Abortions in New York City, 1943–1947," *AJOG* 60 (July 1950): 147; Edwin M. Gold et al., "Therapeutic Abortions in New York City: A 20-Year Review," *AJPH* 55 (July 1965): 966, table 3.

NOTE: Data for 1943 to 1947 are reported as a mean, which I plot for 1945. Data for 1951 to 1962 are reported as totals over three-year intervals. I plot an annual mean at the midpoint year. In the original data for 1951 to 1962, "nonwhite" and "Puerto Rican" are reported separately. Abortion rates for women of color are the weighted average of rates for "nonwhite" and "Puerto Rican."

ing African Americans, Asians, and whites. Therapeutic abortion practices at other hospitals around the country, including those in Chicago, paralleled the practice at Sloane. Hall conducted a national survey of major hospitals and concluded that, "The over-all frequency of therapeutic abortions at 60 outstanding American hospitals is 3.6 times higher on their private services than on their ward services."[43] Municipal hospitals, where the indigent received medical care, performed the fewest therapeutic abortions.[44]

Furthermore, observers noted a pattern of performing abortions for reasons of mental illness more often for private-paying patients than for low-income ward patients. Across the country, Hall reported, physicians treated private patients more liberally. Between 1951 and 1960 at Sloane Hospital, half of the private patients who had therapeutic abortions had them for psychiatric reasons, compared to less than 20 percent of the ward patients.[45] Another physician reported that the "biggest problem" at the university hospitals in Cleveland was abortions performed for "questionable psychiatric reasons, involving members of the medical staff's families."[46]

Middle-class women not only had the necessary ability to pay for consultations, but also enjoyed a more subtle class advantage in gaining the support of their psychiatrists, who were generally of the same class and racial background. Though most women who obtained therapeutic abortions were middle-class and white, the availability of legal abortions to this group should not be overstated. Very few therapeutic abortions were performed.[47] Most middle-class women who had abortions, like low-income women, had illegal abortions.

Dr. Hall pointed to sterilization practices as additional evidence of a double standard in the treatment of low-income patients. When ward patients obtained therapeutic abortions, they were sterilized more than twice as often as private patients.[48] The propensity to sterilize low-income women of color matched the calls by some public officials for forced sterilization of poor, unmarried mothers. These coercive sterilization proposals, based in racist stereotypes and designed to be punitive, were aimed at low-income black women.[49] Some physicians carried out the implied social policies by sterilizing black women without their consent. Not every sterilization was coercive, but the higher incidence in poor and nonwhite populations was cause for concern. The ease with which doctors sterilized poor women, a crucial issue to black feminists and other feminists of color by the 1970s, was already apparent in 1965.[50]

Some physicians and hospitals devised their own coercive steriliza-tion policies as a way to legitimate and limit therapeutic abortions: they insisted that women accept sterilization in exchange. Chicago physi-cians reported in 1939 that when they found therapeutic abortion nec-essary, they preferred to sterilize the woman at the same time in order to avoid performing additional therapeutic abortions in the future. If a woman agreed to an abortion but refused sterilization, the doctors' "general policy" was "to decline to interfere because of the likelihood that the problem will develop again." In an eight-year period at the Chicago Lying-In, 67 percent of the women who had therapeutic abor-tions were sterilized at the same time.[51] Gynecologists around the country agreed to perform abortions only as part of a "package deal," as this policy became known.[52] Media and medical warnings that crim-inal abortions caused sterility came terribly true for some women who had legal abortions in hospitals. Some psychiatrists criticized these ster-ilization policies for being deliberately "punitive" toward women need-ing abortions.[53] At the same time, hospitals restricted access to steril-ization sought by patients.[54] While black women were being sterilized against their will, others who wanted sterilization found it equally im-possible to have their wishes respected.[55]

Both the refusal to sterilize women who sought it and the forced sterilization of others underscore the fundamental medical assumption that reproductive decisions would be made by physicians and the re-jection of patient-defined needs. Furthermore, the contradictory steril-ization policies revealed the medical profession's racial and class identi-fication. Many physicians had adopted a population control view—they believed that low-income women and women of color had "too many" children and should be prevented from having more while affluent white women should not be permitted to avoid childbearing. These at-titudes, coupled with the belief that the medical profession had respon-sibility for reproductive decisions, led many doctors to act on behalf of what they considered best for public policy, rather than on behalf of pa-tients' expressed needs. Plainly, some women refused the package deal and some doctors respected their patients' views. Yet the underlying as-sumptions about medical control over reproductive decisions helped make abuse possible.

Other women took abortion into their own hands. The increased difficulty of locating an abortionist and the skyrocketing prices for abortion surely contributed to the numbers of women who attempted to self-induce their abortions. Douching with soap or bleach was one common and frequently fatal method used by women trying to self-induce abortions. One man who worked in the 1950s at the Chicago Lying-In Hospital, which cared for both white, middle-class patients from the University of Chicago and poor, black patients from the nearby ghetto, recalled seeing young women coming to the hospital who had taken pills or been "injected with lye" to induce abortions. Desperate and low-income women used many of the methods used by previous generations. Some aborted themselves with instruments found at home, including the now infamous coat hanger. One woman described taking ergotrate, then castor oil, then squatting in scalding hot water, then drinking Everclear alcohol. When these methods failed, she hammered at her stomach with a meat pulverizer before going to an illegal abortionist.[56]

The demand for abortion attracted entrepreneurs, and the illegality of abortion meant that the safety and efficacy of various drugs and methods went unregulated. In the early 1950s, sales of a vaginal pill used to induce abortion boomed, and growing numbers of women entered the hospital suffering from vaginal burns. The vaginal pill was the method of destitute women who could not afford to contact a doctor for an abortion but could buy pills. One patient at Cook County Hospital was a twenty-nine-year-old black woman who was described as "extremely pale, cold, and covered with beads of perspiration. . . . [Her] vagina was filled with clots of blood." She told the physicians that she had placed a "grey tablet" in her vagina in order to induce an abortion. When she bled twelve hours later, she believed she had aborted. The hospital treated her, gave her blood transfusions, and, after four days, sent her to the prenatal clinic. The tablet had both injured her and failed to cause an abortion.[57]

Thousands of women with abortion-related complications poured into the nation's hospitals for emergency care every year. Hospitals had entire wards devoted to caring for these patients. In Chicago, the results of the restriction of abortion could easily be seen in Cook County Hospital's wards. In 1939, Cook County Hospital treated over one thousand women for abortion-related complications; twenty years later that number had more than tripled. By 1962, the county hospital reported caring annually for nearly five thousand women with abortion-related complications. (See figure 4.) Though not all of the women who came in had had criminal abortions, physicians believed that most had either induced their own abortions or gone to an abortionist. Population growth alone might have been expected to increase the number

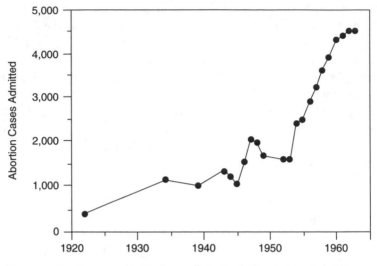

Figure 4. Abortion cases admitted annually to Cook County Hospital, Chicago, 1921–1963.

SOURCES: David S. Hillis, "Experience with One Thousand Cases of Abortion," *Surgery, Gynecology, and Obstetrics* 38 (1924): 83; Augusta Webster, "Management of Abortion at the Cook County Hospital," *AJOG* 62 (December 1951): 1326–1327; Augusta Webster, "Confidential Material Compiled for Joint Commission on Accreditation (June 1964), Obstetrics Department-Accreditation, 1964 folder, box 5, Office of the Administrator, Cook County Hospital Archives, Chicago, Illinois.

NOTE: Although these figures include miscarriages and some therapeutic abortions, physicians believed most of the cases to be the result of illegal abortion.

of cases, but abortionists' access to antibiotics should have mitigated that increase. This hospital's experience was duplicated around the country in hospitals large and small. In the mid-1950s, Los Angeles County Hospital saw over two thousand abortion cases annually. D.C. General's septic abortion ward always had fifteen or twenty extremely ill women in it.[58]

The incredible number of women suffering as a result of illegal abortions had an impact on attendants who knew that abortions could be safely induced. Physicians and nurses at Cook County Hospital saw nearly one hundred women come in every week for emergency treatment following their abortions. Some barely survived the bleeding, injuries, and burns; others did not. The experience at Cook County Hospital suggests the magnitude of the problem of abortion-related complications. Tens of thousands of women every year needed emer-

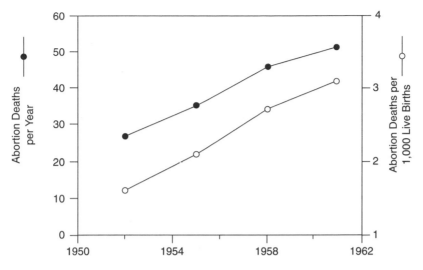

Figure 5. Women's deaths resulting from abortion, New York City, 1951–1962.

SOURCE: Edwin M. Gold et al., "Therapeutic Abortions in New York City, A 20-Year Review," *AJPH* 55 (July 1965): 965, table 1.

NOTE: Data are reported as totals over three-year intervals. I plot an annual mean at the midpoint year.

gency medical attention because of illegal abortion. For health-care providers, this was a problem that was increasingly hard to ignore.

Most disturbing, the number of women who died because of abortion *increased*. New York City data documented the worsening patterns of abortion. Between 1951 and 1962, the absolute number of abortion deaths nearly doubled in this eleven-year period, from twenty-seven deaths per year in the early 1950s to fifty-one per year in the early 1960s. The observed rise in abortion deaths was not simply a function of growing population. When standardized to one thousand live births, the rate of deaths as a result of abortion had practically doubled as well.[59] (See figure 5.)

The risk of dying from an abortion was closely linked to race and class. Nearly four times as many women of color as white women died as a result of abortions. Mortality data revealed the racial inequalities in access to safe abortions. Between 1951 and 1962, the number of abortion-related deaths of women of color more than doubled, from an average of nineteen abortion deaths per year to forty-one. (See figure 6.) In contrast, ten white women died per year because of abortion in the early 1960s. Abortion deaths accounted for half of the maternal deaths

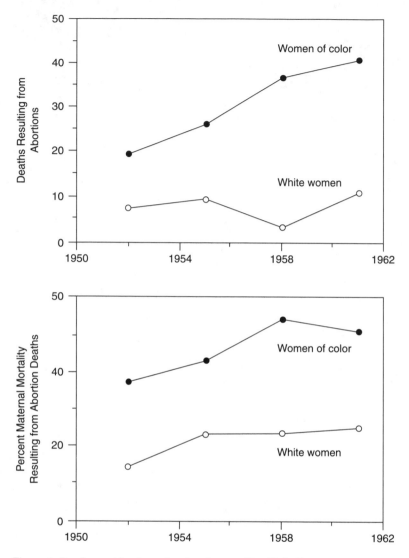

Figure 6. Deaths resulting from abortion, by race, New York City, 1951–1962.

SOURCE: Edwin M. Gold et al., "Therapeutic Abortions in New York City: A 20-Year Review," *AJPH* 55 (July 1965): 965, table 1.

NOTE: Data are reported as totals over three-year intervals. I plot an annual mean at the midpoint year. In the original, "nonwhite" and "Puerto Rican" are reported separately. Abortion rates for women of color are the weighted average of rates for "nonwhite" and "Puerto Rican."

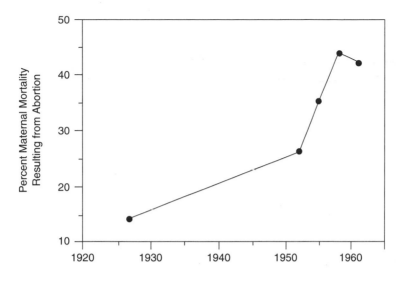

Figure 7. Percent of total maternal mortality resulting from abortion, 1927–1962.
    SOURCES: U.S. Department of Labor, Children's Bureau, *Maternal Mortality in Fifteen States,* Bureau publication no. 223 (Washington, D.C.: Government Printing Office, 1934), 113; Edwin M. Gold et al., "Therapeutic Abortions in New York City: A 20-Year Review," *AJPH* 55 (July 1965): 965, table 1.
    NOTE: The 1927–1928 value is from the Children's Bureau study, which did not include New York. The other values are calculated from the New York City data reported in Gold et al. Data are reported as totals over three-year intervals. I plot an annual mean at the midpoint year.

of women of color, compared to 25 percent of the maternal deaths of white women.[60]

The racial differences in abortion-related deaths and access to safe therapeutic abortions mirrored the racial inequities in health services in general and in overall health. Maternal mortality rates of black women were three to four times higher than those of white women. Black infant mortality was nearly double that of white infant mortality. Furthermore, white Americans could look forward to a longer life expectancy than African Americans. Whites saw physicians more often than African Americans did. Vital statistics revealed how racism took its toll (and how it still does).[61] Abortion contributed to the health problems of low-income women and women of color, but it was only one aspect of fatal inequalities in health care.

Finally, abortion was becoming an increasingly important factor in overall maternal mortality. (See figure 7.) Abortion-related deaths rose as childbirth became safer. At the end of the 1920s, abortion-related deaths accounted for 14 percent of maternal mortality. By the early 1960s, abortion-related deaths accounted for nearly half, or 42.1 percent, of the total maternal mortality in New York City. Furthermore, when skilled practitioners performed this procedure, the mortality rate was lower than that for childbirth.[62] Abortion deaths were almost completely preventable.

Public-health statistics revealed an appalling picture of death and discrimination. Health-care workers and public-health officers observed women dying and thousands more hospitalized as a result of a procedure that could be safe but was not because it was illegal. The illegality of abortion had produced a public-health disaster—especially for low-income and minority women. Maternal mortality had been an important focus of public-health work and a measure of overall health since the early twentieth century. Public-health activists interested in reducing maternal mortality now had to turn their attention to one of the most important causes: illegal abortion.

The results of the criminal status of abortion became plain in the postwar period. Repressive policies designed to control abortion led to a deeply discriminatory and deadly system, a system stamped at every level with the power dynamics of race, class, and gender. Abortion was institutionalized in hospitals in two interrelated structures: the therapeutic abortion committee and the septic abortion ward. While a very small number of women came in through the hospital's front door for scheduled therapeutic abortions, many more abortion patients entered the hospital through the emergency room door. On the one hand, hospital abortion committees approved a few therapeutic abortions, which took place in sterile operating rooms for patients who recovered in private rooms; on the other, hospital abortion wards housed thousands of injured and infected women who had illegal abortions. Class and race defined these hospital spaces: private rooms belonged to a few privileged white women of the middle class; the wards were shared by low-income women of all races, together with some middle-class women who had illegal abortions. Sometimes the patients who were having legal abortions and the patients who needed emergency care stayed in separate sections of the same hospitals, but often they were segregated into different institutions. Private hospitals accepted private patients for therapeutic abortions; public hospitals cared for emergency patients with abortion-related complications. Public policy regarding reproduction had been founded on the assumption that medical men alone, not women, had the right to make decisions about female reproduction. This denial of female autonomy lay at the foundation of the medical system's response to reproduction in general and hospital abortion policy in particular. The discriminatory abortion system was built into the hospital structure.

CHAPTER 8

Radicalization of Reform

The suppression of abortion in the decades immediately preceding *Roe v. Wade* was unique in the history of abortion. That repressive system, and its deadly results, played a crucial role in producing a movement to legalize abortion. The abortion rights movement arose out of the deteriorating conditions of abortion and the frustrations of both women and physicians. As part of their campaign to liberalize state laws, reformers exposed the new and devastating conditions of abortion as intolerable and discriminatory. The social movement to decriminalize abortion drew upon and brought into the open a long-standing acceptance of abortion.

Explanations for the transformation of abortion law that point to media coverage of celebrated abortion cases or changes in medical technology or emphasize the personalities of the Supreme Court justices all simplify the origins of legal and social change. They cannot explain the strength of popular support for legal change. Nor can they explain why members of a socially conservative profession, the medical profession, initiated reform or why the majority of that profession came to support the radical demand for repeal. The abortion cases reached the U.S. Supreme Court as a result of a grassroots movement in which women as well as doctors played a prominent role. The court's decisions arose out of a particularly repressive period and were rooted in both the historical acceptance of abortion and in the contemporary resistance to the law.

The discriminatory and dangerous abortion system bred fear, frustration, and ultimately a movement to change the laws governing abortion. Despite the hazardous character of abortion, women were not the first to articulate publicly and politically their dissatisfaction with the law. In the mid-1950s a small group of physicians and public-health workers initiated the earliest efforts to reform the abortion laws. The hospital system itself, which prevented doctors from providing abortions to patients and forced them to care for the damages resulting from illegal abortions, generated physicians' demands for legal change. Medical reformers soon linked up with leaders in the legal profession, and this professional alliance advocated reform of abortion law. For professionals, the solution to the abortion problem was enlarging the legal space in which physicians could perform abortions.

As women entered the professional abortion discourse they brought their own experiences and insights to bear on political analysis. Feminists retheorized the meaning of abortion. Abortion, as the new feminists analyzed it, was more than an individual need, private crisis, or public-health problem; it was a collective problem for all women. Furthermore, the criminal status of abortion was a fundamental feature of the subordination of women. Feminists found that the assumptions underlying the law and medical practice toward abortion denied women's right to make decisions about their own reproduction, denigrated their moral judgment, and limited their freedom.

Women and professionals looked at the abortion problem from different standpoints, but women, as patients and political actors, moved physicians to a more radical political position. As they had for generations, women insisted that the medical profession listen. Though these "discussions" often took the form of nasty debates, even pickets, much of the medical profession heard the feminist message, just as they had individually heard their individual patients' demands. Now, however, communication and negotiation occurred in public forums between institutions, organizations, and mass movements rather than in conversations in physicians' offices. What had been the private problem of abortion had become political, and what had been the subject of personal discussions had turned into a public debate.

The oppressiveness of the postwar years alone did not produce a movement to legalize abortion, as oppressiveness had not in earlier decades. The changing political context of the period helped produce a mass movement for women's reproductive rights. A movement for abortion rights developed at a time when many in the Civil Rights and anti-war movements mobilized for radical change, a time that gave rise to the second wave of feminism. I examine three phases and several key actors, each representing different groups, with distinctive perspectives: first, the professional movement for reform, composed of physicians and lawyers, which attempted to legislate change; second, the emerging feminist movement, which introduced new meanings of abortion that altered the course of political change; and third, social movement lawyers who challenged the constitutionality of the law and brought together the complaints and claims of physicians, feminists, and low-income women. As a dynamic mass movement in opposition to the existing criminal abortion laws developed, it laid the groundwork for dramatic changes in public policy. The legal challenges framed by Illinois attorneys emphasized the importance of class, race, and gender in abortion. The legal outcome, however, downplayed the significance of race and class in abortion and played up the rights of professionals and female patients.

Professional Reform Measures

Psychiatrists were among the first to question the new structures regulating abortion in the early 1950s. Psychiatrists, the newly liberal and socially activist wing of the medical profession in the postwar period,[1] responded sympathetically to the emotional distress of pregnant women. Their willingness to question the status quo made them early critics of the abortion committee system. Sessions at psychiatry meetings in 1951 and 1952 brought out their frustration. Arthur J. Mandy, a psychiatrist and gynecologist at the Johns Hopkins University, bluntly criticized the therapeutic abortion system as chaotic and discriminatory. Physicians, Mandy declared, found the hospital committee system a "pathetically complicated mess—a hodgepodge of confusion, distortion and duplicity." The lack of clear standards on the indications for therapeutic abortions and the changing policies made the situation "anxiety-provoking" for physicians. The review by hospital committees of honest physicians' recommendations for therapeutic abortion made many of them feel, Mandy reported, like "confirmed criminals."[2]

Hospital restrictions on therapeutic abortion generated resentment among physicians who, as one put it, felt "shackled" by the law. Doctors identified the problem as in the law, not in the structure that had been created by physicians themselves in hospitals under their control.

The monitoring of medical practice delegitimated therapeutic abortion and taught practitioners that they acted on the borderline separating the reputable and the disreputable. Dr. Alan Guttmacher instituted therapeutic abortion committees at two hospitals, yet, he later remarked, those who performed therapeutic abortions had the "haunting feeling that our acts are half-illegal."[3] These doctors soon saw the necessity not of dismantling the hospital committee system, but of changing the law.

Medical and public-health professionals aired the problems of induced abortion in 1955 at a small, unpublicized national conference organized by Planned Parenthood. When Planned Parenthood sponsored this conference on abortion, the organization bravely moved in a new direction. Planned Parenthood, and particularly its medical director, Dr. Mary Steichen Calderone, deserve credit for playing a crucial role in pushing forward a professional movement to reexamine and reform the abortion laws.[4] The organization promised to keep the event quiet.[5] The cloaking of the conference in secrecy is telling: talking about abortion in public scared professionals. The conservatism of the era, both political and sexual, colored the conference. Given that two years earlier one physician had been called to the grand jury as a result of his remarks about abortion at a Planned Parenthood meeting, participants had some reason to worry. Association with abortion could be dangerous. Professionalism did not protect them; instead, it heightened their sense of danger because medical careers depended on good reputations. Conference organizers promised that participants would be quoted only with their permission and could have their "participation deleted" from the published proceedings.[6]

In spite of anxiety about damage to their reputations, the conference participants worked on a joint statement calling for a change in the abortion law, which the majority signed. Professionalism could cut both ways. Professionals worried about protecting their reputations and their social authority, but their status allowed them to speak to controversial matters based on their expertise. "Present laws and mores have not served to control the practice of illegal abortion," their statement began. "To keep on the books, unchallenged, laws that do not receive public sanction and observance," they declared, "is of questionable service to our society." Legal reform was necessary. The participants believed that if current laws were strictly interpreted, most therapeutic abortions would be illegal because they were not induced to "save" a woman's life. The laws should be rewritten to allow doctors

greater legal "latitude" to recommend therapeutic abortions for "psychiatric, humanitarian, and eugenic indications." Liberalizing the abortion laws, the signatories hoped, would expand the practice of legal
therapeutic abortion, lessen the inequality among different classes of
women in access to legal abortion and birth control, and improve the
public health. As a result of the 1955 conference, for the first time in the
United States a group of elite physicians and other professionals collectively advocated reform of the criminal abortion laws.[7]

The 1955 abortion conference was a discussion among professionals,
and the professionals' view of the world shaped their vision of reform.
This is not to say that the efforts initiated by professionals were insignificant, but to point out the boundaries of this conference. Left un-
spoken at these meetings was the question of whether women could
decide for themselves when an abortion was appropriate without having to go through physicians or other intermediaries. The reforms proposed by the group were designed to free physicians from the restraints
of laws and committees and to eliminate the sense that providing therapeutic abortions was a shady, disreputable business. Once the indications for therapeutic abortion had been liberalized, sympathetic physicians would be enabled to help more women who needed abortions.
Women themselves, however, would still have to obtain medical permission for a legal, therapeutic abortion.

Women's rights were left out of the discussion at the conference and
out of the final statement, but it could have been different. The birth
control movement had been founded on the principles of female reproductive and sexual freedom, and feminists in England had extended the
argument to abortion, but Planned Parenthood now advocated birth
control in the name of the family rather than female freedom. Conference participants did not talk about the ALRA in England and its demands for the decriminalization of abortion, though the *Bourne* case
was mentioned and excerpts of the ruling included in an appendix of
the published proceedings.[8] This entire group could not have been ignorant of the ALRA perspective, but they did ignore it. Nonprofessional women did not enter the abortion discourse to speak for themselves until later.

The elite of the legal profession heard the complaints of the medical
profession and identified with them as professionals unnecessarily hampered by the law. In 1959, the year after the publication of the conference proceedings, the prestigious American Law Institute (ALI), made
up of attorneys, judges, and law professors, proposed a model law on

abortion as part of its larger project to standardize American law. As the legal scholar who presented the proposal observed, "The abortion law is out of step with the morals of a substantial, responsible professional group." The ALI's model law clarified the legal exception for therapeutic abortions along the more liberal lines favored by the physicians at the Planned Parenthood conference. It allowed licensed physicians to perform abortions for physical and mental health reasons, fetal defects, or when pregnancy was the result of rape or incest.[9]

The possibility of permitting abortion solely at a woman's request was raised and quickly suppressed. The model law did not allow women and physicians to decide upon abortions without regulation because "it would [not] be sensible to propose a general abortion-at-will statute in this country." Instead, the ALI model law, Leonard Dubin of Philadelphia pointed out, "would go a long way to curing the ill of indefiniteness which has plagued . . . medical practitioners and lawyers trying to advise them." It was hoped that, with the model law, physicians and lawyers would feel less anxiety about therapeutic abortion and, thus, abortions would become more available.[10]

Fearing opposition, the ALI consciously avoided challenging the sexual norms that forbade sex outside of marriage and that treated pregnancy and childbearing as punishment for sexually active unmarried women. The idea of allowing pregnant unmarried women to have abortions provoked a storm. "For us . . . to place the stamp of approval on that," William Marbury explained for the ALI council, "would offend the sensibilities and views of any number of people." This was not about rape, he continued, but about "some girl who goes out and gets herself in trouble and wants to get out of it by an abortion." If the ALI accepted this, it would land in a "great deal of hot water." The speakers expressed little sympathy for the predicament of unmarried women faced with unwanted pregnancies and a great deal of sympathy with a public they assumed to be conservative on the question. The motion to allow abortions in cases of illegitimacy did not receive a second.[11]

The only opposition to the proposed model law on abortion at the 1959 ALI meeting came from a Catholic attorney and a Catholic priest.[12] Like his opponents in the ALI, Illinois attorney Eugene Quay took up abortion as a crucial legal and political question. Quay represented early religious opposition to abortion reform. In 1960 and 1961, he published a lengthy treatise in the *Georgetown Law Journal* in which he alerted Catholic attorneys to the emerging legal movement to liberalize abortion law and provided arguments to fight the ALI reform. The

Catholic Church had played a key role in opposing the birth control movement and would soon lead the fight against legal abortion.[13]

Over the next decade, legal and medical organizations promoted the ALI model law on abortion in state legislatures as well as in the media. In 1960, the Chicago and Illinois Bar Associations advocated legalization of abortion in cases of rape and incest.[14] By 1967, California, Colorado, and North Carolina had passed the model law. The Illinois legislature voted down reform bills in 1967 and 1968. Twenty-eight other states considered similar legislation, and by 1970, twelve states had passed abortion reform measures based on the ALI model law.[15]

The specter of women dying as a result of illegal abortions propelled activists for legal change. Reformers hoped to protect the lives of more women by granting more therapeutic abortions. Data amassed by New York public-health officers had revealed the growing number of deaths resulting from abortion and shown that most of the women who died were African American or Puerto Rican. Public-health professionals joined the earliest calls for reform growing out of the 1955 Planned Parenthood conference. Dr. Alan Guttmacher, who became the most visible national advocate of reform, explained that his belief in the necessity of legal change was the result of having seen women die because of abortions.[16] The memory and mourning of deaths they could not prevent, but that could have been avoided, caused many doctors and other health-care workers to favor reform. On the popular level as well, awareness of tragic deaths generated support for change. For women, death's shadow always lurked when they sought abortions, and they counted themselves among the lucky if they lived through their abortions. As two early supporters of reform in California, Jerome M. Kummer, a physician at UCLA, and Zad Leavy, an attorney and former prosecutor, vividly observed, "We are confronted with a sea of heartache and confusion and the tragic wastage of more than 5,000 deaths per year. . . . How many women must be sacrificed to needless suffering and death," they asked, before the laws were reformed? If the professions did not take the lead in promoting legal change, an "outraged citizenry," they predicted, soon would.[17]

Feminism and Resistance at the Grassroots

Nonprofessional women forged two early alternatives to the professional movement to reform abortion law in the early 1960s.

The Society for Humane Abortion in California was one; "Jane" in Chicago was the other. Both challenged the state in the most fundamental way and made obvious what had long been true: illegal abortions were readily available to thousands, and the state was powerless to stop them. In creating their own illegal abortion networks, the California and Chicago projects circumvented the medical establishment and hinted at the possibility of a health-care system for women run by feminists in competition with the existing medical system. These initiatives were not at first identified as women's liberation efforts—that phrase had not been coined yet. The second wave of feminism, on the verge of breaking, would follow the analysis and activism of these innovative organizers.

One of the earliest nonelite supporters of the reform movement became one of the first critics of the professionals' reform strategy. In 1961, Patricia Maginnis, a San Francisco medical technician, collected petitions in support of a California bill to reform abortion law. She soon recognized, however, the practical and political limitations of reform. First, Maginnis saw that reform laws would not benefit the majority of women seeking abortions, and second, she concluded that writing restrictive "reforms" into law would make it more difficult to further liberalize access to abortion. As early as 1962, she voiced her objection to the type of review boards that the reform laws would institutionalize. Maginnis formed an organization to support reform legislation, but within a few years she and her organization, the Society for Humane Abortion (SHA), rejected reform.[18]

The society put women, rather than physicians, at the forefront. It exposed the medical review committees, which reform measures would make permanent legal institutions, as insulting and humiliating to women. The professionals who initiated the reform movement assumed that physicians would review women's abortion requests. The society criticized such a system. A woman's decision to have an abortion "should not be frustrated and delayed by the complex machinery of legislated abortion committees which sit in judgment of the woman," the SHA argued. "A decision to obtain an abortion should be treated just as any other surgical procedure, as a private matter between a patient and her physician."[19] In an SHA cartoon, a woman asked a psychiatrist, "How much does a psychosis cost for a legal abortion?" Psychiatrists, who had worked to help women obtain abortions, had come to be seen as barriers and were vilified for their role.[20]

The SHA helped radicalize the abortion discourse when it proclaimed abortion as a right and demanded repeal of abortion laws. "The termination of pregnancy," the organization declared, "is a decision which the person or family involved should be free to make as their own religious beliefs, values, emotions, and circumstances may dictate." Furthermore, the group argued, abortions should be available, affordable, and provided in a way that was neither "humiliating nor discriminatory." SHA's perspective would be adopted by women's liberation groups and, ultimately, all sections of the feminist movement.[21] For the first time an American women's organization had framed the problem of abortion in terms of women's right to control their reproduction.[22]

In the mid-1960s, Maginnis created a parallel organization designed to help women obtain illegal abortions. Rather than cultivating friendly hospital abortion committees or teaching women what to say in order to get legal, therapeutic abortions, Maginnis challenged the law by running abortion classes and distributing leaflets on the streets of San Francisco with the names of abortionists in Mexico, Japan, and Sweden. By 1969, SHA's underground arm reported sending twelve thousand women outside the U.S. for abortion. Furthermore, it worked to make women who received referrals politically conscious by requiring them to write letters in support of repeal to their state legislators.[23] The group not only sent women to abortionists, it *regulated* the illegal abortionists.[24] This project turned the tables on the legal abortion system: instead of women having to prove to physicians that they deserved abortions, physician-abortionists had to prove their trustworthiness to potential patients.

Like the SHA in California, what became known as "Jane" in Chicago had roots in a prefeminist era. It grew out of an information network within the Civil Rights and student movements of the mid-1960s. In 1965, Heather Booth found a doctor in the movement who agreed to perform an abortion for the sister of a male friend. Booth was a student at the University of Chicago and an activist; she had participated in sit-ins at Woolworth lunch counters in New York in support of black antisegregation efforts in the South and had registered black voters during Freedom Summer in Mississippi. Like many before her, including Guttmacher and Maginnis, Booth ended up giving out the name of the abortionist repeatedly and was soon overwhelmed by the demand for help and information. Since she was an organizer, Booth set out to find a group of women to take over this necessary work.[25] In 1967, several women active in movement politics created "The Service," which provided abortions to women without questioning the validity of their requests. The group included Hyde Park homemakers and

University of Chicago students. As they gained control over the quality and prices of illegal abortion in Chicago, they formed an alternative, feminist, health-care system. When the activists negotiated with the abortionists to lower the price, they collectively imitated generations of women who had individually bargained with abortionists. They also set up a "scholarship" fund to help low-income women. Jane members initially delivered women to abortionists, but when they realized that some of the "doctors" were not physicians, they decided to learn how to perform abortions themselves.[26]

The Chicago Women's Liberation Union, a citywide coalition, advertised its abortion service through underground newspapers, women's liberation papers, and school papers. When a woman called the union about an abortion, she was given a local telephone number and told to ask for "Jane." After she left a message, a member returned her call, took her medical history, and arranged for her to talk with a counselor, who explained the abortion procedure and told her to go to an apartment called "the Front." There, service members prepared the woman for the procedure, took her temperature, and gave her antibiotics to prevent infections and a leaflet telling her what to do if she had complications. The Front served as a waiting room for the friends, relatives, and lovers who accompanied women seeking abortions, where they could talk or watch TV while snacking on cookies and coffee. From the Front, where by the early 1970s twenty or thirty people might be waiting, members of The Service drove carloads of women to another apartment where a Jane member gave each woman a local anesthetic and performed the dilation and curettage. A counselor held the woman's hand during the procedure. Between 1969 and 1973, Jane provided eleven or twelve thousand abortions, approximately three thousand per year. The women who went to The Service represented every age, racial, and ethnic group and every class. When New York legalized abortion, wealthier women flew there and The Service's clientele changed. As one woman recalled, "about 70 percent were women of color[,] most of whom were living on a subsistence wage or welfare with very poor health care."[27]

This abortion service was similar to other illegal abortion clinics, but different because of its feminist and radical political orientation. Jane was both a health service and a political education project. Not only did Jane eliminate the profit in illegal abortion as it brought abortion under feminist control, it eliminated the judgments of male physicians and the sexual harassment that sometimes occurred. The activists in

The Service provided for women's health needs within an environment designed for women. They sought to empower women through knowledge of their own bodies: during appointments, Jane members provided handmirrors to enable the women to see their cervixes and gave each woman a copy of *Our Bodies, Ourselves*. The activists rejected the authority and distance adopted by physicians as well as the white lab coats; instead they wore jeans and talked with their "patients" as sisters and as equals.[28]

Although The Service expanded beyond the movement, it could be incomprehensible to someone outside the movement that sponsored it. What was an advance for activists in the women's health movement—the rejection of male medical authority and the acquisition of knowledge—disconcerted some patients. One woman later interviewed about Jane had a negative memory of her abortion experience: it took a long time; it was painful; she doubted their skill. That she went to an apartment rather than a hospital or physician's office, that the furniture was shabby, that the abortion was performed in a bedroom, and that the woman who aborted her wore jeans bothered her. Medical offices and white uniforms reassured women that they were getting good medical care; the lack of these symbols suggested that the whole operation was dirty, illegal, and probably dangerous. This woman's negative reaction may have reflected racial and class differences as well as familial religious opposition to abortion. She was an African American going to a mostly white group; she had not graduated from high school, let alone entered college; and her boyfriend's grandmother had been pressuring her to have the baby.[29] An outsider might see the service as a hippie operation and, though essential, distressing despite the counselors and cookies.

The policing of criminal abortion, which received no attention from the professional reformers, figured importantly in the feminist critique of the abortion system. The SHA and Jane warned women of the conventional police methods used for investigating abortion and criticized the surveillance conducted by hospital staff for the state. Every year in the early 1960s, San Francisco hospitals reported to the police over a hundred women who had abortions. Jane members recalled that hospital emergency room staff called police before aiding women in the process of aborting: "Sometimes they would admit a woman and then withhold drugs from her unless she talked."[30] The voluntary policing by medical practitioners helped produce the rage many feminists felt toward the medical profession. Activists advised women who had abortions that they had a right to refuse to answer the questions of police.[31] (See plate 6.)

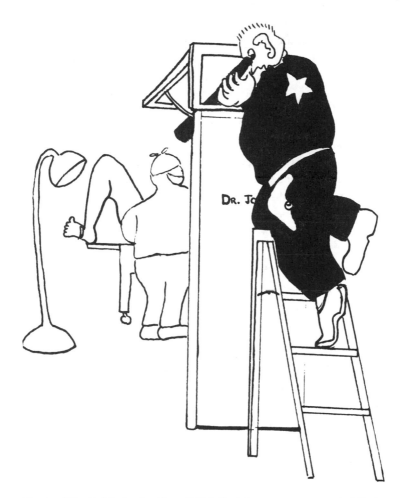

Plate 6. "The D.A.'s Peeping Toms." This feminist cartoon suggests that the investigation and prosecution of abortion provided voyeuristic sexual pleasures for men. It represented the perspective of women who had illegal abortions and feared being discovered and observed by police in precisely this way. Patricia T. Maginnis, *The Abortees' Songbook,* 1969, Positions Papers part 2 folder, WEF. Reproduced with permission of Patricia T. Maginnis and of the C. D. McCormick Library of Special Collections, Northwestern University Library.

By the mid-1960s, women across the country had organized themselves into a number of organizations calling for the equality and liberty of women.[32] Jane and the SHA were formed earlier and became part of this second wave of feminism. Older women active in the 1950s and early 1960s in trade unions and state women's commissions formed NOW, the National Organization for Women, in 1966. NOW emphasized ending sex discrimination in hiring, wages, education, and the media. NOW membership was primarily white, but the stereotypical depiction of NOW as exclusively professional and middle-class is incorrect.[33] At about the same time, poor women—African Americans prominent among them—organized themselves in the National Welfare Rights Organization.[34]

Simultaneously, a group of younger women involved in protest movements ranging from black voter-registration drives in the South to the anti–Vietnam War movement began to examine their dissatisfaction within these movements and to reconsider what the Left had long called "the woman question." In 1967 and 1968, small groups soon named "women's liberation" groups arose separately in a number of cities, including Chicago. These groups generally saw themselves as on the Left, preferred militant tactics to lobbying, and although they had national ties, meetings, and marches, worked locally in decentralized groups. They took up the "personal" issues of relationships between men and women, sexuality, and housework and reanalyzed them as collective and, thus, "political" problems.[35] White women dominated these groups, but women of color, sometimes calling themselves "third-world" feminists, also joined them, and black women's liberation groups arose within radical African American protest organizations as well.[36]

Questions about sexuality were particularly salient for young movement women experiencing the "sexual revolution." As young women shared their experiences in consciousness-raising groups, they identified the power relations embedded in sex. Too many men on the Left had made it plain at national meetings and in more intimate encounters that they regarded women as sex objects who were to serve their sexual pleasures as well as their coffee. Some of these insulting (and later infamous) remarks helped inspire the formation of women's liberation groups. The realization among women that they had been sexually exploited, ignored, or even assaulted, instead of pleasured, fueled discussions. In consciousness-raising groups, women learned together that female sexual pleasure was a political issue—the clitoral orgasm had been denied by medical experts and replaced by the intercourse-directed "vaginal orgasm" that conveniently guaranteed male orgasm. They discussed their fears of unwanted pregnancy and their need for effective, safe birth control and abortion. They analyzed heterosexuality itself as a social construction and reconsidered their attractions to women. Lesbians and gay men "came out" and declared their sexuality with pride. All of these issues added up to a recognition of the contradictions within the new sexual "revolution," but not a retreat from the hope of sexual freedom. These feminists did not want to eliminate sexual freedom in order to avoid having to cope with its difficulties, as advocated by the New Right in the 1970s and 1980s. Their demands pointed to feminist desire to enjoy their sexuality and to make their sexual relations with men or women better.[37]

Abortion was part of this radical feminist analysis of sexual freedom because it had real, material importance in women's lives and because it had symbolic significance. Women had used abortion for generations, but feminists articulated a new analysis of legal, available abortion as fundamental to female freedom. The prohibition of abortion, they argued, forced women to bear children; the state's enforcement of motherhood exemplified the oppression of women. Even though abortion initially divided some groups, feminists across the political spectrum came to support the decriminalization of abortion,[38] just as the diverse organizations which made up the nineteenth-century woman's movement had agreed on voluntary motherhood. The new feminist argument for abortion extended the analyses of earlier feminists. Nineteenth-century feminists rejected involuntary motherhood and agreed on the importance of women's right to refuse the sexual advances of their husbands. Emma Goldman and Sanger went a step further in their analysis of the importance of contraception: without the ability to avoid pregnancy, women could not enjoy (heterosexual) sex or control their own lives.[39] Yet no contraceptive, not even "the pill" introduced in 1960, was 100 percent effective. Furthermore, birth control was hard to get, especially for the unmarried, and some men refused to use it. When women faced unwanted pregnancies, hundreds of thousands of them, married and unmarried, both in the movement and in the mainstream, searched for abortions. Women who never had an abortion needed it as a backup. Abortion was actually used, potentially needed, and representative of women's sexual and reproductive freedom. Each of these meanings underpinned feminist support for legal and accessible abortion.

Feminists not only redefined abortion, they created new tactics. Most important for changing the course of the debate and politics, feminists designated women as the experts on abortion. They rejected the assumption that (almost exclusively) male physicians, religious leaders, philosophers, or politicians had the expertise, authority, or right to decide when an abortion could be performed. At speak-outs, women stood up and declared that they had had illegal abortions. The speak-out was an important political tactic, for it took abortion out of the realm of private secrets and made it an issue that women could talk about in public.[40] This was not the first time that American women discussed abortion—for they had long talked about it at home, at work, and in the offices of doctors, nurses, and midwives—but it was the first time that they admitted their own abortions in political arenas. In openly discussing abortions, women erased the shame and secrecy surrounding abortion. The speak-outs made clear that abortion was not a personal problem, but a problem for all women arising from the double standard. As women shared their stories, they created new knowledge and educated politicians, the medical profession, the judiciary, and the general public about why women needed abortions and the problems of abortion, both illegal and legal.

The emphasis on planning that the birth control movement adopted in the 1940s would haunt the movement to decriminalize abortion. The movement's new name, "Planned Parenthood," implied that *planned* children were better and *unplanned* children undesirable. Exercising such control, however, was a middle-class privilege and virtue.[41] Many, particularly in the working class, did not "plan" their families and did not necessarily regard an unplanned pregnancy or an unplanned child as unwanted. The emphasis on family planning had the unfortunate result of suggesting that everyone should carry out their sex lives and create families in a rational manner and that "accidental" childbearing was reprehensible. This induced guilt (and anger) among middle-class women, who do not always act with foresight but believe that they should, and among low-income women and men, who sense disapproval of their families. Outsiders blamed the children of the poor for their poverty, rather than placing the blame on the economic system or the racism and sexism that denied them well-paid jobs.

Population controllers entered the abortion discourse with a different analysis: they favored legal abortion to combat "overpopulation," a problem they located in low-income and "nonwhite" neighborhoods and third-world countries. As Linda Gordon has pointed out, population control and feminism had different roots. The former was rooted in imperialism and institutionalized in U.S. foreign policy in the 1950s and 1960s to control third-world populations and avert insurrections. The latter was rooted in a desire to combat the oppression of women. Unfortunately, however, the main birth control organization, Planned Parenthood Federation of America, suppressed its feminist origins and joined in the promotion of worldwide population control measures, thus powerfully linking birth control and population control. Population control programs did not emphasize women's rights to make decisions about childbearing, but imposed government-sponsored programs to cut the fertility of the poor. Many new environmentalists picked up the theory of the impending population explosion and embraced population control in the name of protecting the earth from destruction.[42] Demonstrating the popularity of these ideas, in 1970 Senator Robert Packwood (R. Ore.) introduced a bill into Congress to liberalize the abortion laws as a solution to the perceived "population explosion."[43]

At the same time, Planned Parenthood worked to provide birth control services to low-income, urban women of color. Though many low-income black women desperately wanted birth control, the provision of these services often made them feel pressured to accept contraceptives. In Pittsburgh, for example, Planned Parenthood staff advertised their clinic by going door-to-door in poor neighborhoods with the result, said a physician for the NAACP, that many African Americans "feel that they'd better obey 'official suggestions' to visit a birth control clinic or risk losing their monthly welfare check."[44]

Some state officials pushed policies to sterilize poor women. In Illinois, one legislator proposed that welfare recipients be forced "off public aid or undergo sterilization operations if they have more than two children." This legislator did not question the justice of using political power to regulate both the reproduction and the sexual behavior of low-income women. His bill intended to reduce the numbers of the low-income population (and, specifically, if not explicitly, reduce the black population with which welfare had become identified). The bill was defeated, but a message about the official desire to sterilize African Americans had been sent nonetheless.[45]

Urban black nationalists recognized the underlying racism of population controllers and the fears of poor African Americans and renamed birth control, and then abortion, "black genocide." The fear of birth control as a method of racist oppression designed to eliminate this minority population and its political power were mainly located among poor, urban African Americans.[46] Educated African Americans and their organizations had promoted birth control since the early twentieth century, but they too criticized the racism underlying many birth control programs.[47]

Some black nationalists called for the production of more babies, not fewer. One spokesman of an "ultra-militant" New York group (as *Ebony* described him) remarked, "See that sister there? She's having another baby for me. I need an army, and this is how we're going to get it."[48] In the war for black political power, African American women were assigned a role based on their biological capacity and traditional female gender expectations: their job was to reproduce and nurture future soldiers. Black health-care workers pointed out that men feared birth control, not only because of their stated concern about genocide, but because they feared that contraceptives could free female sexuality.[49] Black nationalist men had sexism in common with white men on the Left and the Right.[50]

Feminists of color struggled over these issues with the men of their own racial groups and with white feminists; on the one hand, they fought sexism, on the other, racism. African American and Latina feminists brought the issues of genocide and sterilization to the forefront of feminist attention and rejected the notion that the revolutionary role for black women was to have more babies. "Breeding revolutionaries," Florynce Kennedy commented, "is not too far removed from a cultural past where Black women were encouraged to be breeding machines for their slave masters." The nationalist indictment of contraceptives and abortion as "genocidal" was, Congresswoman Shirley Chisolm believed, "male rhetoric, for male ears." She pointed to the high level of injury and death resulting from illegal abortion among black and Puerto Rican women and advocated legal and accessible birth control and abortion for all.[51]

Third-world feminists made opposition to forced sterilization part of the campaign to repeal the abortion laws. African American women in the Women's National Abortion Action Coalition consistently raised the issue of sterilization abuse. Radical segments of the feminist movement, including the Chicago Women's Liberation Union, heard the charges of black genocide and adopted positions against sterilization abuse. The reproductive rights wing of the abortion movement supported the right to bear children as well as the right to avoid childbearing and demanded all of the services that would make such freedom in childbearing possible.[52] Antiracist and oppositional voices pushed the abortion rights movement to recognize that abortion was not the only issue, but never controlled the movement.

A multitude of groups formed on every level—at the national, regional, state, city, professional, church, and campus levels—to decriminalize abortion. Permanent organizations formed that still exist, and many more ephemeral organizations popped up everywhere. The National Association for the Repeal of Abortion Laws (NARAL) was formed in 1969, and Dr. Ed Keemer became its Midwest vice president.[53] Clergymen from numerous denominations created a national clergy abortion referral service.[54] Women ran an "underground railroad," driving women from southern states to Chicago to get abortions.[55] Students at a Catholic women's college in Chicago formed a chapter of the Women's National Abortion Action Coalition (WONAAC); though the administration opposed them, "several nuns privately expressed their support."[56] In 1970, women's, medical, trade union, socialist, and population control organizations joined under one banner for "Total Repeal of Illinois Abortion Laws."[57]

By 1968, the various branches of the abortion rights movement had adopted the feminist position that the abortion laws had to be repealed. This marked a significant shift in the thinking of the professional movement. Public debate, the new women's movement, and political events pushed doctors, with much of the rest of American society, in directions they previously would not have imagined possible. California passed the ALI model law in 1967, but a year later it was clear that reform was a failure and repeal necessary. The law had made the therapeutic abortion system inflexible. Instead of freeing doctors to perform more therapeutic abortions, reform laws further enchained doctors to the committee system. Where before the legal vagueness enabled different hospital committees to allow therapeutic abortions for a variety of reasons, now the law delineated the acceptable indications and left no room for interpretation. Furthermore, California state officials had initiated a campaign to punish physicians for participating in abortion. Secret investigations resulted in charges against nine physicians. A raid on an abortion clinic revealed that a California doctor referred patients there; Dr. Leon Belous, a public supporter of liberalizing the abortion laws, was prosecuted and convicted in 1968 for referring a woman to that abortion clinic.[58]

Dr. Alan Guttmacher may serve as an example of the transformation of liberal professional thinking. Guttmacher's biography mirrored the political history of abortion. He had been uncomfortable with medical teaching on abortion since the late 1920s, but senior obstetricians silenced his criticism in the 1930s. In the early 1950s, he instituted therapeutic abortion committees, hoping to eliminate the arbitrariness of abortion decisions, only to become frustrated later with the mechanisms he helped create. Guttmacher participated in the professional reform movement at its start and was an outspoken public advocate for legal change since the late 1950s, but until 1968, he opposed repeal as too radical. Both his willingness to challenge abortion policy and his relative slowness to accept the idea of repealing the abortion laws were shaped by his profession. He urged reform because, as an obstetrician, he had seen the horrendous results of the criminal abortion laws, yet his professional assumptions made him prefer limited reform. He was a radical within a conservative specialty. The movement and the results of reform changed his mind. After being appointed by New York Governor Nelson Rockefeller to a state commission on abortion, Guttmacher stopped arguing for halfway reform measures. "I changed my mind and I am in your camp," he told one feminist correspondent who questioned his position; "abortion on demand is the only civilized way to handle the problem."[59]

The medical profession organized to criminalize abortion in the mid–nineteenth century and to oppose those very laws a century later. The nineteenth-century regular medical profession had derived authority by proclaiming its moral superiority and by positioning itself as paternalistic arbiters over female reproductive behavior. A hundred years later, the profession enjoyed enormous social authority.[60] Yet as the abortion laws restricted and monitored medical practice, they undermined medical autonomy. By the late 1960s, esteemed members of the profession no longer needed to attack abortion to prove their purity and could challenge laws promoted by their forebears without having their reputations questioned.

The legalization of abortion gained great medical and popular support in these years. When a Chicago television station made a medical debate on Illinois abortion law reform into a referendum in 1967, the "votes" showed high support for reform.[61] An early survey of New York obstetricians and gynecologists found that an overwhelming majority, 85 percent, supported the ALI model law, and in 1968 the American College of Obstetricians and Gynecologists approved the liberalization of abortion laws along reform lines.[62] Psychiatrists, black medical societies, and the American Public Health Association went further: they supported repeal.[63] The American Public Health Association advocated public funding of abortion to ensure its availability to all women.[64] 1969 polls found that the majority of physicians supported repeal of the criminal abortion laws and the majority of Americans, including most Catholics, believed abortion should be a private decision.[65]

Constitutional Challenges

Young attorneys dedicated to civil liberties and women's rights formulated new legal strategies in their own effort to repeal the criminal abortion laws. Legal teams in many states devised ways to challenge the abortion laws in the courts alongside legislative and protest efforts. Two young women lawyers, Sybille Fritzsche and Susan Grossman, challenged the constitutionality of the Illinois criminal abortion law. The attorneys used a tool adopted by legal activists to make claims for large groups, the class action suit. They formulated an innovative legal strategy that brought together medical professional interests and feminist interests into one class action suit. In linking medical and feminist perspectives, the attorneys wove the disparate and often hostile strands of the movement together and, simultaneously, represented the interests of the two groups who had negotiated the problem of abortion for a century. They constructed a case to speak to the highest levels of the judiciary, which told of the discriminatory nature of the abortion system, the restrictiveness of therapeutic abortion policy, and the dangers women faced as a consequence of the criminal abortion laws. The Illinois case is an example of the crucial strategy, crafted simultaneously by a number of lawyers, that ultimately shaped the U.S. Supreme Court decisions on abortion.[66] The Illinois lawyers shared their briefs with attorneys challenging the abortion laws in other states.[67] The legal arguments formulated by left-leaning feminist lawyers proved to be powerful.

Fritzsche and Grossman were part of "a new generation of lawyers" dedicated to using the law to bring about fundamental social change. The Illinois case, *Doe v. Scott*, began in 1969 when Susan Grossman, a new attorney at the Chicago Legal Aid Bureau, met Sybille Fritzsche at the Chicago office of the American Civil Liberties Union (ACLU). Grossman had gone to Harvard Law School to bring about "social change." At a 1969 summer training session for attorneys beginning to work in legal services to the poor, she was exposed "to the women's liberation movement for the first time close up." Although Grossman considered herself a feminist, these more radical women "intrigued" her and made her think about the problems of poor women. When she learned that September that the California Supreme Court had found the state's nineteenth-century abortion statute unconstitutional in *People v. Belous* (1969), she was spurred to action.[68] One year out of law school, Fritzsche had joined the Chicago ACLU staff, where she worked on free speech and civil rights cases. Although she was "appalled" at the "lack of ambition" among women when she came to the U.S. from Germany in the late 1950s and was one of only three women in a class of 150 at the University of Chicago Law School, she did not identify with the women's liberation movement. Fritzsche's politics were rooted in the European Left.[69] *Belous* prompted lawyers in other states to prepare suits, and several physicians, including Keemer, sought arrest in order to test the constitutionality of abortion laws.[70]

The Illinois challenge grew out of the lawyers' commitment to the poor and to improving the lives of the most oppressed in society. The link between poor people's movements and feminism, evident in this case, has been forgotten. Part of the momentum of the abortion movement lay in the connection that many activists saw between the interests of feminists and the poor. Susan Grossman was a Legal Aid attorney when she proposed challenging the abortion law. "This was *very* radical in 1969," she remarked twenty-five years later; the idea made her supervisor "nervous." The United Charities funded Legal Aid and their supporters included conservatives. Grossman was determined, however, and explained to the board of Chicago Legal Aid why Legal Aid should be involved in this suit. "My feeling from the very beginning," she later explained, "was that the women who were most hurt by the statute were poor women. . . . I felt I was representing the poor women of Illinois." The board approved her participation in the case, but did not allow her to be identified in court documents as a Legal Aid attorney.[71] As hospital and mortality data showed, poor women were hurt the most by the illegality of abortion. Though feminism and the pro-choice movement have been represented as white and middle-class movements, sections of those movements recognized and fought for the interests of low-income women and women of color.[72]

The two colleagues placed class inequality at the forefront of their suit. The case began with two women who wanted legal abortions but were unable to obtain them because physicians feared prosecution under the Illinois law. It highlighted the inequity in access to abortion: one woman was wealthy and eventually went to Great Britain for an abortion; the other was poor and was forced to bear the unwanted baby. The Illinois abortion statute, Fritzsche and Grossman argued, "systematically discriminates against poor women, depriving them of equal access to the treatment available to women of means solely because they are poor." Because women of means could consult with physicians, they explained, they were more likely to gain sympathy and obtain "hospital abortions." If necessary, wealthy women could afford to travel out of state to obtain abortions. The existing laws resulted in "different treatment for different women" and thus violated the equal protection provisions in the constitution.[73]

The lawyers argued for the feminist principle that women had a right to make decisions about whether to carry or terminate their pregnancies. In their brief they forthrightly stated a truth about the meaning of the criminalization of abortion: the law "compel[s] her, against her will, to continue a pregnancy." Forcing a woman to bear an unwanted child forced her to risk her own health and the "quality of her own and her family's life." The state's criminal abortion law, they argued, "represents an impermissible intrusion into her right to her personal integrity and is a deprivation of her personal liberty." Citing the women's suffrage amendment and the Civil Rights Act, they asserted that a woman is "not to be subject to the determination of an individual male such as father or husband," yet the existing law subjected her to male lawmaking and prohibited women from making decisions for themselves.[74] On abortion, Susan Grossman declared during oral arguments, "only the woman must decide."[75]

Finally, the lawyers referred to the right to privacy of women and married couples. In *Griswold v. Connecticut* (1965) the U.S. Supreme Court had concluded that "a zone of privacy" existed in the marital relationship, into which the state could not intrude. The Court found that Connecticut's laws that made birth control illegal violated the constitutional right to privacy. Attorneys seeking to overturn the nation's criminal abortion laws argued that just as the decision to avoid conception through the use of birth control was protected under the right to privacy, so too was the decision to keep or abort a pregnancy. "The mere fact of fertilization," the Illinois team argued, "should not in itself abolish or limit the constitutional right of a woman to decide whether to have a child."[76] *Griswold* was a key case, but the Illinois brief pointed to a tradition of decisions over the previous fifty years that recognized a constitutional right to privacy in family matters ranging from the right to bear children, to send children to private schools, and to interracial marriage.[77]

The Illinois attorneys did not make privacy their primary argument, despite some pressure to do so. Members of the ACLU board wanted Fritzsche to argue the case exclusively on privacy grounds, the preferred argument of feminists. Jody Parsons, one of Jane's founders, advocated this position. (Her presence on the ACLU board illustrates the efforts of different groups to work together.) Fritzsche and Grossman, however, planned to present an array of arguments for overturning the criminal abortion laws as unconstitutional. Having clerked for a federal judge, Grossman understood their conservatism and wanted to provide alternatives that would allow them to select more conservative arguments to reach the same result. As she later explained, "We decided to focus on vagueness . . . and to downpedal the privacy argument."[78]

The innovative aspect of the case created by Grossman and Fritzsche was its attention to the complaints and interests of the medical profession along with those of women of all classes. They argued that the vagueness of the criminal abortion law made it impossible for physicians to practice medicine and serve their patients. They further argued that the laws violated the physician's right to privacy and freedom of speech in the relationship between physician and patient.[79] The legal team brought together Chicago's most prominent academic specialists in obstetrics and gynecology to challenge the Illinois abortion law. The four physician plaintiffs were nationally recognized leaders in their specialty, heads of the obstetrics and gynecology departments at four prestigious Chicago hospitals, and professors and heads of the departments of obstetrics and gynecology at four of Chicago's major medical schools: Northwestern University, Chicago Medical School, University of Illinois Medical Center, and the University of Chicago School of Medicine. Fritzsche and Grossman insisted that, in contrast to the anonymity of the female plaintiffs, the doctors use their names. Doctors Frederick P. Zuspan, David N. Danforth, Charles Fields, and Ralph M. Wynn all signed on to the case.[80] The legal challenge received strong medical support. Over 120 medical school deans and faculty, representing physicians in thirty-four states and Washington, D.C., joined in filing a motion in support of the suit.[81] A group of pediatricians submitted an amicus brief.[82]

Fritzsche and Grossman identified physicians as a class that had an interest in decriminalizing abortion. In recruiting the physicians, the civil liberties lawyers drew upon a growing consensus within the medical profession, but they were not approached by doctors nor were they particularly aware of medical efforts to reform the abortion laws. Fritzsche and Grossman's ideas grew out of an incredible ferment and demand for change that makes the linking of the interests of the medical profession and women in legal reform seem inevitable, but abortion activism was not coordinated. The legal team had thought "very carefully" about who they wanted as representatives of the class and sought out the most prestigious doctors to say, "I should have the freedom to order and do one if I feel it is medically necessary."[83]

The physician plaintiffs expressed the dilemmas and the distress created for doctors by the state abortion laws. Their affidavits and the attorneys' brief spoke to the two problems that had fueled the movement to legalize abortion: the restrictions on physicians' practice of therapeutic abortions, and the deaths and injuries of women that resulted from illegal abortions. Dr. Danforth described cases for which the law did not allow abortions. "Any physician confronted with cases such as these," Danforth confessed, "*reacts with despair and frustration* when he cannot give the woman involved the treatment which in his judgment is medically indicated."[84] Dr. Fields pointed to forty years of experience to explain his support for legalizing abortion. As a resident at Cook County Hospital, he had seen "a large number of septic abortions." His experiences and his patients had "convinced" him "that the woman is usually the best judge of whether a pregnancy should or should not be terminated."[85]

The concerns of these leading physicians spoke to the judges, who were the elite within their own profession. The attached vitas and publication lists surely impressed the judges and impressed upon them the unfairness of forcing reputable professional men to worry about whether their medical decisions conformed with the law. The suit constructed by Fritzsche and Grossman paralleled the drafting of the ALI abortion reform law over ten years earlier. The legal elite then had heard and responded to the complaints of the medical elite and attempted to remove the law from what should have been medical decisions. The plaintiffs in this case implicitly called upon interprofessional respect to raise doubts about the existing law in the minds of the judges.

In January 1971, the federal court held the Illinois abortion law unconstitutional and highlighted both the difficulties faced by reputable doctors and the rights of women. "The treating physician who believes an abortion is medically or psychiatrically indicated," the chief circuit judge explained in the majority opinion, "finds himself threatened with becoming a felon as well as with the possibility of losing his right to practice his profession if he errs in the legal interpretation of a penal statute." The statutory language was unclear and left not only doctors but the courts wondering what was allowed and what not. For these reasons the "void-for-vagueness doctrine" applied.[86] Yet the main reason given for overturning the abortion law was the violation of "fundamental" women's rights. The court found the Illinois statute "an intrusion on constitutionally protected areas. . . . These protected areas are women's rights to life, to control over their own bodies, and to freedom and privacy in matters relating to sex and procreation." Finally, this decision introduced the idea of the trimester system, declaring that "during the early stages of pregnancy—at least during the first trimester—the state may not prohibit, restrict, or otherwise limit

women's access to abortion." The court avoided addressing the problem of class discrimination in access to safe abortions, however.[87]

The lawyers had won—abortion was legal in Illinois. The majority
opinion held that the state could not ban early abortions performed by
licensed physicians in licensed medical centers. Immediately after the
decision, Cook County Hospital received hundreds of phone calls from
poor women seeking abortions. A physician on the ACLU board, Dr.
Marvin Rosner, performed an abortion to establish the right to do so.
Cook County State's Attorney Edward V. Hanrahan and Dr. Bart Heffernan appealed the decision to the U.S. Supreme Court and won an
injunction that stayed the lower court's ruling until the Supreme Court
ruled on the question.[88]

The new era in Illinois lasted just ten days. Abortion was again illegal. Despite the initial victory, the situation was as bad as it had ever
been, and an official backlash against legalization began. As the appeals
on the Illinois case and several others waited to be heard by the U.S.
Supreme Court, women needing abortions found it extremely difficult
to obtain safe abortions. Therapeutic abortions were nearly impossible
to obtain. At Michael Reese Hospital in Chicago a social worker acted
as a gatekeeper and made the first diagnosis: could this woman's condition be considered grounds for a therapeutic abortion? In eighteen
months she interviewed 125 women and rejected two-thirds. In 1970,
eight Chicago hospitals had provided over five hundred therapeutic
abortions. This was a minuscule number compared to the three thousand abortions performed annually by Jane alone and the nearly five
thousand women with abortion complications cared for at Cook
County Hospital. Observers estimated that there were fifty thousand illegal abortions per year in the county and over a million nationwide.[89]

Chicago hospitals had inconsistent policies regarding therapeutic
abortion, as a 1971 study showed. Abortion committees at nine hospitals reviewed ten hypothetical requests for abortions and reached different conclusions in most cases. In hypothetical case number three, the
patient had had rubella, a history that raised the issue of abortions performed because of fetal defects. Six of the Chicago hospitals would allow the abortion in the rubella case and two would not. In case number
four, a minister's daughter had been raped. This case evoked sympathy
for rape and, by identifying the woman as a minister's daughter, assured the committees of the victim's sexual "innocence." Six hospitals
would permit an abortion. In case number eleven, Mrs. A. was described as a woman with five children, tuberculosis, and financial diffi-

culties. She typified the poor woman of the Depression, for whom a therapeutic abortion could be justified on a combination of social, economic, and medical grounds. Only one hospital would deny Mrs. A. a therapeutic abortion for socioeconomic reasons. The study confirmed that suicide attempts, backed up with recommendations by psychiatrists, were the best way to obtain therapeutic abortions in Chicago. All nine hospitals granted a therapeutic abortion for a woman who had attempted suicide "last night." "Different women," the researchers concluded, "are receiving different treatment at different hospitals for precisely the same types of problems," and they questioned the constitutionality of that pattern. The study confirmed the vagueness of the law charged by cocounsel Grossman and Fritzsche.[90]

A few women got legal abortions in Chicago hospitals; others traveled from Chicago to New York for legal abortions. In 1970, Hawaii, Alaska, and New York had decriminalized abortion instead of passing reform bills.[91] When New York legalized abortion, it was a boon for women all over the country. As one woman recalled, a New York abortion clinic treated patients who "had traveled from states such as Mississippi, Arkansas, Michigan and even farther. . . . They spent a lot of time, money and energy to travel to a different state, far away from their homes so that they could be assured of a *safe* abortion."[92] Over 65 percent of the women receiving abortions in New York were from out of state; in 1971 and 1972, thirteen thousand women came from Illinois.[93]

Some of these thousands had been sent to New York by abortion referral services in Chicago. The existence of such services, sponsored by religious and birth control organizations, indicates the depth of political resistance to the criminal abortion laws. In 1966, the Rev. Dr. E. Spencer Parsons, dean of the University of Chicago's Chapel, had started Chicago's Clergy Consultation Service on Problem Pregnancies. The Baptist minister's involvement in abortion grew out of his earlier work to legalize birth control in Massachusetts.[94] The Chicago service was part of a national ecumenical effort in opposition to the criminal abortion laws. Each woman met with a minister or rabbi who listened to her predicament and gave her an abortion referral; some found the counseling helpful and no doubt others thought it paternalistic. In 1970, the clergy service helped seventy-five hundred women get abortions outside of Illinois. After Planned Parenthood's referral service discovered it could help fewer than half of the callers, the two services joined as one.[95] In one month in 1971, the combined service referred almost 750 women to New York for legal abortions. Nearly equal numbers of the women were married and unmarried. Of the women referred, 70 percent were white, 23 percent black, 43 percent Catholic, and 20 percent low-income. Within months, however, the service could not meet demand because low-income women could not afford the cost of travel and clinics refused to lower their fees.[96]

The story of Doris B., a twenty-six-year-old black woman in Chicago, underlines the inherent limitations of legalization in one faraway state and of local efforts to provide abortions for low-income women who sought them. Even though the referral service and Jane tried to help all Chicago women who needed abortions, some low-income women never found either organization. The "tragic event" was, her friend later wrote, "well-etched in my memory." Doris B. had four children and depended on welfare to care for them. "It was a constant struggle to provide for these children," her friend recalled, "and she felt that another child was more than she could endure." Doris B. considered going to New York, but poverty "made that impossible. Doris chose the 'cheaper' illegal alternative in Chicago." She died from septicemia following her illegal abortion in 1972, and her children became orphans.[97] The uneven development of legalization contributed to Doris B.'s death. Legalization of abortion in a few states was an advance, but it still left most women in most states facing the dangers of illegal abortion. An underground feminist abortion service willing to help anyone, including those who could pay nothing, could not reach and serve everyone.

Meanwhile, the Cook County state's attorney was on a crusade of his own to signal physicians and others that he personally would not tolerate the practice of abortion in his city. The suppression of abortion had become newly politicized. "Physicians were very afraid. It was known," Fritzsche vividly recalled, "that Hanrahan was going to enforce this law and people were really afraid."[98] Chicago authorities investigated a rabbi working with the clergy consultation service as a suspect of "an abortion ring" and searched his university offices.[99] At the urging of then Illinois house majority leader Henry Hyde, Hanrahan called the clergy consultation service's founder before the grand jury, demanding that he name the abortionists he knew. Rev. Spencer Parsons refused to testify, claiming the right of clergy to confidentiality.[100] Official harassment did not stop the abortion referral service.

In January 1972, one year after the *Doe v. Scott* victory, the Illinois Supreme Court dealt the abortion rights movement a blow. As a counterattack to the abortion rights movement, Hanrahan had appealed a

Chicago therapeutic abortion case to the state supreme court. A juvenile court had allowed a suicidal teenage ward of the state to have an abortion on psychiatric grounds. For the first time, the court ruled on the medical indications for therapeutic abortion. In *People ex rel. Hanrahan v. White,* the court concluded that the law did not allow therapeutic abortion for suicidal intentions.[101] The *Hanrahan* case was a defeat for the abortion rights movement and threatened women's access to therapeutic abortions in Illinois. The state's attorney's vigorous pursuit of this unique case warned physicians and hospitals that prosecutors might challenge their therapeutic abortion practices.

Police stepped up their arrests of abortion activists at about the same time. Several months after the *Hanrahan* ruling, Chicago police raided Jane. Police took nearly fifty people to the police station for questioning, brought three women in the middle of being aborted to a hospital, and arrested seven Jane members. Local police had ignored Jane, but officers in another district raided them in response to a complaint. Jane activists had counted on their friendly relations with the police to protect them; given that police regularly harassed protesters, their trust seems politically naive.[102] Florida officials arrested and prosecuted Shirley Wheeler for having an abortion, a shocking move, and in 1971 she was convicted of manslaughter.[103] Ten days before a Michigan referendum on the state's abortion laws, Dr. Keemer, a visible proponent of repeal and a NARAL officer, was raided. He, his assistants, and a dozen patients were arrested and jailed for abortion.[104]

The raid on Jane advertised the organization to the public and simultaneously drove it further underground. Supporters on the Left began raising money to bail out and defend the Jane women and wore buttons declaring "Free the Abortion Seven." Like other illegal abortionists raided in the postwar period, Jane adopted clandestine measures to protect itself. The process, one member recalled, became "much more nerve-wracking" for the women seeking abortions. They eliminated the Front and instead, "We'd pick people up in public places, on street corners, and take them to the place where they were going to have the abortion and counsel them just before it." The group refrained from returning to blindfolds, a protection abolished when members began doing abortions.[105]

Unlike women and men caught in the abortion raids of the 1940s and 1950s, the Jane members had the support of a political movement. By then that movement had been transformed from a small, professional reform effort to a mass movement with organizations big and small across the country. Advocates of the legalization of abortion ranged from the elite to the newest members of the medical and legal professions, to a multiplicity of religious denominations, to the most militant of feminists and leftists. Activists had strong popular support for bringing the laws governing abortion into line with actual practice and with a popular morality that accepted women's rights to control their reproduction. That broad-based movement to decriminalize abortion brought about the 1973 U.S. Supreme Court decisions in *Roe v. Wade* and *Doe v. Bolton,* and as a result, the charges against Chicago's "Abortion Seven" were dropped and Keemer's earlier conviction erased.[106]

On January 22, 1973, the U.S. Supreme Court found the nation's century-old criminal abortion laws and the new reform laws unconstitutional because they violated the rights of women and the rights of physicians. The Supreme Court decisions in *Roe v. Wade* and *Doe v. Bolton*[107] put women and doctors together at the center of abortion, the two groups who had negotiated the terrain of legal and illegal abortion for generations and who had come to find the laws intolerable. The medical profession had played a key role in making reproductive policy since the nineteenth century; for the first time, the state recognized women's role and rights in reproductive policy. *Roe v. Wade* declared that the right of privacy included "a woman's decision whether or not to terminate her pregnancy." The majority opinion described abortion as a medical decision and recognized the right of physicians to practice medicine without undue interference. In the first trimester of pregnancy, "the attending physician, in consultation with his patient, is free to determine, without regulation by the State, that, in his medical judgment, the patient's pregnancy should be terminated."[108] The history of the relationship between medicine and women shaped the political movement, public policy, and Supreme Court decisions.

In a companion opinion, *Doe v. Bolton,* the Supreme Court declared the hospital therapeutic abortion committee system, devised in the 1940s and 1950s and institutionalized in reform laws, unconstitutional. Though often overlooked since, this decision was as important as *Roe.* The Court held in *Doe v. Bolton* that policies designed to restrict access to abortion, such as those in the Georgia reform statute, violated the rights of women to health care and of physicians to practice. In March 1973, the Illinois Supreme Court found the Illinois criminal abortion statute, originally passed in 1867, to be unconstitutional.[109]

The U.S. Supreme Court rejected, however, the crucial argument that the nation's abortion laws were discriminatory.[110] The constitutional challenges framed by activist attorneys had emphasized the importance of class, race, and gender in abortion.[111] The class inequities under the framework of legalized abortion arose not from the women's movement or the cases presented to the Court, but from the Court's unwillingness to address economic inequality.

The Court's decisions were less than what feminists had wanted, because they left abortion in the hands of physicians, because women's rights were "balanced" against the rights of the state and limited by a technologically determined "viability" of the fetus, and because the inequities of class were ignored. However, the acknowledgment of women's rights to make decisions about their own bodies and reproduction independently of men was a significant advance. Winning legal abortion was a victory—as important as winning suffrage or equal pay for equal work. *Roe v. Wade* and *Doe v. Bolton* ended an era of illegal abortion. These decisions, with all of their limitations, represented a transformation in the status of women in American society.

Epilogue:
Post-*Roe*, Post-*Casey*

The legalization of abortion brought immediate benefits to women. Open access to legal abortion replaced the world of illegal abortion. After *Roe v. Wade,* women in the United States could look in a phone book for a physician-abortionist. Abortion clinics made the procedure widely available.[1] State and federal programs extended coverage of abortion to low-income women. Legal, safe abortions became accessible to women across class and race, rather than the privilege of a few. In Chicago, two abortion clinics opened and Cook County Hospital and a handful of other hospitals began providing a small number of abortions. The publication of abortion providers and their office hours on the front page of a Chicago weekly illustrated the changed legal climate.[2] The legalization of abortion freed women from the fear of police raids and arrests and from wondering whether the "Dr." was in fact a skilled doctor or a "butcher." The abortion committee system was dismantled. Legal abortion was safe, safer than normal childbirth.[3]

Making abortion legal improved public health: overall maternal mortality dropped dramatically. In New York City, maternal mortality fell 45 percent the year after the state legalized abortion. "In 1971," city health officials reported, "New York City experienced its lowest maternal mortality rate on record." California and North Carolina reported similar improvement.[4] Septic abortion wards closed. As a public-health measure, the legalization of abortion represented an improvement in maternal mortality that ranks with the invention of antisepsis and antibiotics.[5] In countries where abortion remains illegal, abortion is a significant contributor to maternal morbidity and mortality.[6] The open availability of safe abortions in the U.S. benefited in particular low-income women and women of color, who had had the least access to skilled practitioners and were most likely to be injured or die as a result of illegal abortion. In New York City, over half the women who had abortions after legalization belonged to minority groups.[7]

The legalization of abortion strengthened patients' rights. The recognition of a fundamental right of women to make decisions about pregnancy reinforced the rights of patients to be protected against co-ercive medical treatment and to make decisions regarding their own medical care. Women's reproductive rights challenge male supremacy uniquely, but patients' rights and reproductive rights alike challenge medical authority. Both seek greater medical and legal acknowledgment of patients' decision making and autonomy. Yet this is not simply a battle between doctors and patients, because, as we have seen, the medical profession is not uniform in its thinking or practice. Indeed, this study has uncovered a long tradition of physicians listening to and learning from patients and treating health care as a partnership. A significant segment of the medical profession prefers a more egalitarian, rather than authoritarian, mode of physician-patient relations.

Contemporary disputes over living wills, the right to die, and the right to refuse treatments against medical advice, as well as abortion, all attest to continuing conflict among Americans about patients' rights, appropriate use of technology, and the proper way to live and die. The battles reveal sharp division over both how to respond to difficult issues in medical care and who should make these decisions. Our society is in the midst of a deep philosophical and political struggle over whether there are absolute answers to medical dilemmas that shall be applied to all citizens—whether those answers come from medical, state, or religious authorities—or whether a democratic society must accommodate a multiplicity of moral viewpoints and allow individuals to make difficult (and differing) decisions for themselves.

Finally, the legalization of abortion strengthened civil liberties. As the state pressed the medical profession into investigating illegal abortion, due process rights guaranteed citizens under the Constitution were eroded. When doctors and hospital staff questioned patients at the behest of the state, physicians became police, patients became suspects. Medical surveillance of patients—whether for the progress of pregnancy, the use of illegal drugs, or the presence of stigmatized infectious diseases such as HIV—compromises constitutional protections against unreasonable search and seizure by the state as well as the rights to bodily integrity and privacy. Furthermore, the acceptance of this policing function by medical personnel diminishes respect for patients, damages patient confidentiality, and threatens the health of the patients they serve. As public-health professionals understand, making it dangerous to present a particular malady to health-care workers results in people delaying or avoiding care and risking their lives in order to avoid punitive measures. Using health-care professionals to serve as the state's investigators is dangerous public policy.

A backlash in reaction to the expansion of women's reproductive rights and sexual freedom, nurtured by the Catholic Church, Protestant fundamentalists, and the New Right, developed into an intense minority movement in the 1980s and 1990s. The denial of public funding for abortions for low-income women and federal employees was the first defeat of the coalition that won *Roe v. Wade*. Illinois Congressman Henry Hyde sponsored the restrictive "Hyde Amendment" passed by Congress in 1977. Abortion opponents have succeeded in creating a new discourse, given the fetus new meaning as a human "life," and labeled abortion "murder." Furthermore, the antiabortion movement has projected a fetal "voice" to compete with and discredit the voices of real, live women, a group that only recently spoke of its experiences in public, political arenas. The fetus has been used to shift the debate away from women and their narratives about the crimes of illegal abortion.[8] Silencing the political voice of women, however, is only one aspect of a far-reaching project. The antiabortion discourse has overshadowed interdenominational religious opinion that supports legal abortion,[9] and the antiabortion movement has organized to prevent the practice of legal abortion. The picketing of clinics and the homes of abortion providers and patients has become routine; a climate of hatred has fostered bombings of clinics and assassinations of physicians and clinic personnel.[10] The related assault on lesbians and gays harms the feminist struggle for female sexual independence. The New Right has pushed forward a conservative political agenda hostile to feminism, sexual freedom, freedom of speech and religion, and civil rights.[11]

The women whose reproductive rights are most abridged and vulnerable to attack are teenagers and low-income women. The New Right expresses particular hostility toward sexually active teenage girls, whom they perceive as beyond parental, specifically paternal, control.[12] This is a change; the plight of pregnant single women garnered the greatest sympathy at the turn of the century and evoked sympathy among many reformers in the 1960s. Single women were then perceived as victims; today's antiabortion movement blames them for being sexual actors. Conservative attacks on "welfare"[13] and abortion are related, for both seek to control women and their reproduction. The efforts to dismantle welfare and to require that minors notify their parents or obtain their consent for abortion are both intended to hurt young women and to punish them for their sexual behavior. In calling for an end to Aid to Families with Dependent Children (AFDC), or for mandatory sterilization or contraception for poor women, conservatives attempt to stop one group of women (stereotyped as poor black women) from bearing children. In restricting abortion use, they attempt to force a different group (middle-class white women) to bear children. The racial stereotypes obscure the fact that both black and white women use legal abortion and social assistance; few are teenagers. Conservatives hope that making pregnancy a punishment for sex will make young (white) women either forego sex or enter marriage. Sexism, racism, and elitism are embedded in the twin assault on welfare and abortion.

Neither welfare benefits nor access to legal abortion guarantees reproductive rights. Real reproductive freedom for women requires that all women, regardless of race, class, age, sexual orientation, or marital status, be able to avoid unwanted childbearing through the use of contraception and abortion *and* be able to bear children without being stigmatized, impoverished, or compelled to give up their education, employment, or children.

If *Roe v. Wade* were to be overturned and abortion made illegal again, the history of when abortion was a crime suggests that the results would be dire indeed. The practice of abortion might dip in response to pressure, but it would not stop. Women would once again besiege physicians and other health-care workers with requests for abortion. Enforcement of new criminal statutes would no doubt be patterned on the old system. State authorities would again expect medical personnel to assist the state by reporting, interrogating, and physically examining women suspected of having abortions; police would revive the practice of raiding abortionists' offices and capturing women. Any woman who miscarried would be treated as a potential criminal and subjected to medical examination, which could include internal "viewing" via ultrasound. Medical mistreatment of women would become routinized as the health-care system became further enmeshed in the state's law enforcement apparatus. If abortion is made illegal, some women will die; many more will be injured. The old abortion wards will have to be reopened, a public-health disaster recreated. Making abortion hard to obtain will not return the United States to an imagined time of virginal brides and stable families; it will return us to the time of crowded septic abortion wards, avoidable deaths, and the routinization of punitive treatment of women by state authorities and their surrogates.

However, the past will not be duplicated in every detail if abortion is again made illegal, for the historical circumstances differ. In the last twenty-five years, abortion has been politicized in new ways. We can anticipate the "private" enforcement of the laws by the antiabortion troops that now harass abortion providers and women who seek abortion.[14] Women could be routinely prosecuted and imprisoned for having abortions, which they were not during the era of illegal abortion.[15]

It is not impossible to imagine women in the United States being subjected to constant state surveillance of their reproductive systems similar to that recently experienced in Romania.[16] The monitoring of female menstrual cycles, investigation of miscarriages, and the transformation of prenatal care from checkups to checks that all pregnancies are progressing to term are conceivable in the United States. With the rise of an antiabortion movement that proclaims the primacy of the fetus, prenatal care and medical thinking have already moved in the direction of putting the fetus ahead of the pregnant woman. Too often pregnant women are perceived as vessels for ensuring the best outcome of a future child. The obsessive focus on the behavior of pregnant women allows Americans to overlook the social and economic roots of this country's high infant mortality rates as well as the general population's difficulty in improving its eating habits or eliminating smoking and alcohol and drug abuse. Some women have been charged with "child abuse" of a fetus in utero; others have been surgically delivered by cesarean section against their will. Predictably, it is mostly low-income women, minority women, or women who hold religious views different from those of their doctors who have been charged or forced to undergo such surgery.[17]

Discounting the rights of pregnant women weakens everyone's rights as patients. If a pregnant woman cannot reject a cesarean section—whether for religious, political, or personal reasons—then any woman can be forced to submit to procedures deemed necessary for the fetus; any patient can be forced to comply with treatments deemed essential by medical personnel. This society rejects the sacrifice of one person in order to save another considered more important; an organ may be donated voluntarily, for example, but donations may not be obtained through coercion. Reproductive rights are based on the same principle: women cannot be required to sacrifice their own health and lives in order to produce babies.

It seems unlikely that the U.S. Supreme Court will overturn *Roe* and *Doe* outright, but *Roe v. Wade* may be so thoroughly gutted by judicial and legislative action that it will be meaningless. In *Webster v. Reproductive Health Services* (1989) and *Planned Parenthood v. Casey* (1992) the justices "preserved" *Roe* on thin grounds.[18] Feminists should look carefully and not be fooled into thinking that abortion is still legal if it isn't. If legal abortion is so restricted that it is available only to rich women or to women whose lives are endangered by pregnancy or to women pregnant as a result of rape,[19] then abortion should be declared, in truth, illegal. Most women who have abortions now, as during the era of illegal abortion, do not fit these categories. Defending abortion on these grounds narrows the definition of reproductive rights and does an injustice to the majority of women. Even when abortion was illegal, there were always some legal, therapeutic abortions, and at certain moments, therapeutic indications were broadly defined. If legal abortion becomes available in only a few states or cities or only to wealthy women, whether as a result of law or successful anti-abortion harassment campaigns, then the situation will match the pre-*Roe* era of illegal abortion.

As a result of the attack on legal abortion and the deference of elected officials and health-care providers to the minority leading the attack, the present increasingly resembles the pre-*Roe* period. One of the features of illegal abortion at its most restrictive was the inequity in access to safe abortions along racial and class lines. Although contraception and abortion are essential components of women's health care—and have demonstrably improved maternal mortality and morbidity in the United States—coverage of these necessary services is not uniform. Many private health insurance plans do not cover the abortions women need, though they cover sterilization procedures and delivery services.[20] Federally funded health care for government employees and for low-income people is perennially politicized; at the most it covers abortions only when pregnancy threatens the life of the "mother"[21] or when pregnancy results from rape or incest. A handful of states cover abortion services for low-income women, though much of this coverage is restrictive.[22] Place of residence is an increasingly crucial determinant of abortion availability. Today about one third of

American women cannot locate an abortion provider in their own county. In over 80 percent of American counties—and virtually all rural counties—no one is providing (legal) abortions. Some states have only one provider.[23] Having to travel long distances makes abortion impossible for some women, expensive and arduous for others.

A small group of doctors has shouldered the responsibility of providing abortions and, though their work has shielded others from persistent requests, they have received little public support from their profession. An appallingly small number of physicians are being trained in abortion; in 1991 to 1992, only 12 percent of the programs for residents in obstetrics and gynecology routinely taught first trimester abortions.[24] As medical educators fail to teach new doctors this basic procedure, the profession implicitly teaches other lessons: young doctors learn not only that abortion, though legal, is less than honorable, but that they need not listen to the expressed needs of women in particular or patients in general.

Hospitals have not re-formed therapeutic abortion committees, but state legislatures, with the sanction of the Supreme Court, have erected new barriers to abortion, including waiting periods, mandatory "counseling" invented to deter women from abortion, and parental notification or permission requirements. In *Casey* the Court found only the requirement that husbands be notified of abortions to be an "undue burden" to women seeking to exercise their right to abortion. *Doe v. Bolton*, which found measures designed to prevent women and their doctors from carrying out a decision to abort to be unconstitutional, has been quietly overturned. Furthermore, *Webster* and *Casey* eliminate the trimester system outlined in *Roe* (prohibiting state interference in the first trimester of pregnancy and limiting regulation in the second). In these recent cases, the Court has given greater prominence to "potential life" throughout pregnancy.[25] Most discouraging, illegal abortionists are in business again; women are dying again because of illegal abortions. They tend to be low-income women, women of color, or minors trying to avoid parental notification requirements.[26] Perhaps we have not yet reverted to the pre-*Roe* years, but we are close.

However, as forceful as the backlash against legal abortion is, it has not succeeded in erasing the advances in reproductive freedom. Indeed, the strength of the reaction may serve as a rough measure of both the radical implications of legal abortion and the strength of feminism.[27] In contrast to the image achieved by the opponents of abortion, the majority of Americans support legal abortion. Furthermore, that support has gotten stronger over time, and the proportion of Americans who believe abortion should be illegal in all circumstances has fallen to less than 15 percent.[28] There are positive signs of growing activism and renewed alliances at both the local and national levels in support of abortion and reproductive rights. Physicians and health-care organizations have begun providing abortions in defiance of the New Right; physician assistants in Montana and Vermont are already filling the gap in abortion providers, and some nurse-practitioners and nurse-midwives have expressed willingness to do the same.[29] The Accreditation Council for Graduate Medical Education is trying to rectify the de-skilling that has occurred among doctors by requiring training in abortion for future specialists in obstetrics and gynecology.[30] After a twelve-year hiatus, Cook County Hospital recently began providing abortions for low-income patients.[31] New pharmaceutical methods of inducing early abortions are being found and tested.[32] Following years of harassment of patients and providers at clinics, state and federal measures have been passed to protect clinic access.[33] African American women are increasingly visible in the movement for reproductive rights; their organizations enlarge the focus and bring to public attention the need for health care and respectful nonracist treatment as well as legal abortion.[34] National organizations such as NOW and Planned Parenthood work for both welfare and abortion rights. Feminist organizations that sometimes avoided the issue of teenagers' access to abortion now actively oppose parental notification requirements.

The legalization of abortion was a positive development for all women, not just those who seek abortions. Legal abortion represents an expansion of women's actual ability to control their reproduction, their sexuality, and their lives. The very availability of legal abortion provides a measure of freedom and control even for women who never use it, both because it can be counted on as a backup and because it symbolizes female sexual autonomy. The legal right to abortion sends the message to all women (and to men) that women have power over their own lives and are not controlled by men, the state, or the church. Finally, the ability to avoid motherhood helps to create new meanings for motherhood and fatherhood—as chosen and desirable life experiences rather than roles forced on women and men, willing or unwilling. The restriction or reversal of abortion rights sends the opposite message: women cannot be trusted to make moral decisions about children and family, but must be overseen and regulated by men; procreation is a state mandate not a choice; women's lives, sexuality, and bodies are not their own.

The affirmation of women's right to decide whether to terminate or carry a pregnancy to term was rooted in more than a century of subterranean belief and behavior. The transformation of law that began in the mid-1960s and culminated in *Roe* and *Doe* grew out of women's longstanding demand for abortion and ability to communicate, first to individual doctors in private conferences and then to society as a whole in public arenas, their need for abortion. The movement to decriminalize abortion built upon a century of physician-patient relationships in which doctors listened to women and helped them obtain abortions. When feminists called for "Abortion on Demand," they echoed generations of individual women before them. As the women's movement articulated a sense of women's right to control their reproduction, they brought into the open what had been popularly accepted for generations and gave it new meaning as a human right. In so doing, they transformed the abortion discourse. For the first time, public discussion of abortion included the perspective of the millions of women who needed and had abortions.

Women themselves had taken abortion out of the private and into the public. Women's reproductive rights were never protected or guaranteed in the private sphere; they had to be brought into the public, political sphere to win recognition. Despite the personal dangers of being publicly exposed and associated with the crime of abortion, women made the private secrets of their lives public knowledge in order to change policy and improve the lives of women and girls. "Private" discussion of abortion with selected physicians, relatives, friends, and others had allowed some women to obtain abortions while protecting them from public exposure. But keeping these matters private simultaneously sustained the illegal and stigmatized status of abortion. Women's right to "privacy" in matters of sexuality and procreation, a key concept underlying the legalization of abortion, was won only through public debate, political organizing, coalition building, and collective action.

Note on Sources

The core of the research for *When Abortion Was a Crime* was in medical and legal sources. *The Index Catalogue of the Library of the Surgeon General's Office* guided me to the medical literature for the period covered by this book. Because the *Index* misses some items, I systematically examined every issue of several journals to locate all the articles, correspondence, and notices related to abortion in them. The bibliography includes these selected journals but not the dozens of other journals and periodicals consulted or the more than one thousand medical, legal, and popular articles analyzed for this book.

A special issue of *Illinois Libraries* 63 (April 1981) is a helpful guide to Chicago area medical archives. The American Medical Association's Historical Health Fraud Collection (HHFC), containing materials collected since 1906, is particularly valuable. In the HHFC I found a series of files on abortion, which included abortion advertisements, correspondence about abortion, and several hundred newspaper clippings. The collection is national in scope, but sources concentrate on Chicago, where the AMA headquarters is located. The collection has since been reorganized, but the notes should enable future researchers to locate sources used.

Rather than focusing on legal treatises, statutes, or judicial opinions alone, I searched for original criminal trial and lower-level court records on abortion. I collected all of the Illinois Supreme Court and Appellate Court opinions on cases that addressed abortion from 1867 to 1973 (ninety-one published opinions). Any case appealed to these higher courts is preserved in perpetuity by the state. In Illinois, the transcripts of these original criminal trials and all other materials are held in the Illinois State Archives in Springfield. I examined case files for forty cases appealed to the Illinois Supreme Court. These case files (Record Series 901) contain verbatim transcripts of the original trial, which could run to five hundred pages or more, briefs, affidavits, exhibits, and all other material presented to the court of appeal. In the notes, the published opinion is referred to by its name, and the associated legal records held in the Illinois State Archives are referred to as the Transcript of a particular case. Trials that ended with an acquittal or were not appealed were not transcribed, which makes the cases available for analysis somewhat unusual. Yet the supreme and appellate court case files show standard procedures, and they are supplemented with many other sources.

Judicial opinions alerted me to another important set of legal records: coroner's inquests into the deaths of women who died following abortions. With a list of names of women who had died as a result of abortion in Chicago and approximate dates of death obtained through research in court opinions and in newspaper clippings found in the HHFC, I searched for the Cook County coroner's inquests into these deaths. Inquests are public records held at the Cook County Medical Examiner's Office in Chicago; coroner's records for other cities and counties may be held in archives. Medical examiner records can be located only by name and date of death, not by cause of death. The only way to locate every abortion death investigated by the Cook County coroner would be to go through the entire series of inquests in order to find the one hundred or fewer inquests into abortion per year. This would be a daunting task; in 1928 alone, there were over nine thousand inquests.* A randomized study of abortion cases investigated by the coroner would yield little or no data. I examined fifty-two transcripts of Cook County coroner's inquests into women's deaths resulting from abortion and requested an additional thirty-one cases for which no transcript could be located. Two were found in criminal trial transcripts.

The Municipal Reference Collection in the Chicago Public Library is an important resource for historians of Chicago. There I researched Chicago, Cook County, and Illinois statutes; the annual reports of the Cook County Coroner's Office, Chicago police, Chicago and Illinois health departments; and other government documents. I was unable to gain access to records of the Cook County State's Attorney's Office, which prosecuted abortion cases, or the Chicago Police Department. Records available at the Cook County Circuit Court contained minimal information, and it was often unclear whether a particular case concerned abortion or some other violation. Historians can surely locate published state statutes, state appellate and supreme court opinions, and the files for cases appealed to the highest court of each state, but local government documents can vary significantly and be held in a variety of locations. For Illinois, see the *Descriptive Inventory of the Archives of the State of Illinois* and *A Summary Guide to Local Government Records in the Illinois Regional Archives.*

The Women's Ephemera Collection, held in the Northwestern University Library's C. D. McCormick Library of Special Collections, proved to be an invaluable source on the movement to decriminalize abortion in the 1960s and

---

*Samuel A. Levinson, "History and Progress of the Scientific Work of the Cook County Coroner's Office," *Proceedings of the Institute of Medicine of Chicago* 12 (November 15, 1939): 470.

early 1970s. This collection, amassed at the time, contains newsletters, flyers, reports, and newspaper clippings about the grassroots women's liberation movement, with a particular emphasis on Chicago. In addition, the library holds runs of newsletters and newspapers, including the *SHA Newsletter* and the *WONAAC Newsletter*. Archival collections that were consulted but did not yield material for this study are not included in the bibliography.

Abbreviations

ACLU	American Civil Liberties Union
AHA	American Hospital Association
AJO	*American Journal of Obstetrics and Diseases of Women and Children*
AJOG	*American Journal of Obstetrics and Gynecology*
AJPH	*American Journal of Public Health*
ALI	American Law Institute
ALRA	Abortion Law Reform Association
AMA	American Medical Association
BCR	*Birth Control Review*
HHFC	Historical Health Fraud Collection, AMA
JAMA	*Journal of the American Medical Association*
JNMA	*Journal of the National Medical Association*
NARAL	National Association for the Repeal of Abortion Laws (1969–1973)
	National Abortion Rights Action League (1973–1993)
	National Abortion and Reproductive Rights Action League (1994–present)
NOW	National Organization for Women
NYT	*New York Times*
SHA	Society for Humane Abortion
SHSW	State Historical Society of Wisconsin
WEF	Women's Ephemera Folders, C.D. McCormick Library of Special Collections, Northwestern University Library
WMJ	*Woman's Medical Journal*
WONAAC	Women's National Abortion Action Coalition

Notes

Introduction

1. On the legal status of abortion, see James C. Mohr, *Abortion in America: The Origins and Evolution of National Policy, 1800–1900* (New York: Oxford University Press, 1978); Linda Gordon, *Woman's Body, Woman's Right: Birth Control in America,* rev. and updated (1976; reprint, New York: Penguin Books, 1990), 49–61, 402–416; Michael Grossberg, *Governing the Hearth: Law and the Family in Nineteenth-Century America* (Chapel Hill: University of North Carolina Press, 1985), 155–195; Rosalind Pollack Petchesky, *Abortion and Woman's Choice: The State, Sexuality, and Reproductive Freedom,* rev. ed. (1984; reprint, Boston: Northeastern University Press, 1990), 67–138; Carroll Smith-Rosenberg, *Disorderly Conduct: Visions of Gender in Victorian America* (New York: Oxford University Press, 1985), 217–244; Kristin Luker, *Abortion and the Politics of Motherhood* (Berkeley: University of California Press, 1984).

2. Barbara Welter, "The Cult of True Womanhood," *American Quarterly* 18 (summer 1966): 151–174; Nancy F. Cott, *The Bonds of Womanhood: "Woman's Sphere" in New England, 1780–1835* (New Haven: Yale University Press, 1977); Carroll Smith-Rosenberg, "Female World of Love and Ritual: Relations between Women in Nineteenth-Century America," *Signs* 1 (1975): 1–29.

3. See two critiques and reviews of the field of women's history, Nancy A. Hewitt, "Beyond the Search for Sisterhood: American Women's History in the 1980s," *Social History* 10 (October 1985); reprint in *Unequal Sisters: A Multi-Cultural Reader in U.S. Women's History,* edited by Ellen Carol DuBois and Vicki L. Ruiz (New York: Routledge, 1990), 1–14; Linda K. Kerber, "Separate Spheres, Female Worlds, Women's Place: The Rhetoric of Women's History," *Journal of American History* 75 (June 1988): 9–39. For collections of recent scholarship on the history of women of color and working-class women, see DuBois and Ruiz, *Unequal Sisters;* Ava Baron, ed., *Work Engendered: Toward a New History of American Labor* (Ithaca: Cornell University Press, 1991); and

the pathbreaking collection by Gerda Lerner, ed., *Black Women in White America: A Documentary History* (New York: Random House, 1972).

4. The key work generating intellectual thought and debate on the public sphere is Jürgen Habermas, *The Structural Transformation of the Public Sphere: An Inquiry into a Category of Bourgeois Society,* translated by Thomas Burger with Frederick Lawrence (Cambridge, Mass.: MIT Press, 1989). For a collection of recent scholarship, see Craig Calhoun, ed., *Habermas and the Public Sphere* (Cambridge, Mass.: MIT Press, 1992). For feminist thinking, see Nancy Fraser, *Unruly Practices: Power, Discourse, and Gender in Contemporary Social Theory* (Minneapolis: University of Minnesota Press, 1989); Mary P. Ryan, *Women in Public: Between Banners and Ballots, 1825–1880* (Baltimore: Johns Hopkins University Press, 1990); Judith R. Walkowitz, *City of Dreadful Delight: Narratives of Sexual Danger in Late-Victorian London* (Chicago: University of Chicago Press, 1992); Linda K. Kerber, "A Constitutional Right to Be Treated Like American Ladies: Women and the Obligations of Citizenship," in *U.S. History as Women's History: New Feminist Essays,* edited by Linda K. Kerber, Alice Kessler-Harris, and Kathryn Kish Sklar (Chapel Hill: University of North Carolina Press, 1995), 17–35.

5. This cooperative relationship may have been particularly significant for public health and women's lives. Linda Gordon, *Heroes of Their Own Lives: The Politics and History of Family Violence, Boston, 1880–1960* (New York: Viking, 1988); Molly Ladd-Taylor, *Mother-Work: Women, Child Welfare, and the State, 1890–1930* (Urbana: University of Illinois Press, 1994); Robyn L. Muncy, *Creating a Female Dominion in American Reform, 1890–1935* (New York: Oxford University Press, 1990); Jane Lewis, *The Politics of Motherhood: Child and Maternal Welfare in England, 1900–1939* (London: Croom Helm, 1980); Judith Walzer Leavitt, *The Healthiest City: Milwaukee and the Politics of Health Reform* (Princeton: Princeton University Press, 1982), 190–213; Susan L. Smith, *Sick and Tired of Being Sick and Tired: Black Women's Health Activism in America, 1890–1950* (Philadelphia: University of Pennsylvania Press, 1995).

6. For examples of earlier feminists' views of medicine, see Ann Douglas Wood, "'The Fashionable Diseases': Women's Complaints and Their Treatment in Nineteenth Century America," in *Clio's Consciousness Raised: New Perspectives on the History of Women,* edited by Mary S. Hartman and Lois Banner (New York: Harper and Row, 1974), 1–22; and the critical response by Regina Morantz, "The Lady and Her Physician," in Hartman and Banner, *Clio's Consciousness Raised,* 38–53. See also Adrienne Rich, *Of Woman Born: Motherhood as Experience and Institution* (New York: W. W. Norton, 1976); Barbara Ehrenreich and Deirdre English, *For Her Own Good: 150 Years of the Experts' Advice to Women* (Garden City, N.Y.: Doubleday, 1978). For a different view, see Judith Walzer Leavitt, *Brought to Bed: Childbearing in America, 1750–1950* (New York: Oxford University Press, 1986).

7. For other patient-focused histories, see Leavitt, *Brought to Bed;* Roy Porter, ed., *Patients and Practitioners* (Cambridge: Cambridge University Press, 1985); Mary E. Fissell, *Patients, Power, and the Poor in Eighteenth-Century Bristol* (Cambridge: Cambridge University Press, 1991).

8. On police, see Eric H. Monkkonen, *Police in Urban America, 1860–1920*

(New York: Cambridge University Press, 1981); Roger Lane, *Policing the City: Boston 1822–1885* (Cambridge: Harvard University Press, 1967). On prisons, see Lawrence M. Friedman and Robert V. Percival, *The Roots of Justice: Crime and Punishment in Alameda County, California, 1870–1910* (Chapel Hill: University of North Carolina Press, 1981), 288–309; Estelle B. Freedman, *Their Sisters' Keepers: Women's Prison Reform in America, 1830–1930* (Ann Arbor: University of Michigan Press, 1981); David J. Rothman, *The Discovery of the Asylum: Social Order and Disorder in the New Republic* (Boston: Little, Brown and Co., 1971).

On marriage, divorce, and women's property rights, see Kerber, "A Constitutional Right to Be Treated Like American Ladies"; Nancy F. Cott, "Giving Character to Our Whole Civil Polity: Marriage and the Public Order in the Late Nineteenth Century," in Kerber, Kessler-Harris, and Sklar, *U.S. History as Women's History*, 107–121; Grossberg, *Governing the Hearth;* Marylynne Salmon, *Women and the Law of Property in Early America* (Chapel Hill: University of North Carolina Press, 1986); Norma Basch, *In the Eyes of the Law: Women, Marriage, and Property in Nineteenth-century New York* (Ithaca: Cornell University Press, 1982); D. Kelly Weisberg, *Property, Family, and the Legal Profession,* vol. 2 of *Women and the Law: A Social Historical Perspective* (Cambridge, Mass.: Schenkman Publishing, 1982). On women and crime, see D. Kelly Weisberg, *Women and the Criminal Law,* vol. 1 of *Women and the Law: A Social Historical Perspective* (Cambridge, Mass.: Schenkman Publishing, 1982); Mary E. Odem, *Delinquent Daughters: Protecting and Policing Adolescent Female Sexuality in the United States, 1885–1920* (Chapel Hill: University of North Carolina Press, 1995); Anna Clark, *Women's Silence, Men's Violence: Sexual Assault in England, 1770–1845* (New York: Pandora Press, 1987).

9. James C. Mohr, *Doctors and the Law: Medical Jurisprudence in Nineteenth-Century America* (New York: Oxford University Press, 1993); Mohr, *Abortion in America;* Charles E. Rosenberg, *The Trial of the Assassin Guiteau: Psychiatry and Law in the Gilded Age* (Chicago: University of Chicago Press, 1968); Michael Clark and Catherine Crawford, eds., *Legal Medicine in History* (Cambridge: Cambridge University Press, 1994).

10. James Willard Hurst, *The Growth of American Law: The Law Makers* (Boston: Little, Brown and Co., 1950). For overviews of American legal history, see Lawrence M. Friedman, *A History of American Law,* 2d ed. (New York: Simon and Schuster, 1985); Kermit L. Hall, *The Magic Mirror: Law in American History* (New York: Oxford University Press, 1989).

11. Histories of courts in action include Stanton Wheeler et al., "Do the 'Haves' Come out Ahead? Winning and Losing in State Supreme Courts, 1870–1970," *Law and Society Review* 21 (1987): 403–445; Robert A. Silverman, *Law and Urban Growth: Civil Litigation in the Boston Trial Courts, 1880–1900* (Princeton: Princeton University Press, 1981); Hendrik Hartog, "The Public Law of a County Court; Judicial Government in Eighteenth Century Massachusetts," *The American Journal of Legal History* 20 (1976): 282–329.

12. Michel Foucault, *Discipline and Punish: The Birth of the Prison,* translated by Alan Sheridan (1975; reprint, New York: Vintage Books, 1979), 111, 108.

13. The state criminal abortion laws did not change at all or only in nonsubstantive ways for a century; Mohr, *Abortion in America,* 224–225. In Illi-

nois, the legislature amended the law to prohibit advertising of abortion in 1919 and, in 1961, clarified that an attempted abortion, even if the woman was not pregnant, would be considered abortion. Illinois, *Laws of Illinois,* 1919, pp. 427–428, sec. 6; Illinois, *Laws of Illinois,* 1961, p. 2027.

14. Kristin Luker argues that there was medical consensus on therapeutic abortion for a century until about 1960 when new technology broke that consensus apart and disagreement erupted within the medical profession and, then, the public. I disagree with this interpretation. Luker, *Abortion and the Politics of Motherhood,* 54–91.

15. Addison Niles, "Criminal Abortion," in *Transactions of the Twenty-First Anniversary Meeting of the Illinois State Medical Society* (Chicago: Fergus Printing, 1872), 99; James Foster Scott, "Criminal Abortion," *American Journal of Obstetrics and Diseases of Women and Children* (hereafter cited as *AJO*) 33 (January 1896): 77. On the pluralism and ambiguity of American law, see Hendrik Hartog, "Pigs and Positivism," *Wisconsin Law Review* 1985, no. 4 (1985): 899–935.

16. John T. Noonan Jr., "An Almost Absolute Value in History," in *The Morality of Abortion: Legal and Historical Perspectives,* edited by John T. Noonan Jr. (Cambridge, Mass.: Harvard University Press, 1970), 1–59.

17. A survey of the guides to religious periodicals shows this to be true. The small number of articles on abortion published in religious magazines were overwhelmed by those on birth control. The *Catholic Periodicals Index,* for example, lists 155 citations to articles on birth control and only 6 on abortion in 1930–1933. In 1961–1962, there were 111 articles on birth control and 28 on abortion. The *Index to Religious Periodical Literature* lists in one ten-year period, 1949–1959, only 6 articles on birth control and 3 on abortion. Not until 1971–1972 did the index cite more articles on abortion than on birth control. I am grateful to Rose Holz and Lynne Curry for collecting and tabulating this data.

18. On religious opinion in response to the birth control movement, see David M. Kennedy, *Birth Control in America: The Career of Margaret Sanger* (New Haven: Yale University Press, 1970), 136–171.

19. Gordon, *Woman's Body, Woman's Right,* 5–10; Glanville Williams, *The Sanctity of Life and the Criminal Law* (New York: Knopf, 1957), 148–152, 192–197; Ronald L. Numbers and Darrel W. Amundsen, *Caring and Curing: Health and Medicine in the Western Religious Traditions* (New York: Macmillan, 1986), 31, 50, 87, 156–157. Most of the essays in *Caring and Curing* address only current attitudes toward abortion, suggesting that until recently, most sects showed little interest in abortion.

20. Luker, *Abortion and the Politics of Motherhood,* chap. 3.

21. For a helpful discussion of Foucault, poststructural analysis, and feminist critiques, see Walkowitz, *City of Dreadful Delight,* 1–13. Michel Foucault, *An Introduction,* vol. 1 in *The History of Sexuality,* translated by Robert Hurley (1976; reprint, New York: Random House, 1978). Joan Wallach Scott has become known as the strongest advocate for poststructural analysis of women's history; see *Gender and the Politics of History* (New York: Columbia University Press, 1988). For a debate, see Linda Gordon and Joan Scott in *Signs* 15 (summer 1990): 848–860. For another critique of the emphasis on linguistics, see

bell hooks, *Talking Back: thinking feminist, thinking black* (Boston, Mass.: South End Press, 1989), 35–41.

22. My discussion of abortion in common law and its criminalization relies most on Mohr, *Abortion in America*.

23. Ibid., 10, chap. 1; Angus McLaren, *Reproductive Rituals: The Perception of Fertility in England from the Sixteenth Century to the Nineteenth Century* (London: Methuen, 1984), 102–103, 108–109, 188 n. 98.

24. McLaren, *Reproductive Rituals*, 188 n. 98; Williams, *The Sanctity of Life and the Criminal Law*, 149–152, 197.

25. Mohr, *Abortion in America*, 3–45; Charles E. Rosenberg, "The Therapeutic Revolution: Medicine, Meaning, and Social Change in Nineteenth-Century America," in *The Therapeutic Revolution: Essays in the Social History of American Medicine*, edited by Morris J. Vogel and Charles E. Rosenberg (Philadelphia: Temple University Press, 1970), 3–26.

26. Quotation as cited in Julia Cherry Spruill, *Women's Life and Work in the Southern Colonies* (1938; reprint, New York: W. W. Norton, 1972), 325–326. Mohr, *Abortion in America*, chap. 1, 58–66; McLaren, *Reproductive Rituals*, 103–105. On abortion methods worldwide, see Edward Shorter, *A History of Women's Bodies* (New York: Basic Books, 1982), 177–224.

27. Cornelia Hughes Dayton uncovered this case and the phrase, "Taking the Trade: Abortion and Gender Relations in an Eighteenth-Century New England Village," *William and Mary Quarterly* 48 (January 1991): 1, 24–25; McLaren, *Reproductive Rituals*, 106–107.

28. Mohr, *Abortion in America*, 20–25; Illinois, *Revised Code*, 1827, sec. 46, p. 131.

29. Mohr, *Abortion in America*, 22, 24.

30. Ibid., 47–59, 70–71; Smith-Rosenberg, *Disorderly Conduct*, 225–227.

31. Mohr, *Abortion in America*, 86–94.

32. Ibid., 147–225. On the Jacksonian period, the status of the regular profession, and Irregulars, see Richard Harrison Shryock, *Medical Licensing in America, 1650–1965* (Baltimore: Johns Hopkins University Press, 1967); Ronald L. Numbers, "The Fall and Rise of the Medical Profession," in *Sickness and Health in America: Readings in the History of Medicine and Public Health*, edited by Judith Walzer Leavitt and Ronald L. Numbers, 2d ed., rev. (Madison: University of Wisconsin Press, 1985), 185–205; William G. Rothstein, *American Physicians in the Nineteenth Century: From Sects to Science* (Baltimore: Johns Hopkins University Press, 1972); Norman Gevitz, ed., *Other Healers: Unorthodox Medicine in America* (Baltimore: Johns Hopkins University Press, 1988). Regulars presented abortion as an Irregular practice, but Homeopaths essentially shared their antiabortion position. See, for example, Edwin M. Hale, *The Great Crime of the Nineteenth Century* (Chicago: C. S. Halsey, 1867).

33. Daniel Scott Smith, "Family Limitation, Sexual Control, and Domestic Feminism in Victorian America," *Feminist Studies* 1 (winter-spring 1973): 40–57; Robert V. Wells, "Family History and Demographic Transition," *Journal of Social History* 9 (fall 1975): 1–9.

34. Mohr, *Abortion in America*, 166–168. Quotation from Horatio Robinson Storer, *Why Not? A Book for Every Woman* (Boston: Lee and Shepard,

1868); reprinted as *A Proper Bostonian on Sex and Birth Control* (New York: Arno Press, 1974), 85.

35. Quotation from Horatio Robinson Storer, *Is It I? A Book for Every Man* (Boston: Lee and Shepard, 1868); reprinted as *A Proper Bostonian on Sex and Birth Control*, 134; Smith-Rosenberg, *Disorderly Conduct*, 224–228, 236–239; Mohr, *Abortion in America*, 107–108, 168–170.

36. Mary Roth Walsh, *"Doctors Wanted: No Women Need Apply": Sexual Barriers in the Medical Profession, 1835–1975* (New Haven: Yale University Press, 1977), 109–118; Virginia G. Drachman, *Hospital with a Heart: Women Doctors and the Paradox of Separatism at the New England Hospital, 1862–1969* (Ithaca: Cornell University Press, 1984).

37. On the anxieties about sexuality woven into the use of anesthesia and obstetrics, see Mary Poovey, *Uneven Developments: The Ideological Work of Gender in Mid-Victorian England* (Chicago: University of Chicago Press, 1988), 24–50; Martin S. Pernick, *A Calculus of Suffering: Pain, Professionalism, and Anesthesia in Nineteenth-Century America* (New York: Columbia University Press, 1985), 61–62. On the expectation that female physicians would care for female patients and treat them differently, see M. Walsh, *Doctors Wanted*, 93–95, 115–116; Regina Markell Morantz-Sanchez, *Sympathy and Science: Women Physicians in American Medicine* (New York: Oxford University Press, 1985).

38. On medical concern about the morality of obstetrics and gynecology, see M. Walsh, *Doctors Wanted*, 113; Virginia G. Drachman, "The Loomis Trial: Social Mores and Obstetrics in the Nineteenth Century," in *Childbirth: The Beginning of Motherhood, Proceedings of the Second Motherhood Symposium* (Madison, Wis.: Women's Studies Research Center, 1982), reprint in Leavitt, *Women and Health in America*, 166–174.

39. On prostitution, see Carroll Smith-Rosenberg, "Beauty, the Beast, and the Militant Woman: A Case Study in Sex Roles and Social Stress in Jacksonian America," *American Quarterly* 23 (1971): 562–584, reprint in Smith-Rosenberg, *Disorderly Conduct*, 109–128; Judith R. Walkowitz, *Prostitution and Victorian Society: Women, Class, and the State* (New York: Cambridge University Press, 1980); Ruth Rosen, *The Lost Sisterhood: Prostitution in America, 1900–1918* (Baltimore: Johns Hopkins University Press, 1982). On antislavery, see Jean Fagan Yellin, *Women and Sisters: The Anti-Slavery Feminists in American Culture* (New Haven: Yale University Press, 1989); Gerda Lerner, *The Grimké Sisters from South Carolina: Rebels against Slavery* (Boston: Houghton Mifflin, 1967). On temperance, see Barbara Leslie Epstein, *The Politics of Domesticity: Women, Evangelism, and Temperance in Nineteenth-Century America* (Middletown, Conn.: Wesleyan University Press, 1981). On voluntary motherhood, see Gordon, *Woman's Body, Woman's Right*, chap. 5. On ninteenth-century women's sense of moral superiority as a source of activism, see Lori D. Ginzberg, *Women and the Work of Benevolence: Morality, Politics, and Class in the Nineteenth-Century United States* (New Haven: Yale University Press, 1990). On the women's movement as a whole, see Ellen Carol DuBois, *Feminism and Suffrage: The Emergence of an Independent Women's Movement in America, 1848–1869* (Ithaca: Cornell University Press, 1978); Eleanor Flexner, *Century of Struggle: The Woman's Rights Movement in the United States*, rev. ed. (1959; reprint Cambridge, Mass.: Belknap Press of Harvard University Press, 1975).

40. Storer, *Why Not?*, 76, 83.

41. Ibid., 32.

42. Ibid., 34–35, 69–70, 84.

43. Mohr, *Abortion in America*, 200–225.

44. On Comstockery, see Gordon, *Woman's Body, Woman's Right*, 24, 164–166, 208–209; Brodie, *Contraception and Abortion in Nineteenth-Century America*, 257–258, 263–266, 281–288.

45. On the state laws in general, see Mohr, *Abortion in America*, 29–30. Only one statement has been uncovered to explain why the state of Illinois passed this new criminal abortion law in early 1867: "Mr. Green explained that the reason for the introduction of the bill," the *Illinois State Journal* reported, "was that there was now no law on this subject in this state." "Illinois Legislature, Introduction of Bills," *Springfield, Illinois State Journal*, February 8, 1867, p. 1; Illinois, *Journal of the Senate*, 1867, p. 1107; Illinois, *Journal of the House of Representatives*, 1867, p. 689. Quotations from Illinois, *Public Laws of Illinois*, 1867, p. 89, and Illinois, *Public Laws of Illinois*, 1872, p. 369. The Illinois State Medical Society Papers, Illinois State Historical Library, Springfield, Illinois, yielded no further information on the passage of this law in Illinois.

46. Ellen Ross, *Love and Toil: Motherhood in Outcast London, 1870–1918* (New York: Oxford University Press, 1993). The time it took for physicians to accept their own role in spreading infection via their hands and to change their own behavior is the classic example of the sometimes slow pace of change in medicine; Erwin H. Ackerknecht, *A Short History of Medicine*, rev. ed. (1955; Baltimore: Johns Hopkins University Press, 1992), 187–191.

47. Research included examining every issue of the *Journal of the National Medical Association*, vol. 1 (1901) to vol. 65 (1973); a survey of African American periodical literature, indexed in *Index to Periodical Articles by and about Negroes*, 1943–1972 and *Index to Periodical Articles by and about Blacks*, 1973; and research in archival collections.

48. James Gilbert, *Perfect Cities: Chicago's Utopias of 1893* (Chicago: University of Chicago Press, 1991); Harold M. Mayer and Richard C. Wade, with the assistance of Glen E. Holt, *Chicago: Growth of a Metropolis* (Chicago: University of Chicago Press, 1969); Bessie Louise Pierce, *The Rise of a Modern City, 1871–1893*, vol. 3 of *A History of Chicago* (New York: Knopf, 1957); Emmett Dedmon, *Fabulous Chicago* (New York: Random House, 1953); Thomas N. Bonner, *Medicine in Chicago, 1850–1950: A Chapter in the Social and Scientific Development of a City*, 2d ed. (1957; reprint, Urbana: University of Illinois, 1991).

49. Records that would give precise quantitative answers to questions about the practice of abortion do not exist. We will never know exactly how many abortions were performed or how many women died as a result of their abortions; nor will we ever be able to determine the proportion of the female population who had abortions or the proportion of practitioners who performed them. Social surveys and aggregate data that became available in medical literature in the 1930s help make it possible to estimate answers to these types of questions. Sources are discussed further in the text and in the note on sources.

50. On the related history of pregnancy, childbirth, and contraception, see Leavitt, *Brought to Bed*; Richard W. Wertz and Dorothy C. Wertz, *Lying-In: A History of Childbirth in America* (New York: Schocken Books, 1979); Gordon,

Woman's Body, Woman's Right; Kennedy, *Birth Control in America;* James Reed, *From Private Vice to Public Virtue: The Birth Control Movement and American Society Since 1830* (New York: Basic Books, 1978); Ellen Chesler, *Woman of Valor: Margaret Sanger and the Birth Control Movement in America* (New York: Simon and Schuster, 1992). On the centrality of reproduction to society and history, see Frederick Engels, *The Origin of the Family, Private Property, and the State* (1884; reprint, New York: International Publishers, 1972); Mary O'Brien, *The Politics of Reproduction* (Boston: Routledge, 1981).

Chapter 1.   An Open Secret

1. Dr. A. S. Warner's office was at 3236 West Polk Street. Inquest on Frances Collins, May 7, 1920, case no. 161–5–20, Medical Records Department, Cook County Medical Examiner's Office, Chicago, Illinois.

2. Ibid.

3. I have identified 111 women in the Chicago area who had abortions between 1880 and 1930. Most were white and working class. Of 73 for whom there is information available on their marital status, the majority were married (45, or 63 percent). This is not based on a random sample and cannot be universalized. Other historians have also noted the importance of abortion to working-class women. Linda Gordon, *Woman's Body, Woman's Right: Birth Control in America,* rev. and updated (1976; reprint, New York: Penguin Books, 1990), 144; James C. Mohr, *Abortion in America: The Origins and Evolution of National Policy* (Oxford: Oxford University Press, 1978), 243.

4. For examples of the use of silence as a metaphor for the history of abortion, see Patricia Miller, *The Worst of Times* (New York: Harper Collins, 1993), 6–7; Kristin Luker, *Abortion and the Politics of Motherhood* (Berkeley: University of California Press, 1984), 40. On the liberatory aspects of speaking, see bell hooks, *Talking Back: thinking feminist, thinking black* (Boston, Mass.: South End Press, 1989), 10–18; Adrienne Rich, *On Lies, Secrets, and Silence: Selected Prose, 1966–1978* (New York: W. W. Norton, 1979). For a recent collection showing the fruitfulness of this theoretical conceptualization, Elaine Hedge and Shelley Fisher Fishkin, eds., *Listening to Silences: New Essays in Feminist Criticism* (New York: Oxford University Press, 1994).

5. The focus on the past as silencing and speaking as liberatory overdraws the oppressiveness of the past, the transformations of the late 1960s, and the freedoms of the present. My critique of this silencing trope is similar to the critique made recently by queer theorists of the tendency in lesbian-gay history to present a history of progress from marginalization or invisibility to coming out. See Henry Abelove, "The Queering of Lesbian/Gay History," *Radical History Review* 62 (spring 1995): 44–57; Lisa Duggan, "'Becoming Visible: The Legacy of Stonewall,' New York Public Library, June 18-September 24, 1994," *Radical History Review* 62 (spring 1995): 193. The entire spring issue of *Radical History Review* is titled "The Queer Issue: New Visions of America's Lesbian and Gay Past."

6. "The bonds of womanhood" was Sarah Grimké's phrase and is the title

of Nancy F. Cott's book, *The Bonds of Womanhood: "Woman's Sphere" in New England, 1780–1835* (New Haven: Yale University Press, 1977), 1. See also Carroll Smith-Rosenberg, "Female World of Love and Ritual: Relations between Women in Nineteenth-Century America," *Signs* 1 (1975): 1–29; Judith Walzer Leavitt, *Brought to Bed: Childbearing in America, 1750 to 1950* (New York: Oxford University Press, 1986), 4–7. For a debate and critiques of this idea see Nancy Cott, Mari Jo Buhle, Temma Kaplan, Gerda Lerner, and Carroll Smith-Rosenberg, "Politics and Culture in Women's History: A Symposium," *Feminist Studies* 6:1 (1980): 26–62; Denise Riley, *"Am I That Name?" Feminism and the Category of "Women" in History* (Minneapolis: University of Minnesota Press, 1988). I do not suggest that the biological experiences of being female create "natural" bonds among all women, overcoming social differences by race, class, age, and so on, but these shared female experiences helped define womanhood and could, at moments, create sympathies across social boundaries.

7. The coroner's physician discovered during the autopsy that she had had an ectopic pregnancy, which her physicians, not surprisingly, had not discerned. The preeminent obstetrician Joseph B. DeLee reported that it was rare for a physician to diagnose ectopic pregnancy. The ectopic pregnancy was a contributing factor in Collins's death, but all of Collins's efforts were directed at aborting her pregnancy and that is what I concentrate on here. Edward H. Hutton, "Doctor's Statement Blank," Inquest on Collins; Joseph B. DeLee, *The Principles and Practice of Obstetrics*, 2d ed., rev. (Philadelphia: W. B. Saunders, 1916), 399.

8. As cited in Gordon, *Woman's Body, Woman's Right*, 493 n. 23.

9. For the estimate by Dr. C. S. Bacon, see "Chicago Medical Society. Regular Meeting, Held Nov. 23, 1904," *JAMA* 43 (December 17, 1904): 1889; quote from J. Henry Barbat, "Criminal Abortion," *California State Journal of Medicine* 9 (February 1911): 69.

10. Marie E. Kopp, *Birth Control in Practice: Analysis of Ten Thousand Case Histories of the Birth Control Clinical Research Bureau* (1933; reprint, New York: Arno Press, 1972), 124; Katharine Bement Davis, *Factors in the Sex Life of Twenty-Two Hundred Women* (1929; reprint, New York: Arno Press, 1972), xi–xiii, 20, 21; Gilbert Van Tassel Hamilton, *A Research in Marriage* (New York: Albert and Charles Boni, 1929), 134, 133.

11. U.S. Department of Labor, Children's Bureau, *Maternal Mortality in Fifteen States*, Bureau Publication No. 223 (Washington D.C.: Government Printing Office, 1934), 108, 112–113; Calvin Schmid, *Social Saga of Two Cities: An Ecological and Statistical Study of Social Trends in Minneapolis and St. Paul* (Minneapolis: Minneapolis Council of Social Agencies, 1937), 410–411. I am grateful to Elizabeth Lockwood for sharing the Schmid study with me. Isabella V. Granger, "Birth Control in Harlem," *Birth Control Review* (hereafter cited as *BCR*) 22 (May 1938): 92; J. W. Walker in Val Do Turner, "Fertility of Women," *Journal of the National Medical Association* (hereafter cited as *JNMA*) 5 (October-December 1913): 250; Caroline Hadley Robinson, *Seventy Birth Control Clinics: A Survey and Analysis Including the General Effects of Control on Size and Quality of Population* (Baltimore: Williams and Wilkins, 1930), 66–67.

12. Regine K. Stix, "A Study of Pregnancy Wastage," *The Milbank Memorial*

Fund Quarterly 13 (October 1935): 351–352. For examples of Catholic women in Chicago who had abortions, see Inquest on Frauciszka Gawlik, February 19, 1916, case no. 27–3–1916, Medical Records Department; Inquest on Mary Colbert, March 25, 1933, case no. 7–4–1933, Medical Records Department.

13. Frederick J. Taussig, *Abortion, Spontaneous and Induced: Medical and Social Aspects* (St. Louis: C. V. Mosby, 1936), 26.

14. James Foster Scott, "Criminal Abortion," *AJO* 33 (January 1896): 80; Schmid, *Social Saga of Two Cities,* 410; Jerome E. Bates and Edward S. Zawadzki, *Criminal Abortion: A Study in Medical Sociology* (Springfield, Ill.: Charles C. Thomas, 1964), 44–45. Newspapers can be misleading. After examining abortion coverage in the *New York Times* and abortion case histories in the medical literature, James Mohr concluded that after 1880 abortion became the practice of unwed women. Mohr, *Abortion in America,* 240–244.

15. Press and court interest in unmarried women and men are discussed further in later chapters of this volume.

16. Mary A. Dixon-Jones, "Criminal Abortion—Its Evils and Its Sad Consequences," *Woman's Medical Journal* (hereafter cited as *WMJ*) 3 (August 1894): 34; Dr. J. R. Gardner in Inquest on Ellen Matson, November 19, 1917, case 330–11–1917, Medical Records Department.

17. Marie Hansen in Inquest on Mary Schwartz, May 21, 1934, case no. 340–5–1934, Medical Records Department.

18. "Prevention or Abortion, Which?" *BCR* 7 (May 1923): 127.

19. Dr. B. Liber, "As a Doctor Sees It," *BCR* 2 (February-March 1918): 10; "Prevention or Abortion—Which?" *BCR* 7 (July 1923): 182. A midwife used this phrase in 1888, "Infanticide," *Chicago Times,* December 13, 1888, p. 2.

20. Frank Mau in Inquest on Catherine Mau, March 12, 1928, case 390–3–1928, Medical Records Department.

21. Clara Taylor, "Observations of a Nurse," *BCR* 2 (June 1918), 13; see also Mary A. Dixon-Jones, "Criminal Abortion—Its Evils and Its Sad Consequences" continued, *WMJ* 3 (September 1894): 62, 63.

22. "Two Pertinent Remarks," *Chicago Times,* December 30, 1888, p. 4; A.B.C., "Does Public Opinion in the United States Sanction Abortion?" *Medical Critic and Guide* 23 (1920): 71. I suspect that "A.B.C." was William J. Robinson, an advocate of birth control and early advocate for legalized abortion. He was the editor of the *Medical Critic and Guide* and wrote most of its articles. Entry for William J. Robinson in *The National Cyclopaedia of American Biography Being the History of the United States,* vol. 35 (New York: James T. White and Co., 1949), 546; Gordon, *Woman's Body, Woman's Right,* 170–176.

23. Joseph Taber Johnson, "Abortion and its Effects," *AJO* 33 (January 1896): 86–97, quotation on 91. See also Scott, "Criminal Abortion," 72–86.

24. E. S. McKee, "Abortion," *AJO* 24 (October 1891): 1333.

25. Henry O. Marcy in J. H. Carstens, "Education as a Factor in the Prevention of Criminal Abortion and Illegitimacy," *JAMA* 47 (December 8, 1906): 1890; John G. Clark in Edward A. Schumann, "The Economic Aspects of Abortion," *American Journal of Obstetrics and Gynecology* (hereafter cited as *AJOG*) 7 (April 1924): 485.

26. Gordon, *Woman's Body, Woman's Right,* 36; Susan E. Cayleff, "Self-

Help and the Patent Medicine Business," in *Women, Health, and Medicine in America: A Historical Handbook,* edited by Rima D. Apple (New York: Garland Publishing, 1990), 311–336; Leavitt, *Brought to Bed,* chap. 4. On self-medication in the early twentieth century, see Ronald L. Numbers, *Almost Persuaded: American Physicians and Compulsory Health Insurance, 1912–1920* (Baltimore: Johns Hopkins University Press, 1978), 2–3.

27. Denslow Lewis, "Facts Regarding Criminal Abortion," *JAMA* 35 (October 13, 1900): 944.

28. Anne Burnet, "Abortion as the Exciting Cause of Insanity, *WMJ* 9 (November 1899): 400. On the germ theory and antiseptic procedure, see Charles E. Rosenberg, *The Care of Strangers: The Rise of America's Hospital System* (New York: Basic Books, 1987), 137–150; Gert H. Brieger, "American Surgery and the Germ Theory of Disease," *Bulletin of the History of Medicine* 40 (March-April 1966): 135–145.

29. Barbara Brookes, *Abortion in England, 1900–1967* (London: Croom Helm, 1988), 23, 37; quotation in "Hard Facts," *BCR* 4 (June 1920): 16. Regine Stix found that one illegal abortion (of 686) was performed by a neighbor, "A Study of Pregnancy Wastage," 360 n. 14.

30. Dixon-Jones, "Criminal Abortion" (September 1894), 60–61.

31. Inquest on Matson. Matson's aunt remarked that she and Matson's mother had advised against an abortion. Whether this remark was true or a comment made to avoid trouble with the authorities, neither aunt nor mother abandoned her.

32. Inquest on Colbert.

33. Joan Jacobs Brumberg, "'Ruined Girls': Changing Community Responses to Illegitimacy in Upstate New York, 1890–1920," *Journal of Social History* 18 (winter 1984): 247–272, quotation on 248.

34. Dixon-Jones, "Criminal Abortion" (August 1894), 36.

35. Inquest on Ester Reed, June 9, 1914, case no. 73771, Medical Records Department. Although Emma Alby denied having done anything "wrong," her parents were convinced she was pregnant and took her to a physician for an abortion. Inquest on Emma Alby, September 11, 1915, case no. 141–10–1915, Medical Records Department.

36. Inquest on Gawlik; Brumberg, "'Ruined Girls,'" 248–249, 250, 258; John D'Emilio and Estelle B. Freedman, *Intimate Matters: A History of Sexuality in America* (New York: Harper and Row, 1988), 187, 259. On neighborhood policing of unmarried women's sexual behavior, Joanne Meyerowitz, "Sexual Geography and Gender Economy: The Furnished Room Districts of Chicago, 1890–1930," *Gender and History* 2 (autumn 1990): 277.

37. "Queries and Minor Notes. Maternities for the Unmarried," *JAMA* 43 (July 2, 1904): 42.

38. Dr. Henry Fitzbutler founded the Louisville National Medical College. This is from the recollections of his grandson. Case 14, "Research Projects, The Negro Family in the U.S., Documents on Higher Class Families in Chicago," folder 13, box 131–81, E. Franklin Frazier Papers, used with the permission of the Manuscript Division, Moorland-Spingarn Research Center, Howard University, Washington D.C. On black hospitals, see Vanessa Northington Gamble,

Making a Place for Ourselves: The Black Hospital Movement, 1920–1945 (New York: Oxford University Press, 1995).

39. Brumberg, "'Ruined Girls'," 260; Elizabeth Karsen Lockwood, "The Fallen Woman, the Maternity Home, and the State: A Study of Maternal Health Care for Single Parturients, 1870–1930" (master's thesis, University of Wisconsin, Madison, 1987); Regina G. Kunzel, *Fallen Women, Problem Girls: Unmarried Mothers and the Professionalization of Social Work, 1890–1945* (New Haven: Yale University Press, 1993). By 1904, mandatory breastfeeding was an "established policy" among Illinois charitable maternities for the unwed, "Maternities for the Unmarried," 42.

40. Kunzel, *Fallen Women, Problem Girls,* 68–69, 81.

41. Women's wages were based on the (false) assumption that women did not support themselves or their families because they had husbands or fathers who supported them. This discussion is drawn from Joanne Meyerowitz's excellent survey of women's wages in the early twentieth century, *Women Adrift: Independent Wage Earners in Chicago, 1880–1930* (Chicago: University of Chicago Press, 1988), 33–38. See also Alice Kessler-Harris, *Out to Work: A History of Wage-Earning Women in the United States* (New York: Oxford University Press, 1982), 230, 258, 262–263.

42. Linda Gordon, *Heroes of Their Own Lives: The Politics and History of Family Violence, Boston, 1880–1960* (New York: Viking Penguin, 1988), 92–95, 98, 107–109, 112–113.

43. Inquest on Collins. See also Inquest on Mary Baxter Moorhead, November 29, 1926, case no. 371–11–1926, Medical Records Department.

44. Inquest on Mary Schwartz.

45. Inquest on Mau. See also Inquest on Rosie Kawera, June 15, 1916, case no. 152–5–1916, Medical Records Department.

46. The second visit is recorded in the Transcript of *People v. Anna Heissler,* 338 Ill. 56 (1930), Case Files, vault no. 44783, Supreme Court of Illinois, Record Series 901, Illinois State Archives, Springfield, Illinois.

47. Inquest on Collins; Inquest on Emily Projahn, October 10, 1916, case no. 26–12–1916, Medical Records Department; Inquest on Elsie Golcher, February 15, 1932, case no. 225–2–32, Medical Records Department; Inquest on Carolina Petrovitis, March 21, 1916, case no. 234–3–1916, Medical Records Department.

48. Laurel Thatcher Ulrich, *A Midwife's Tale: The Life of Martha Ballard, Based on Her Diary, 1785–1812* (New York: Knopf, 1990). On women in immigrant neighborhoods, see Elizabeth Ewen, *Immigrant Women in the Land of Dollars: Life and Culture on the Lower East Side, 1890–1925* (New York: Monthly Review Press, 1985).

49. Ellen Ross notes a sense of "community obligation" among poor London mothers who automatically helped each other with child care. Ellen Ross, *Love and Toil: Motherhood in Outcast London, 1870–1918* (New York: Oxford University Press, 1993), 134–135; Leavitt, *Brought to Bed,* 87–108, 202–203, 208.

50. In eleven cases found through coroner's records, boyfriends helped their unmarried lovers obtain abortions. For example, Inquest on Anna Johnson, May 27, 1915, case no. 77790, Medical Records Department; Inquest on

Mary Nowakowski, April 4, 1935, case no. 80–5–1935, Medical Records Department; Inquest on Mary L. Kissell, August 3, 1937, case no. 300–8–1937, Medical Records Department; Dorothy Dunbar Bromley and Florence Haxton Britten, *Youth and Sex: A Study of 1300 College Students* (New York: Harper and Brothers Publishers, 1938), 262. On dating, see Meyerowitz, *Women Adrift*, 101–106; Kathy Peiss, *Cheap Amusements: Working Women and Leisure in Turn-of-the-Century New York* (Philadelphia: Temple University Press, 1986), 54–55, 108–110.

51. Inquests on Matson, Colbert, Nowakowski, Kissell.

52. Charley Morehouse in Inquest on Matson.

53. See, for example, Statement of Patrick O'Connell in 1907 Inquest on Nellie Walsh included in Transcript of *People v. Beuttner,* 233 Ill. 272 (1908), Case Files, vault no. 30876, Supreme Court of Illinois, Record Series 901.

54. John Harris in Inquest on Anna Marie Dimford, September 30, 1915, case no. 75–11–1915, Medical Records Department.

55. Testimony of Fred Corderay in Inquest on Alma Heidenway, August 21, 1918, case no. 232–8–1918, Medical Records Department. He denied having a sexual relationship with Heidenway.

56. Testimony of Edward Dettman and Annie Cullinan in Inquest on Colbert.

57. Meyerowitz, *Women Adrift,* 118–123.

58. For example, see Joan M. Jensen, "The Death of Rosa: Sexuality in Rural America," *Agricultural History* 67 (fall 1993): 1–12; I am grateful to Daniel Schneider for showing me this article. See also Catharine MacKinnon, "The Male Ideology of Privacy: A Feminist Perspective on the Right to Abortion," *Radical America* 17 (July-August 1983): 23–35 and the responses by Rosalind Pollack Petchesky, "Abortion as 'Violence against Women': A Feminist Critique," *Radical America* 18 (March-June 1984): 64–68; Carole Joffe, "Comments on MacKinnon," *Radical America* 18 (March-June 1984): 68–69.

59. How to assess the female experience of heterosexuality has been a source of crucial debate among feminists. The role of pornography in women's oppression and legal measures to repress it have been especially controversial. See the proposed antipornography ordinance in Andrea Dworkin and Catharine A. MacKinnon, *Pornography and Civil Rights: A New Day for Women's Equality* (n.p., 1988). For analyses of feminist thought on sexual pleasure and danger today and in the nineteenth century, see Carole S. Vance, ed. *Pleasure and Danger: Exploring Female Sexuality* (Boston: Routledge and Kegan Paul, 1984); Ellen Carol DuBois and Linda Gordon, "Seeking Ecstasy on the Battlefield: Danger and Pleasure in Nineteenth-Century Feminist Sexual Thought," *Feminist Studies* 9 (spring 1983): 7–25.

60. Edward A. Balloch, "Criminal Abortion," *AJO* 45 (February 1902): 238.

61. Although Hoffmann may have miscarried, her abortion and death were investigated by the coroner as a criminal abortion. Inquest on Milda Hoffmann, May 29, 1916, case no., 342–5–1916, Medical Records Department. On the rape of young, unmarried women, see Mary E. Odem, *Delinquent Daughters: Protecting and Policing Adolescent Female Sexuality in the United States, 1885–1920* (Chapel Hill: University of North Carolina Press, 1995).

62. Inquest on Edna M. Lamb, February 19, 1917, case no. 43–3–1917, Medical Records Department.

63. Inquest on Petrovitis.

64. Ross, *Love and Toil,* 112–118; Leavitt, *Brought to Bed,* 95. But husbands did sometimes assist; see the illustration of labor in early Virginia in Leavitt, 105.

65. Inquest on Collins; Inquest on Mau.

66. Burnet, "Abortion as the Exciting Cause of Insanity," 401.

67. Gordon, *Woman's Body, Woman's Right,* 102–103, 106, 121–122.

68. Testimony of Earnest Projahn in Inquest on Projahn.

69. Testimony of Earnest Projahn, written statement of Emily Projahn in Inquest on Projahn.

70. Testimony of Dr. C.W. Mercereau and Dr. Garford D.E. Haworth in Inquest on Projahn.

71. Gordon, *Woman's Body, Woman's Right,* chaps. 9, 4.

72. For example, John C. Vaughan, "Birth Control Not Abortion," *BCR* 6 (September 1922): 183; "Birth Control and Abortion," *BCR* 8 (July 1924): 202; "Ten Good Reasons for Birth Control," *BCR* 13 (January 1929), no page no.

73. "Prevention or Abortion—Which?" (July 1923), 182.

74. Rachelle Yarros, "Birth Control Clinics in Chicago," *BCR* 12 (December 1928): 354–355. I have calculated the percentage from figures provided in the article.

75. Kate Simon, *Bronx Primitive: Portraits in a Childhood* (New York: Harper and Row, 1982), 70. I am grateful to Joyce Follet for bringing Simon's book to my attention.

76. The editor further commented, "In the case of many of the opponents of Birth Control this misapprehension is deliberately made . . . to discredit the cause. In other cases it arises out of ignorance." "Prevention or Abortion—Which?" (July 1923), 181.

77. These were constant themes. For example, see "Hard Facts," 16; Margaret Sanger, "Why Not Birth Control Clinics in America?" *BCR* 3 (May 1919): 10; "A Desperate Choice," *BCR* 9 (March 1925): 78; Margaret Sanger, *Motherhood in Bondage* (1928; reprint, Elmsford, N.Y.: Maxwell Reprint, 1958), 394–410. A political challenge to the birth control movement's perspective on abortion did not develop as it did in England nor did a movement for legalization. See Brookes, *Abortion in England,* 79–80, 87; and chapter 5 of this volume.

78. "Letters from Women," Letter No. 10, *BCR* 2 (April 1918): 12; "How Would You Answer This Woman?" *BCR* 5 (March 1921): 14.

79. "Letters from Women," Letter No. 17 and Letter No. 16, *BCR* 2 (June 1918): 12.

80. Ross, *Love and Toil,* 99; Rima D. Apple, *Mothers and Medicine: A Social History of Infant Feeding, 1890–1950* (University of Wisconsin Press, 1987), chap. 6.

81. "A Desperate Choice," 78.

82. Leavitt, *Brought to Bed,* chap. 1.

83. "Appeals from Mothers," *BCR* 6 (August 1922): 150.

84. "Appeals from Mothers," p. 151. See also "Letters from Women," Letter no. 2, *BCR* 2 (January 1918): 13.

85. The Cook County Coroner's report for 1918–1919 showed that the great majority of women who died due to abortions (some of them miscarriages) were married, over 80 percent, and that over half of the women had children already. Most of the mothers had two children or more. Cook County Coroner, *Biennial Report, 1918–1919,* p. 78, Municipal Reference Collection, Chicago Public Library, Chicago, Illinois.

86. See Barbara Katz Rothman's insightful discussion of pregnancy and motherhood, *Recreating Motherhood: Ideology and Technology in a Patriarchal Society* (New York: W. W. Norton, 1989), esp. 106–108.

87. For example, "Letters from Women" (January 1918), 13; "Unemployment," *BCR* 15 (May 1931): 131.

88. Louise Kapp Howe, *Moments on Maple Avenue: The Reality of Abortion* (1984; New York: Warner Books, 1986), 90–91, 117–118, 121–126.

89. "But What Can I Do?" *BCR* 11 (November 1927): 296.

90. Testimony of Lt. William P. O'Brien in Inquest on Mau.

91. These were not all illegal abortions, *Biennial Report, 1918–1919,* 78.

92. See the video, *Motherless: A Legacy of Loss from Illegal Abortions,* produced by Barbara Attie, Janet Goldwater, and Diane Pontius, Filmmakers Library, New York; and interviews with orphans in Miller, *The Worst of Times,* 39–47, 48–57, 237–241.

93. "Letters from Women," Letter no. 14, *BCR* 2 (May 1918): 12.

94. The mother described herself as having "born and raised 6 children." This example illustrates changing norms. Women who grew up in large families themselves adopted the new smaller family norm promoted by the birth control movement. "'Why?'" *BCR* 2 (December 1918): 6.

95. "Hard Facts. Jennie K.," *BCR* 3 (November 1919): 15.

96. Inquest on Margaret Winter, November 13, 1916, case no. 274–11–1916, Medical Records Department.

97. Simon, *Bronx Primitive,* 21, 25, 73; Ross, *Love and Toil,* 148–154.

98. "Letters from Women," Letter No. 17, *BCR* 2 (June 1918): 12. See also "Prevention or Abortion—Which?" (July 1923), 182.

99. Stix, "A Study of Pregnancy Wastage," 357–359; Gebhard et al., *Pregnancy, Birth and Abortion* (New York: Harper and Brothers and Paul B. Hoeber Medical Books, 1958), 114, 120, 109–110, table 54.

100. Gordon, *Woman's Body, Woman's Right,* chap. 8; James Reed, *From Private Vice to Public Virtue: The Birth Control Movement and American Society Since 1830* (New York: Basic Books, 1978), 45; "A Connecticut Physician's Letter," *BCR* 5 (September 1921): 15.

101. Susan J. Kleinberg, "Technology and Women's Work: The Lives of Working Class Women in Pittsburgh, 1870–1900," *Labor History* 17 (winter 1976): 58–72.

102. "Letters from Women," Letter no. 1 (January 1918): 13; Ross, *Love and Toil,* 98–99; on wife-beating in America, Gordon, *Heroes of Their Own Lives,* 250–288.

103. "Letters from Women," Letter no. 1 *BCR* 2 (January 1918), 13.

104. "Prevention or Abortion—Which?" (July 1923), 182; "Prevention or Abortion, Which?" (May 1923), 127. See also "'A Damnably Cruel Dilemma,'" *BCR* 3 (July 1919): 17.

105. Frank A. Stahl, "Some Expressions of Abortive Attempts at Instrumental Abortion," *JAMA* 31 (December 31, 1898): 1560–1561.

106. Maximilian Herzog, "The Pathology of Criminal Abortion," *JAMA* 34 (May 26, 1900): 1310–1311; J. E. Lackner, "Serological Findings in 100 Cases, Bacteriological Findings in 50 Cases, and a Resume of 679 Cases of Abortion at the Michael Reese Hospital," *Surgery, Gynecology, and Obstetrics* 20 (1915): 537; Lewis, "Facts Regarding Criminal Abortion," 945. J. L. Andrews reported the use of knitting needles, rubber catheters, and slippery elm to induce abortions, in "The Greatly Increased Frequency of the Occurrence of Abortion, as Shown by Reports from Memphis Physicians: An Essay on the Causes for the Same," *Transactions of the Medical Society of Tennessee* 72 (1905): 126–127. In 1928 a Cook County Hospital physician reported from patient histories that women used "catheters . . . orange sticks, hairpins, cotton ball, a substance called slippery elm." Dr. Gertrude Engbring in Transcript of *People v. Heissler* (1930); George Erety Shoemaker, "Septicemia from Self-Induced Abortion," *AJO* 35 (June 1897): 637; "Tetanus Follows Attempt to Abort with Chicken Feather," *JAMA* 84 (February 7, 1925): 470.

107. G. D. Royston, "A Statistical Study of the Causes of Abortion," *AJOG* 76 (October 1917): 571–572, quotation on 573.

108. Royston, "Statistical Study," 572–573; Dr. Gertrude Engbring in Transcript of *People v. Heissler* (1930).

109. Bessie Louise Pierce, *The Rise of a Modern City,* vol. 3. of *A History of Chicago* (New York: Knopf, 1957), 188.

110. John S. Haller, *American Medicine in Transition, 1840–1910* (Urbana: University of Illinois Press, 1981), 267–270.

111. Addison Niles, "Criminal Abortion," *Transactions of the Twenty-First Anniversary Meeting of the Illinois State Medical Society* (Chicago: Fergus Printing, 1872), 100; Calvin Schmid reported on 109 abortion deaths in Minneapolis between 1927 and 1936 and found that the catheter was used in 29 cases, slippery elm in 18, in *Social Saga of Two Cities,* 411. "Propaganda for Reform. Chichester's Diamond Brand Pills," *JAMA* 56 (May 27, 1911): 1591.

112. Dr. Frederick D. Newbarr, Detroit, to Editor, July 21, 1920, Abortifacient File, Historical Health Fraud Collection of the AMA (hereafter cited as HHFC), AMA, Chicago, Illinois. See B. E. Ellis, M.D., Indianapolis, to *JAMA,* November 10, 1923, Abortifacient File, HHFC.

113. Ling's office was at 1909 Archer Avenue in Chicago. Letter to AMA from Chicago, August 22, 1922, Abortifacient File, HHFC.

114. Inquest on Anna P. Fazio, February 14, 1929, case no. 217–2–1929, Medical Records Department.

115. Quotations from A.B.C., "Does Public Opinion in the United States Sanction Abortion?," 61, 64.

Chapter 2.   Private Practices

1. "Infanticide," *Chicago Times,* December 15, 1888, pp. 1, 5.

2. Coverage related to the abortion exposé appeared in the *Chicago Times* through January 23, 1889.

3. "The Evil and the Remedy," *Chicago Times,* December 13, 1888, p. 4.

4. Paul Starr, *The Social Transformation of American Medicine* (New York: Basic Books, 1982), 79–144; William G. Rothstein, *American Physicians in the Nineteenth Century: From Sects to Science* (Baltimore: Johns Hopkins University Press, 1972); Thomas Neville Bonner, *Medicine in Chicago: A Chapter in the Social and Scientific Development of a City, 1850–1950,* 2d ed. (1957; reprint, Urbana: University of Illinois, 1991).

5. One physician estimated in 1913 that no more than 13 percent of sick patients were treated in the hospital and not until 1938 did approximately half of all births take place in the hospital, as cited in Charles E. Rosenberg, *The Care of Strangers: The Rise of America's Hospital System* (New York: Basic Books, 1987), 316; Judith Walzer Leavitt, *Brought to Bed: Childbearing in America, 1750–1950* (New York: Oxford University Press, 1986), 171–195, 269; Morris J. Vogel, *The Invention of the Modern Hospital: Boston, 1870–1930* (Chicago: University of Chicago Press, 1980); Rosemary Stevens, *American Medicine and the Public Interest* (New Haven: Yale University Press, 1971), 80–82, 145.

6. Thomas Goebel, "American Medicine and the 'Organizational Synthesis': Chicago Physicians and the Business of Medicine, 1900–1920," *Bulletin of the History of Medicine* 68 (winter 1994): 639–663; Donald E. Konold, *A History of American Medical Ethics* (Madison: State Historical Society for the Department of History, University of Wisconsin, 1962), 11–12, 57–67, 75.

7. Bessie Louise Pierce, *The Rise of a Modern City, 1871–1893,* vol. 3 of *A History of Chicago* (New York: Knopf, 1957), 166, 408–409, 418–419, 408 n. 47.

8. On this idea, see Peter Fritzsche, *Reading Berlin 1900* (Cambridge, Mass.: Harvard University Press, 1996).

9. Emmett Dedmon, *Fabulous Chicago* (New York: Random House, 1953), 73–94; 135–147.

10. Frank Luther Mott, *American Journalism: A History of Newspapers in the United States Through 250 Years, 1690–1940* (New York: Macmillan, 1941), 436–443; Michael Schudson, *Discovering the News: A Social History of American Newspapers* (New York: Basic Books, 1978), 70–74, 86; Norma Green, Stephen Lacy, and Jean Folkerts, "Chicago Journalists at the Turn of the Century: Bohemians All?" *Journalism Quarterly* 66 (winter 1989): 815–816; Judith R. Walkowitz, *City of Dreadful Delight: Narratives of Sexual Danger in Late-Victorian London* (Chicago: University of Chicago Press, 1992), 81–134.

11. Justin E. Walsh, *To Print the News and Raise Hell!, A Biography of Wilbur F. Storey* (Chapel Hill: University of North Carolina Press, 1968), chap. 8 and 216–217.

12. "The Evil and the Remedy," *Chicago Times,* December 13, 1888, p. 4; "Doctors Who Advertise," *Chicago Times,* December 16, 1888, p. 4; "Hercules and the Doctor," cartoon, *Chicago Times,* December 16, 1888, p. 9; "Moral Aids Needed," *Chicago Times,* December 18, 1888, p. 4; "A Noble Work," *Chicago Times,* December 23, 1888, p. 4.

13. Text accompanying cartoon, "It Out-Herods the Days of Herod," *Chicago Times,* December 19, 1888, p. 4.

14. See the cartoons, "It Out-Herods the Days of Herod," *Chicago Times,* December 19, 1888, p. 4; "Hercules and the Baby," *Chicago Times,* December 21, 1888, p. 4; Mott, *American Journalism,* 438–439.

15. "Infanticide," *Chicago Times,* December 12, 1888, p. 1; "The Evil and the Remedy," *Chicago Times,* December 13, 1888, p. 4; "Infanticide," *Chicago Times,* December 15, 1888, p. 5.

16. "Infanticide," *Chicago Times,* December 12, 1888, p. 1.

17. "Infanticide," *Chicago Times,* December 13, 1888, p. 1; "The Evil and the Remedy," *Chicago Times,* December 13, 1888, p. 4.

18. "The Sunday Times," *Chicago Times,* December 15, 1888, p. 4; "To the Readers of 'The Times,'" *Chicago Times,* December 19, 1888, p. 4; "Triple Sheet," *Chicago Times,* December 22, 1888, p. 4.

19. "Infanticide," *Chicago Times,* December 13, 1888, p. 1.

20. "Infanticide," *Chicago Times,* December 15, 1888, p. 1.

21. "Infanticide," *Chicago Times,* December 14, 1888, pp. 1–2. For other examples of midwives who refused to perform abortions, see the Vice Commission of Chicago, *The Social Evil in Chicago, A Study of Existing Conditions with Recommendations by the Vice Commission of Chicago* (1911; reprint, New York: Arno Press, 1970), p. 225; Inquest on Mary L. Kissell, August 3, 1937, case no. 300–8–1937, Medical Records Department.

22. "Infanticide," *Chicago Times,* December 15, 1888, p. 1.

23. See, for example, the sketch of five female portraits, "For the Doctors," which asked, "Guess which one of the above is the 'girl reporter?'" and the sketch "A Souvenir," both in *Chicago Times,* December 21, 1888, p. 4; Editorial from the *St. Louis Republic* reprinted in "Talk About 'The Times,'" *Chicago Times,* December 23, 1888, p. 4. Interest in the reporters themselves was typical of the era, Schudson, *Discovering the News,* 65, 69.

24. "Infanticide," *Chicago Times,* December 18, 1888, pp. 1–2.

25. "Infanticide," *Chicago Times,* December 20, 1888, p. 5.

26. "Infanticide," *Chicago Times,* December 17, 1888, p. 5.

27. "Infanticide," *Chicago Times,* December 21, 1888, p. 1. On Clark Street, Emmett Dedmon, *Fabulous Chicago* (New York: Random House, 1953), 140, 144–145.

28. "Professional Abortionists," *JAMA* 11:26 (December 29, 1888): 913; Wilhelm Becker, "The Medical, Ethical, and Forensic Aspects of Fatal Criminal Abortion," *Wisconsin Medical Journal* 7 (April 1909): 624–626.

29. Thirty-one of the thirty-four physicians who agreed to perform abortions can be identified; of these, twenty-two were Regulars. Of the forty-eight who agreed to help in some fashion, forty-two can be identified. Thirty-three, or over two-thirds of the total, were Regulars. At least twenty-one belonged to a medical society, including some Irregular societies, and twenty-one belonged to none. I am grateful to Rose Holz and Lynne Curry for collecting and tabulating this biographical information. Biographical information located in *Medical and Surgical Register of the United States* (Detroit: R. L. Polk, 1886 and 1890 editions); *McDonald's Illinois State Medical Directory: A Complete List of Physicians in the State* (Chicago: J. Newton McDonald, 1891); *Connorton's Directory of Physicians, Dentists, and Druggists of Chicago, Including Suburbs in Cook County* (Chicago: J. Newton McDonald, 1889).

30. "Infanticide," *Chicago Times,* December 16, 1888, p. 9; "Infanticide," *Chicago Times,* December 18, 1888, p. 2; J. H. Etheridge to Editor, *Chicago Times,* December 18, 1888, p. 5.

31. "Infanticide," *Chicago Times*, December 18, 1888, p. 2; Walkowitz, *City of Dreadful Delight*, 212–214.

32. "Awake! Arise!" *Chicago Times*, January 2, 1889, p. 4. I counted over sixty-five letters to the editor of the *Chicago Times* from doctors in the two-week period of the exposé. For example, Benjamin Miller to Editor, *Chicago Times*, December 21, 1888, p. 3.

33. "Infanticide," *Chicago Times*, December 17, 1888, p. 1; "Infanticide," *Chicago Times*, December 20, 1888, p. 1; "Infanticide," *Chicago Times*, December 22, 1888, p. 1; "From the Girl Reporter," *Chicago Times*, December 23, 1888, p. 9.

34. Council Minutes, December 17, 1888, vol. 1887–1892, pp. 104–105, Chicago Medical Society Records, Archives and Manuscripts Department, Chicago Historical Society, Chicago, Illinois. Jacob Franks and see William T. Thackerey in "The Doctors Will Investigate," *Chicago Times*, December 18, 1888, p. 2. The *Times* reported that 250 people attended this meeting.

35. Quotation by Etheridge in "Infanticide," *Chicago Times*, December 18, 1888, p. 2; Council Minutes, December 17, 1888, vol. 1887–1892, p. 105, Chicago Medical Society Records.

36. Council Minutes, January 7, 1889, vol. 1887–1892, pp. 108–112, Chicago Medical Society Records; "Thurston Is Expelled," *Chicago Times*, January 8, 1889, p. 1.

37. Bonner, *Medicine in Chicago*, 64–67, 84–103; *Connorton's Directory*, 31–53, 61–67.

38. "Professional Abortionists," 913; Dr. J. W. Hervey to Editor, *JAMA* 12 (January 12, 1889): 69.

39. Others have made similar observations. Norman Himes, *Medical History of Contraception* (1936; reprint, New York: Gamut Press, 1963), 282; Linda Gordon, *Woman's Body, Woman's Right: Birth Control in America*, rev. and updated (1976; reprint, New York: Penguin Books, 1990), 167–168.

40. Regina Markell Morantz-Sanchez, *Sympathy and Science: Women Physicians in American Medicine* (New York: Oxford University Press, 1985), 188–189, 220; James C. Mohr, *Abortion in America: The Origins and Evolution of National Policy, 1800–1900* (New York: Oxford University Press, 1978), 161; Mary Roth Walsh, *"Doctors Wanted: No Women Need Apply": Sexual Barriers in the Medical Profession, 1835–1975* (New Haven: Yale University Press, 1977), 145.

41. "Seeking the Remedy," *Chicago Times*, January 5, 1889, p. 8; "Infanticide," *Chicago Times*, December 16, 1888, p. 9. Dr. Emilie Siegmund agreed to perform an abortion, "Infanticide," *Chicago Times*, December 15, 1888, p. 1.

42. "Infanticide," *Chicago Times*, December 19, 1888, p. 7. Letters from P. Curran, M.D., and Birney Hand, M.D., confirmed that most women seeking abortions were married, in "Infanticide," *Chicago Times*, December 22, 1888, p. 5.

43. "Infanticide. Retrospective Thoughts," *Chicago Times*, December 25, 1888, p. 1.

44. "Bring the Husbands to Book," *Chicago Times*, December 28, 1888, p. 1; "Seeking the Remedy," *Chicago Times*, January 5, 1889, p. 5. See also "A Vigorous Letter from a Woman Physician," *Chicago Times*, December 16, 1888,

p. 9. On nineteenth-century feminists' views, see Mohr, *Abortion in America,* 111–113; Gordon, *Woman's Body, Woman's Right,* chap. 5.

45. Reprint from Galesburg, Illinois, in "Talk About 'The Times,'" *Chicago Times,* December 23, 1888, p. 4; partial reprint of paper by Dr. H. H. Markham, "Seeking the Remedy, Duty of the Doctors," *Chicago Times,* January 1, 1889, p. 3.

46. Reprint from *Chicago Medical Visitor* in "Infanticide in Chicago," *Chicago Times,* January 23, 1889, p. 4; "The Infanticide Revelations," *JAMA* 12 (January 12, 1889): 55.

47. "The Infanticide Revelations," 56.

48. "He Did His Full Duty," *Chicago Times,* December 22, 1888, p. 5.

49. "Infanticide," *Chicago Times,* December 12, 1888, p. 1; "The Cream City Needs Just Such a Cleansing," Letter from Milwaukee, *Chicago Times,* December 22, 1888, p. 5; "The Devilish Crime Is Not Confined to Chicago," *Chicago Times,* December 22, 1888, p. 5; "An Adjunct to the Remedy," Letter from Monticello, Illinois, *Chicago Times,* December 31, 1888, p. 5.

50. Inez C. Philbrick, "Social Causes of Criminal Abortion," *Medical Record* 66 (September 24, 1904): 491; Henry W. Cattell, "Some Medico-Legal Aspects of Abortion," *Bulletin of the American Academy of Medicine* 8 (1907): 339; Earnest F. Oakley, "Legal Aspect of Abortion," *AJOG* 3 (January 1922): 38.

51. Illinois, *Public Laws of Illinois,* 1867, p. 89.

52. See chapter 8 of this volume.

53. For historical analyses of the interplay between society and disease definition and treatment, see Joan Jacobs Brumberg, *Fasting Girls: The Emergence of Anorexia Nervosa as a Modern Disease* (Cambridge: Harvard University Press, 1988); Allan M. Brandt, *No Magic Bullet: A Social History of Venereal Disease in the United States Since 1880,* expanded ed. (New York: Oxford University Press, 1987); Charles E. Rosenberg, *The Cholera Years: The United States in 1832, 1849, and 1866* (Chicago: University of Chicago Press, 1962).

54. Peter J. O'Callaghan and Charles B. Reed in "Chicago Medical Society. Regular Meeting Held Nov. 23, 1904," *JAMA* 43 (December 17, 1904): 1890; Christian Johnson, "Therapeutic Abortion," *St. Paul Medical Journal* 9 (1907): 240, 241–242; Ronald L. Numbers, "A Note on Medical Education in Wisconsin," in *Wisconsin Medicine: Historical Perspectives,* edited by Ronald L. Numbers and Judith Walzer Leavitt (Madison: University of Wisconsin Press, 1981), 183.

55. Indications that necessitated abortion in order to preserve the pregnant woman's life included diseases of the kidneys, chronic heart or respiratory disease, eclampsia, cancers of the rectum, uterus, and breast, severe cases of rheumatism, contracted pelvis, uterine cysts, placenta previa, and pernicious anaemia. W. C. Bowers, "Justifiable Artificial Abortion and Induced Premature Labor," *JAMA* 33 (September 2, 1899): 568–569; E. S. McKee, "Abortion," *AJO* 24 (October 1891): 1333–1334; Frank A. Higgins, "The Propriety, Indications and Methods for the Termination of Pregnancy," *JAMA* 43 (November 19, 1904): 1531–1533.

56. Quotation from Bowers, "Justifiable Artificial Abortion," 569; phrase from R. C. Brown, "Vomiting," *Cyclopedia of Medicine,* edited by George Mor-

ris Piersol, vol. 12 (Philadelphia: F. A. Davis, 1935), 945. On vomiting in the nineteenth century, see Joseph Taber Johnson, "The Mechanical Treatment of the Vomiting of Pregnancy," *JAMA* 6 (March 13, 1886): 285. On the cure for this condition, see Paul Titus, "Hyperemesis Gravidarum: Treatment by Intravenous Injections of Glucose and Carbohydrate Feedings," *JAMA* 85 (August 15, 1925): 488–493, as cited in Kristin Luker, *Abortion and the Politics of Motherhood* (Berkeley: University of California Press, 1984), 55, 275 n. For continuing discussion, see Henricus J. Stander, *Williams Obstetrics: A Textbook for the Use of Students and Practitioners,* 7th ed., a revision and enlargement of the text originally written by J. Whitridge Williams (New York: D. Appleton-Century, 1936), 521. The Children's Bureau found that vomiting remained an important indication for therapeutic abortions in the late 1920s, U.S. Department of Labor, Children's Bureau, *Maternal Mortality in Fifteen States,* Bureau publication no. 223 (Washington, D.C.: Government Printing Office, 1934), 108.

57. Paul Titus, "A Statistical Study of a Series of Abortions Occurring in the Obstetrical Department of the Johns Hopkins Hospital," *AJO* 65 (June 1912): 960–961; Taussig, *Abortion, Spontaneous and Induced: Medical and Social Aspects* (St. Louis: C. V. Mosby, 1936), 281–282, see table on 282; Irving K. Perlmutter, "Analysis of Therapeutic Abortions, Bellevue Hospital 1935–1945," *AJOG* 53 (June 1947): 1012.

58. Joseph B. DeLee, *The Principles and Practice of Obstetrics,* 2d ed. (Philadelphia: W. B. Saunders, 1916), 1045; E. A. Weiss, "Some Moral and Ethical Aspects of Feticide," *AJO* 67 (January 1913): 76, 73; Walter B. Dorsett, "Criminal Abortion in Its Broadest Sense," *JAMA* 51 (September 19, 1908): 957. See also Edward P. Davis, "Therapeutic Abortion," *Therapeutic Gazette* 43 (June 15, 1919): 389–390.

59. "Is Abortion Justifiable in the Insane Pregnant?" *JAMA* 38 (January 4, 1902): 69; Response in "Queries and Minor Notes. Is Abortion Justifiable in the Insane Pregnant?" *JAMA* 38 (January 18, 1902): 213. R. Finley Gayle commented that "older physicians" had aborted women for eugenic reasons in "The Psychiatric Consideration of Abortion," *Southern Medicine and Surgery* 91 (April 1929): 251. On eugenics, see Gordon, *Woman's Body, Woman's Right,* 118–132; Mark H. Haller, *Eugenics: Hereditarian Attitudes in American Thought* (New Brunswick, N.J.: Rutgers University Press, 1963), 95–143.

60. "Pregnancy from Rape Does Not Justify Abortion," *JAMA* 43 (August 6, 1904): 413.

61. "Therapeutic Abortion," *JAMA* 92 (February 16 1929): 581.

62. H. Douglas Singer, "Mental Disease and the Induction of Abortion," *JAMA* 91 (December 29, 1928): 2042–2044; Gayle, "The Psychiatric Consideration of Abortion," 252–254.

63. "Pregnancy and Contracted Pelvis," *JAMA* 38 (February 8, 1902): 433.

64. Ibid. Professor H. J. Boldt believed that the patient with contracted pelvis should decide whether to have an abortion or a cesarean section. H. J. Boldt, "The Treatment of Abortion," *JAMA* 46 (March 17, 1906): 791.

65. Judith Walzer Leavitt, "The Growth of Medical Authority, Technology, and Morals in Turn-of-the-Century Obstetrics," *Medical Anthropology Quarterly* 1 (September 1987): 230–255; Carey Culbertson, "Therapeutic Abortion

and Sterilization," *The Surgical Clinics of Chicago* 1 (1917): 608; Evelyn Fine, "'Belly Ripping Has Become a Mania': A History of the Cesarean Section Operation in Twentieth Century America" (master's thesis, University of Wisconsin, Madison, Department of the History of Science, 1982), 4–6, 8–12, 42.

66. On choosing the family physician, George Rosen, *The Structure of American Medical Practice, 1875–1941,* edited by Charles E. Rosenberg (Philadelphia: University of Pennsylvania Press, 1983), 22. Quotations from Becker, "Medical, Ethical, and Forensic Aspects," 624; E. F. Fish, "Criminal Abortion," *Milwaukee Medical Journal* 17 (April 1909): 107–108. See also Dorsett, "Criminal Abortion in Its Broadest Sense," 958.

67. "The Case of Robert Thompson," *JAMA* 92 (February 16, 1929): 579. Similar networks in Chicago are analyzed further in chapter 5 of this volume.

68. For examples, "Medicolegal. Revocation of License for Conviction of Offense Involving Moral Turpitude," *JAMA* 68 (February 10, 1917): 485; "Medical News. INDIANA. Sentenced for Illegal Operation," *JAMA* 93 (July 13, 1929): 125.

69. Judith Walzer Leavitt has similarly argued for the importance of analyzing nineteenth-century rural medical practice in terms of its location within the domestic domain in "'A Worrying Profession': The Domestic Environment of Medical Practice in Mid-Nineteenth-Century America," *Bulletin of the History of Medicine* 69 (spring 1995): 1–29.

70. Kate Simon, *Bronx Primitive: Portraits in a Childhood* (New York: Harper and Row, Perennial Library, 1982), 68–70, quotation on 70. From the context, I conclude that this doctor practiced during the 1920s, perhaps into the 1930s and longer. See also B. Liber, "As a Doctor Sees It," *BCR* 2 (February-March 1918): 10.

71. Becker, "The Medical, Ethical, and Forensic Aspects of Fatal Criminal Abortion," 624.

72. In this particular case, Aiken was convicted but appealed his case to the state Supreme Court of Illinois, which reversed the conviction and remanded it back. I do not know if he was retried. *Aiken v. the People,* 183 Ill. 215 (1899); Transcript of *Aiken v. the People,* 183 Ill. 215 (1899), Case Files, vault no. 8105, Supreme Court of Illinois, Record Series 901.

73. Denslow Lewis, "Facts Regarding Criminal Abortion," *JAMA* 35 (October 13, 1900): 945; Mary Dixon-Jones, "Criminal Abortion—Its Evil and Its Sad Consequences," continued, *WMJ* 3 (September 1894): 66; W. W. Parker, "In Opposition to Woman Doctors in Insane Asylums," *JAMA* 22 (March 31, 1894): 479.

74. Rudolph W. Holmes in "Symposium on Criminal Abortion," *JAMA* 43 (December 17, 1904): 1891; "Criminal Advertisements," *JAMA* 37 (August 10, 1901): 393. Post Office officials used classified advertisements to investigate and prosecute midwives and doctors for abortion advertising in 1912. Dr. Margaret Livingston had advertised herself as a "specialist for diseases of women." See Govt. Ex. 9 in *U.S. v. Margaret Livingston,* November 22, 1912, Case no. 5084, Criminal Docket Book no. 8 (Criminal Case Files), Northern District of Illinois, Eastern Division, Record Group 21, Records of the District Courts of the United States, National Archives—Great Lakes Region, Chicago, Illinois. For

examples of nineteenth-century advertisements, see Mohr, *Abortion in America,* 51, 52, 54, 56, 57.

75. See Charlotte G. Borst, *Catching Babies: The Professionalization of Childbirth, 1870–1920* (Cambridge, Mass.: Harvard University Press, 1995).

76. I have identified sixty-one abortionists in the Chicago area between 1890 and 1930. Thirty-eight were physicians, twenty-three midwives.

77. Grace Abbott, "The Midwife in Chicago," *The American Journal of Sociology* 20 (March 1915): 687. Nationally, midwives had delivered half the country's babies in 1900, but only 15 percent by 1930. Leavitt, *Brought to Bed,* 12, graph; Judy Barrett Litoff, *American Midwives: 1860 to the Present* (Westport, Conn.: Greenwood Press, 1978), 141.

78. In the St. Louis study, a large proportion of the abortions were self-induced (thirty, or 36 percent). I calculated the percentages from the data presented in table 1 in Royston. G. D. Royston, "A Statistical Study of the Causes of Abortion," *AJOG* 76 (October 1917): 573.

79. Marie E. Kopp, *Birth Control in Practice: Analysis of Ten Thousand Case Histories of the Birth Control Clinical Research Bureau* (1933; reprint, New York: Arno Press, 1972), table 8.

80. Jerome E. Bates and Edward Zawadzki, appendix C in *Criminal Abortion: A Study in Medical Sociology* (Springfield, Ill.: Charles C. Thomas, 1964), 202. In the last decade of this study, it is unlikely that any midwives would still have been practicing, but, unfortunately, the authors did not break down their findings by decade.

81. Caroline Hedger reported that 57 of 363 Chicago midwives (or 6 percent, my calculation) were "suspected of practicing abortion." F. Elisabeth Crowell investigated 500 New York midwives in 1906 and found 176 midwives who had been convicted of abortion or agreed to perform one (35 percent, my calculation) and suspected over half the midwives practiced abortion. The 1908 study of Chicago midwives found 49 out of 223 midwives who "agreed to operate" and concluded that "at least one-third should be classified as criminal." The Baltimore study found almost one third of the midwives (48 of 150) were "suspected of criminal practice." A 1912 study of Massachusetts found that 5 percent (5 of 91) of the midwives were suspected of performing abortions. Caroline Hedger, "Investigation of 363 Midwives in Chicago," *Transactions of the American Association for the Study and Prevention of Infant Mortality* 3 (1912): 264, table 3; F. Elisabeth Crowell, "The Midwives of New York," *Charities and the Commons* 17 (January 1907): 667–677, reprint in Judy Barrett Litoff, *The American Midwife Debate: A Sourcebook on Its Modern Origins* (New York: Greenwood Press, 1986), 44; Rudolph W. Holmes et al., "The Midwives of Chicago," *JAMA* 50 (April 25, 1908): 1347–1348; Mary Sherwood, "The Midwives of Baltimore," *JAMA* 52 (June 19, 1909): 2010; James Lincoln Huntington, "Midwives in Massachusetts," *Boston Medical and Surgical Journal* 167 (October 17, 1912): 547.

82. Recorded statement of Emily Projahn and testimony of Earnest Projahn, Inquest on Emily Projahn, October 10, 1916, case no. 26–12–1916, Medical Records Department.

83. Of twenty-one cases where it can be determined where the operation

occurred, all but three took place in the physician's office (which in some cases was the doctor's home). The other three were induced in hospitals run by the doctor.

84. Inquest on Viola Koepping, June 7, 1929, case no. 246–6–29, Medical Records Department.

85. *People v. Rongetti* 331 Ill. 581 (1928), p. 584; "Woman Confesses Murder of Baby," *Chicago Daily News,* [July] 1928, Abortionists Files, HHFC. See also Joseph G. Stern in *Chicago Tribune,* January 10, 1929, Abortionists Files, HHFC.

86. There are twenty cases with information on fees paid to Chicago doctors for abortions between 1890 and 1930. The average fee stated to prospective patients would be higher than what doctors actually received.

87. Inquest on Ester Reed, June 9, 1914, case no. 73771, Medical Records Department.

88. McKee, "Abortion," 1334; Frank A. Higgins, "The Propriety, Indications, and Methods for the Termination of Pregnancy," *JAMA* 43 (November 19, 1904): 1533; Frederick J. Taussig, *The Prevention and Treatment of Abortion* (St. Louis: C. V. Mosby, 1910), 91–121; Taussig, *Abortion,* 352–354, 322–340.

89. Ten Chicago physicians who performed abortions used instruments of some kind, perhaps uterine sounds to open the cervix or curettes to scrape out the uterus. For illustrations of instruments, see Taussig, *The Prevention and Treatment of Abortion,* 78, 92, 120.

90. Inquest on Edna Lamb, February 19, 1917, case no. 43–3–1917, Medical Records Department.

91. Catherine Heidman as quoted by Harry Golcher in Inquest on Elsie Golcher, February 16, 1932, case no. 225–2–32, Medical Records Department.

92. Of thirty-eight identified abortion providers in the Chicago area, twenty-seven are identified as Regulars. Five of these physicians had graduated from irregular schools, but each of them was identified as a Regular in the directory published by the AMA. I have therefore counted them as Regulars, but even if they were subtracted, the majority of the physician-abortionists in this sample would still be Regulars. That Homeopaths and Eclectics now considered themselves Regulars and the AMA described them as such, despite their education, demonstrates the process of consolidation of all sects into Regulars in the early twentieth century. Biographical data found in *American Medical Directory* 1912–1940 (Chicago: American Medical Association); *Polk's Medical and Surgical Register of the United States* (1896); Chicago Medical Society, *History of Medicine and Surgery and Physicians and Surgeons of Chicago* (Chicago: Biographical Publishing, 1922).

93. Mary Elizabeth Fiorenza, "Midwifery and the Law in Illinois and Wisconsin, 1877 to 1917" (master's thesis, University of Wisconsin, Madison, 1985), 35–36. Holmes et al., "The Midwives of Chicago," 1346, 1347, table 1. The African American population in Chicago before World War I was small; in 1913 African Americans made up only 2.5 percent of Chicago's population. Louise DeKoven Bowen, "The Colored People of Chicago" (Juvenile Protective Association, 1913) Jane Addams Collection, reel 54, Department of Special Collections, The University Library, University of Illinois-Chicago.

94. Inquest on Rosie Kawera, June 15, 1916, case no. 152–5–1916, Medical Records Department.

95. "Infanticide," *Chicago Times,* December 13, 1888, p. 1.

96. On the issue of refusing male physicians during childbirth, see Abbott, "The Midwife in Chicago," 685.

97. Inquest on Kawera; Inquest on Frauciszka Gawlik, February 19, 1916, case no. 27–3–1916, Medical Records Department. On this issue, see Abbott, "The Midwife in Chicago," 684–685; Litoff, *American Midwives,* 27–30; Eugene Declerq, "The Nature and Style of Practice of Immigrant Midwives in Early Twentieth-Century Massachusetts," *Journal of Social History* 19 (1985): 113–129. In *Catching Babies,* Charlotte Borst points out the preference of immigrant women for doctors who were either foreign-born themselves or children of the foreign-born and who understood their culture and language.

98. Hedger, "Investigation of 363 Midwives in Chicago," 264, table 3; Jane Pacht Brickman, "Public Health, Midwives, and Nurses, 1880–1930" in *Nursing History: New Perspectives, New Possibilities,* edited by Ellen Condliffe Lagemann (New York: Teacher's College Press, 1983), 71. I have calculated the average fee for an abortion charged by the midwives from the figures given in the 1910 report. The fees ranged from $10 to $50. Chicago Vice Commission, *The Social Evil in Chicago,* 225–227.

99. There were twelve cases with information on fees paid to midwives for abortions between 1900 and 1930. The range was $4 to $35, and the most frequent fee was $25.

100. Inquest on Kawera; *People v. Wyherk,* 347 Ill. 28 (1931), p. 30; Inquest on Matilda Olson, April 30, 1918, case no. 289–4–1918, Medical Records Department. On check-ups by midwives, see Hedger, "Investigation of 363 Midwives in Chicago," 264; Litoff, *American Midwives,* 28–29.

101. Chicago Vice Commission, *The Social Evil in Chicago,* 225; Inquest on Esther Stark, June 12, 1917, case no. 65–6–1917, Medical Records Department. Also see Inquest on Bertha Dombrowski, February 23, 1917, case no. 223–3–1917, Medical Records Department; Holmes et al., "The Midwives of Chicago," 1349.

102. Chicago Vice Commission, *The Social Evil in Chicago,* 225–227.

103. First quotation is in Holmes et al., "The Midwives of Chicago," 1349. Last quotation is in testimony of Robert Crelly in Inquest on Kissell. See also Abbott, "The Midwife in Chicago," 691; *People v. Patrick,* 277 Ill. 210 (1917), p. 212; "Officials Plan Fight to Curb Abortion Evil," n.p., June 7, 1915, Abortionists Files, HHFC.

104. Quotations from Transcript of *People v. Wyherk,* 347 Ill. 28 (1931) Case Files, vault no. 45804, Supreme Court of Illinois, Record Series 901; Styskal in Inquest on Margaret B. Winter, November 13, 1916, case no. 274–11–1916, Medical Records Department; Haisler in Inquest on Catherine Mau, March 12, 1928, case no. 390–3–1928, Medical Records Department.

105. Litoff, *American Midwives,* 139. For a table showing the national distribution of midwives, see Louis S. Reed, *Midwives, Chiropodists, and Optometrists: Their Place in Medical Care* (Chicago: University of Chicago Press, 1932), 5–6, 67, table 1A.

106. *Cook County Coroner's Quadrennial Report, 1908–1922,* p. 20, Municipal Reference Collection.

107. *Maternal Mortality in Fifteen States,* 103.

108. Transcript of *People v. Hagenow,* 236 Ill. 514 (1908), Case Files, vault no. 31202, Supreme Court of Illinois, Record Series 901; *People v. Hagenow,* 334 Ill. 341 (1929). I do not know how long Hagenow was in prison, but in 1907 she had been convicted and sentenced to twenty years imprisonment (a conviction upheld by the Illinois State Supreme Court).

109. On maternal mortality see Irvine Loudon, "Maternal Mortality: 1880–1950. Some Regional and International Comparisons," *Social History of Medicine* 1 (August 1988): 186, figure A, 210–211; Joyce Antler and Daniel M. Fox, "The Movement toward a Safe Maternity: Physician Accountability in New York City, 1915–1940," *Bulletin of the History of Medicine* 50 (1976): 569–595, reprint in *Sickness and Health in America: Readings in the History of Medicine and Public Health,* edited by Judith Walzer Leavitt and Ronald L. Numbers (Madison: University of Wisconsin Press, 1978), 375–376, 386. For a different view of how trends in maternal mortality changed over time, see Edward Shorter, *A History of Women's Bodies* (New York: Basic Books, 1982), 130–138, 193–195.

110. The 14 percent figure is the sum of abortions categorized in the study as "induced," which includes both self-induced abortions and "criminal" abortions induced by others (11 percent), and those counted as "type not reported" (3 percent) because the researchers suspected that the latter were also induced abortions. It is a mistake to assume as some scholars have that illegal abortions were responsible for the total proportion of maternal deaths assigned to abortion (25 percent), because this total includes deaths following spontaneous abortions, or miscarriages (8 percent), and deaths following therapeutic abortions (3 percent). These latter figures show the dangers of medical intervention. The report discusses the problem of physicians curetting when they should not. Furthermore, it is incorrect to assume that all septic abortion cases were illegal abortions, because physicians responding to spontaneous abortions or performing therapeutic abortions also introduced infections and caused deaths. Finally, the international classification list of maternal mortality cannot be relied upon either because of the way it assigned abortions to other causes and included cases that should not have been. The handful of "certified" criminal abortions were assigned to "homicide." *Maternal Mortality in Fifteen States,* 103–115.

111. Dorothy Reed Mendenhall, "Prenatal and Natal Conditions in Wisconsin," *Wisconsin Medical Journal* 15 (March 1917): 353, as cited in Leavitt, *Brought to Bed,* 56–57, 231 n; Antler and Fox, "The Movement toward a Safe Maternity," 381; Charles R. King, "The New York Maternal Mortality Study: A Conflict of Professionalization," *Bulletin of the History of Medicine* 65 (winter 1991): 482, 484, 489; Shorter concludes that midwives and doctors were "about equally septic" in attending deliveries, in *A History of Women's Bodies,* 137. Loudon finds that home deliveries tended to be safer, whether by M.D. or midwife, than hospital deliveries, in "Maternal Mortality," 219–221.

112. Cook County data in "Officials Plan Fight to Curb Abortion Evil," June 7, 1915, no name of newspaper, Abortionists Files, HHFC; Becker, "The Medical, Ethical, and Forensic Aspects of Fatal Criminal Abortion," 620; Calvin Schmid, *Social Saga of Two Cities: An Ecological and Statistical Study of*

Social Trends in Minneapolis and St. Paul (Minneapolis: Minneapolis Council of Social Agencies, 1937), 410–411.

113. Taussig, *Abortion,* 222–238, quotation on 225–226. Taussig believed nonphysicians to be more responsible for infections. Taussig summarizes the history of the debate around curetting as a treatment for miscarriage and criminal abortion cases on pages 156–158. Specialists disagreed over whether or not to intervene and whether to use the curette or other methods. Some believed too many general practitioners lacked gynecological expertise, yet actively intervened in all abortion cases with the curette. H. J. Boldt, "The Treatment of Abortion," *JAMA* 46 (March 17, 1906): 792; Discussion of Frederick J. Taussig, "What Shall We Teach the General Practitioner Concerning the Treatment of Abortion?" *JAMA* 52 (May 8, 1909): 1530–1531.

114. Lester C. Hall in Frank A. Higgins, "The Propriety, Indications, and Methods for the Termination of Pregnancy," 1534. The experience of abortion in the Soviet Union, which legalized abortion in 1920, showed that abortion could be safe. Paul Lublinsky, "Birth Control in Soviet Russia," *BCR* 12 (May 1928): 143; Frederick J. Taussig, "The Abortion Problem in Russia," *AJOG* 22 (July 1931): 134–139.

115. Rosemary Stevens, *American Medicine and the Public Interest* (New Haven: Yale University Press, 1971), 78–82, 96, 127–128; Ronald L. Numbers, *Almost Persuaded: American Physicians and Compulsory Health Insurance, 1912–1920* (Baltimore: Johns Hopkins University Press, 1978), 4–5; Leavitt, *Brought to Bed,* 163–168.

116. Others have made this argument about attendants during childbirth; Antler and Fox, "The Movement toward a Safe Maternity," 375–392; Leavitt, *Brought to Bed,* chap. 6; King, "The New York Maternal Mortality Study," 484, 489–491. Today, legal abortion is much safer than childbirth. The Centers for Disease Control reported that the risk of a woman dying as a result of childbirth was seven times higher than the risk of a woman who had an abortion. Cited in Rosalind Pollack Petchesky, *Abortion and Woman's Choice: The State, Sexuality, and Reproductive Freedom,* rev. ed. (1984; reprint Boston: Northeastern University Press, 1990), 310.

Chapter 3.   Antiabortion Campaigns, Private and Public

1. Joseph Taber Johnson, "Abortion and Its Effects," *AJO* 33 (January 1896): 86–97; James Foster Scott, "Criminal Abortion," *AJO* 33 (January 1896): 72–86, discussion, 128–132.

2. The phrase is Kristin Luker's, *Abortion and the Politics of Motherhood* (Berkeley: University of California Press, 1984), chap. 3–5.

3. On specialists, see Charlotte G. Borst, "The Professionalization of Obstetrics: Childbirth Becomes a Medical Specialty," in *Women, Health, and Medicine in America: A Historical Handbook,* edited by Rima D. Apple (New York: Garland Publishing, 1990), 197–216; Frances E. Kobrin, "The American Midwife Controversy: A Crisis of Professionalization," in *Women and Health in America: Historical Readings,* edited by Judith Walzer Leavitt (Madison: University of Wisconsin Press, 1984), 318–326.

4. The section was renamed several times after it was formed in 1860. Harold Speert, *Obstetrics and Gynecology in America: A History* (Chicago: American College of Obstetricians and Gynecologists, 1980), 115–116.

5. J. Milton Duff, "Chairman's Address," *JAMA* 21 (August 26, 1893): 292; C. S. Bacon, "The Legal Responsibility of the Physician for the Unborn Child," *JAMA* 46 (June 30, 1906): 1981–1984; Walter B. Dorsett, "Criminal Abortion in Its Broadest Sense," *JAMA* 51 (September 19, 1908): 957–961; H. G. Wetherill, "Retrospection and Introspection: Our Opportunities and Obligations," *Transactions of the Section on Obstetrics and Diseases of Women of the American Medical Association* (1911), 17–31.

6. See the introduction, this volume; James C. Mohr, *Abortion in America: The Origins and Evolution of National Policy, 1800–1900* (New York: Oxford University Press, 1978), 78, 147–170.

7. Duff, "Chairman's Address," 292.

8. James C. Mohr has also examined the attempts to suppress abortion in Chicago in the 1900s, "Patterns of Abortion and the Response of American Physicians, 1790–1930," in Leavitt, *Women and Health in America*, 119–120.

9. Meeting of January 12, 1904, Council Minutes, 1903–1905, vol. 19, Chicago Medical Society Records, Archives and Manuscripts Department, Chicago Historical Society, Chicago, Illinois. For biographical information, see Rudolph W. Holmes, Deceased Physician Master File, AMA; Charles Sumner Bacon, Deceased Physician Master File; C. S. Bacon, "Failures of Midwives in Asepsis," *JAMA* 28 (February 6, 1897): 247; Charles B. Reed, Deceased Physicians Master File.

10. This is based on my reading of the *Journal of the National Medical Association* (*JNMA*) from 1909 through 1973, vol. 1–65. For black women seeking abortions from black doctors, see J. W. Walker in discussion of Val Do Turner, "Fertility of Women," *JNMA* 5 (October-December 1913): 250. For an antiabortion article, see Barnett M. Rhetta, "A Plea for the Lives of the Unborn," *JNMA* 7 (July-September 1915): 292.

11. Charles B. Reed, "Therapeutic and Criminal Abortion," *Illinois Medical Journal* 7 (January 1905): 27.

12. Mary A. Dixon-Jones, "Criminal Abortion—Its Evils and Its Sad Consequences," *WMJ* 3 (August 1894): 34–38, quotation on 34; Mary A. Dixon-Jones, "Criminal Abortion—Its Evils and Its Sad Consequences" continued, *WMJ* 3 (September 1894): 61, quotation on 60; remark of A. McDermid in George J. Engelmann, "The Increasing Sterility of American Women," *JAMA* 37 (October 5, 1901): 896–897.

13. E. E. Hume in C. J. Aud, "In What Per Cent, Is the Regular Profession Responsible for Criminal Abortions, and What is the Remedy?" *Kentucky Medical Journal* 2 (September 1904): 100; William McCollum called for "missionary work" in this area in "Criminal Abortion," *JAMA* 26 (February 8, 1896): 258.

14. Dr. Stuver in Minnie C. T. Love, "Criminal Abortion," *Colorado Medicine* 1 (1903–1904): 60.

15. "Chicago Medical Society. Regular Meeting, Held Nov. 23, 1904. Symposium on Criminal Abortion," *JAMA* 43 (December 17, 1904): 1891. See also J. L. Andrews, "The Greatly Increased Frequency of the Occurrence of Abor-

tion, as Shown by Reports from Memphis Physicians: An Essay on the Causes for the Same," *Transactions of the Tennessee State Medical Association* 72 (1905): 136.

16. C. P. McNabb and others in Andrews, "The Greatly Increased Frequency of the Occurrence of Abortion," 139–142. In the 1888 investigation of abortion in Chicago, many physicians suggested that the woman marry, for example, Dr. J. Harvey, "Infanticide," *Chicago Times,* December 21, 1888, p. 1.

17. Meeting of January 12, 1904, Chicago Medical Society Records; "Chicago Medical Society. Regular Meeting, Held Nov. 23, 1904. Symposium on Criminal Abortion," 1889; Meeting of October 1905, Council Minutes, October 1905-July 1907, vol. 20, Chicago Medical Society Records. Apparently this event did not attract local press; neither the *Chicago Tribune,* November 20–26, 1904, nor the *Chicago Record-Herald,* November 21–26, 1904, covered it.

18. Frederick J. Taussig, *The Prevention and Treatment of Abortion* (St. Louis: C. V. Mosby, 1910), 79. For discussions of the contemporary importance of the deployment of fetal images, see Rosalind Petchesky, "Fetal Images: The Power of Visual Culture in the Politics of Reproduction," *Feminist Studies* 13 (summer 1987): 263–292; Barbara Duden, *Disembodying Women: Perspectives on Pregnancy* (Cambridge, Mass.: Harvard University Press, 1993).

19. For example, "Little Jane's Tragedy Typical of Hundreds Who Disappear Here," *Chicago Examiner,* March 3, 1918; Abortionists Files, HHFC.

20. David M. Kennedy, *Birth Control in America: The Career of Margaret Sanger* (New Haven: Yale University Press, 1970), 191.

21. Phrase in Frank H. Jackson, "Criminal Abortion. Its Prevalence, Results, and Treatment," *AJOG* 58 (October 1908): 663; and Palmer Findley, "The Slaughter of the Innocents," *AJOG* 3 (January-June 1922): 36.

22. Wilmer Krusen, "The Indications for Therapeutic Abortion, with Consideration of the Rights of the Unborn Child," *The Therapeutic Gazette* 34 (March 15, 1910): 163.

23. Duff, "Chairman's Address," 292.

24. Jackson, "Criminal Abortion," 662, 663, 669. On private efforts and calls to purge the profession, see McCollum, "Criminal Abortion," 259; Aud, "In What Per Cent," 96.

25. Edward W. Pinkham, "The Treatment of Septic Abortion, with a Few Remarks on the Ethics of Criminal Abortion," *AJO* 61 (March 1910): 420; Meetings of Jan 9, 1912 and March 12, 1912, Council Minutes, October 1911-June 1912, vol. 25, Chicago Medical Society Records.

26. Meeting of January 10, 1911, Council Minutes, 1911–1912, vol. 25, Chicago Medical Society Records.

27. "Chicago Medical Society. Regular Meeting, Held Nov. 23, 1904. Symposium on Criminal Abortion," 1891; Report of Dr. Rudolph Holmes, Meeting of October 9, 1906, Council Minutes, October 1905-July 1907, vol. 20, Chicago Medical Society Records.

28. Report of Dr. Parkes, Meeting of January 9, 1912, 55–56, Chicago Medical Society Records.

29. On antiabortion activities in Philadelphia and New York, see Henry W.

Cattell, "Some Medico-Legal Aspects of Abortion," *Bulletin of the American Academy of Medicine* 8 (1907): 338–340, quotation on 339. See chapter 4 for analysis of coroner's inquests.

30. Report of Dr. Holmes, Meeting of October 9, 1906, Chicago Medical Society Records; Meeting of December 13, 1906, Board of Trustees Minutes, May 1903–07, vol. 14, Chicago Medical Society Records.

31. J. Henry Barbat, "Criminal Abortion," *California State Journal of Medicine* 9 (February 1911): 69.

32. For numerous examples of correspondence between physicians, businesses, government agencies, and the Bureau of Investigation, see Abortifacient Files, HHFC.

33. B. O. Halling Report on AMA Bureau of Investigation, July 14, 1938, Bureau of Investigation File, HHFC; W. L. Taggart, Trial Attorney for Federal Trade Commission to AMA, August 24, 1937, Abortifacient Files, HHFC. The Los Angeles County Medical Association and the AMA's Bureau of Investigation worked with California district attorneys, Board of Medical Examiners, and special agents in the 1934 to 1940 investigation and prosecution of the "Pacific Coast Abortion Ring," Pacific Coast Abortion Ring File, HHFC.

34. Comment by R. W. Holmes in Dorsett, "Criminal Abortion in Its Broadest Sense," 960.

35. Report of Dr. Carey Culbertson, Meeting of January 10, 1911, Chicago Medical Society Records.

36. Report of Dr. Parkes, Meeting of January 9, 1912, p. 53, Chicago Medical Society Records.

37. Resolution proposed in Dorsett, "Criminal Abortion in Its Broadest Sense," 958–959; *JAMA Proceedings of the Fifty-Ninth Annual Session Held at Chicago* (June 1–5, 1908): 40–41, 45, quotations on 40.

38. Kobrin, "The American Midwife Controversy," 318–326; Judy Barrett Litoff, *American Midwives: 1860 to the Present* (Westport, Conn.: Greenwood Press, 1978).

39. F. Elisabeth Crowell, "The Midwives of New York," *Charities and the Commons* 17 (January 1907): 667–677; reprint, in Judy Barrett Litoff, ed., *The American Midwife Debate: A Sourcebook on Its Modern Origins* (New York: Greenwood Press, 1986), 45.

40. Charles R. King, "The New York Maternal Mortality Study: A Conflict of Professionalization," *Bulletin of the History of Medicine* 65 (winter 1991): 476–480; Speert, *Obstetrics and Gynecology in America;* Judith Walzer Leavitt, *Brought to Bed: Childbearing in America, 1750–1950* (New York: Oxford University Press, 1986), chaps. 2, 6, 7; Litoff, *The American Midwife Debate,* 6–7.

41. King, "New York Maternal Mortality Study," 483–485, 495.

42. Brickman alone noted that the charge of abortion was a way to degrade midwives; Jane Pacht Brickman, "Public Health, Midwives, and Nurses, 1880–1930," in *Nursing History: New Perspectives, New Possibilities,* edited by Ellen Condliffe Lagemann (New York: Teacher's College, Columbia University Press, 1983), 69. For an overview of the history of midwives, see Judy Barrett Litoff, "Midwives and History," in Apple, *Women, Health, and Medicine in America,* 443–458. On midwife practices, see Charlotte G. Borst, *Catching Babies: The Professionalization of Childbirth, 1870–1920* (Cambridge, Mass.: Harvard Uni-

versity Press, 1995); Eugene R. Declercq, "The Nature and Style of Practice of Immigrant Midwives in Early Twentieth Century Massachusetts," *Journal of Social History* 19 (1985): 113–129. On African American midwives, see Susan L. Smith, "White Nurses, Black Midwives, and Public Health in Mississippi, 1920–1950," *Nursing History Review* 2 (1994): 29–49; Ruth C. Schaffer, "The Health and Social Functions of Black Midwives on the Texas Brazos Bottom, 1920–1985," *Rural Sociology* 56 (spring 1992): 89–105; Molly Ladd-Taylor, "'Grannies' and 'Spinsters': Midwife Education Under the Sheppard-Towner Act," *Journal of Social History* 22 (1988): 255–275; Debra Anne Susie, *In the Way of Our Grandmothers: A Cultural View of Twentieth-Century Midwifery in Florida* (Athens: University of Georgia Press, 1988); Sharon A. Robinson, "A Historical Development of Midwifery in the Black Community: 1600–1940," *Journal of Nurse-Midwifery* 29 (July-August 1984): 247–250.

43. On the Progressive Era, see Alan Dawley, *Struggles for Justice: Social Responsibility and the Liberal State* (Cambridge, Mass.: Belknap Press of Harvard University Press, 1991); Noralee Frankel and Nancy S. Dye, eds., *Gender, Class, Race, and Reform in the Progressive Era* (Lexington: University Press of Kentucky, 1991); Paul Boyer, *Urban Masses and Moral Order in America, 1820–1920* (Cambridge, Mass.: Harvard University Press, 1978), 123 292; Robert Wiebe, *The Search for Order, 1877–1920* (New York: Hill and Wang, 1967).

44. Rudolph W. Holmes et al., "The Midwives of Chicago," *JAMA* 50 (April 25, 1908): 1347, 1346; see also Edward A. Ayers et al., "Report of the Committee on 'The Practice of Obstetrics by Midwives,'" *Medical Record* 44 (December 9, 1893): 767; Thomas Darlington, "The Present Status of the Midwife," *AJO* 63 (May 1911): 874; Ralph Waldo Lobenstine, "The Influence of the Midwife upon Infant and Maternal Morbidity and Mortality," *AJO* 63 (May 1911): 878; Kobrin, "The American Midwife Controversy."

45. Robyn Muncy, *Creating a Female Dominion in American Reform, 1890–1935* (New York: Oxford University Press, 1991); Molly Ladd-Taylor, "Hull House Goes to Washington: Women and the Children's Bureau," in Frankel and Dye, *Gender, Class, Race, and Reform in the Progressive Era*, 110–126; Thomas Neville Bonner, *Medicine in Chicago, 1850–1950: A Chapter in the Social and Scientific Development of a City*, 2d ed. (1957; Urbana: University of Illinois Press, 1991), 84–107.

46. Ruth Rosen, *The Lost Sisterhood: Prostitution in America, 1900–1918* (Baltimore: Johns Hopkins University Press, 1982); Allan M. Brandt, *No Magic Bullet: A Social History of Venereal Disease in the United States Since 1880*, expanded ed. (New York: Oxford University Press, 1987); Joanne J. Meyerowitz, *Women Adrift: Independent Wage Earners in Chicago, 1880–1930* (Chicago: University of Chicago Press, 1988); Kathy Peiss, *Cheap Amusements: Working Women and Leisure in Turn-of-the-Century New York* (Philadelphia: Temple University Press, 1986); Mary E. Odem, *Delinquent Daughters: Protecting and Policing Adolescent Female Sexuality in the United States, 1885–1920* (Chapel Hill: University of North Carolina Press, 1995); Linda Gordon, *Woman's Body, Woman's Right: Birth Control in America*, rev. and updated (1976; reprint, New York: Penguin Books, 1990), chap. 7; John D'Emilio and Estelle B. Freedman, *Intimate Matters: A History of Sexuality in America* (New York: Harper and Row, 1988), 171–235.

47. Eliza H. Root, "The Status of Obstetrics in General Practice," in *Transactions of the First Pan-American Medical Congress,* part 1 (Washington, D.C.: Government Printing Office, 1895), 901–904. I learned of this event through an entry in *Women in Medicine: A Bibliography of the Literature on Women Physicians,* edited by Sandra L. Chaff et al. (Metuchen, N.J.: Scarecrow Press, 1977), 293.

48. Root, "The Status of Obstetrics in General Practice," 904–905.

49. Ibid., 904. On Stevenson, see Regina Markell Morantz-Sanchez, *Sympathy and Science: Women Physicians in American Medicine* (New York: Oxford University Press, 1985), 232–233.

50. Ella M. S. Marble, "The First Pan-American Medical Congress—Some of the Women Who Took Part," *WMJ* 1 (October 1893): 199.

51. Morantz-Sanchez, *Sympathy and Science,* 47–65, 216–228.

52. Letter from Sarah Hackett Stevenson, *Chicago Times,* December 23, 1888, p. 11; Elizabeth Jarrett, "The Midwife or the Woman Doctor," *Medical Record* 54 (October 22, 1898): 610–611. See also Georgina Grothan, "Evil Practices of the So-Called Midwife," *Omaha Clinic* 7 (1895–1896): 175–180. A handful of physicians, female and male, defended midwives or advocated their training. Comments of Dr. Mary Putnam Jacobi as recorded in "Special Meeting, January 31, 1898. Discussion on Proposed Legislation against Midwives," *Medical Record* 53 (February 5, 1898): 210; Litoff, *American Midwives,* 34–37.

53. Litoff notes that few historians of midwifery ever suggested that the campaign to control midwives was a plot of male physicians against women, though others have summarized the history in this way. Litoff, "Midwives and History," 446–447, 451. Robyn Muncy and Molly Ladd-Taylor discuss the relationship between reformers and midwives at later dates; Muncy, *Creating a Female Dominion,* 115–119; Ladd-Taylor, " 'Grannies' and 'Spinsters,' " 255–275.

54. Mohr, *Abortion in America,* 94–95, 102–118, 168–169, 188, 216; Rosalind Pollack Petchesky, *Abortion and Woman's Choice: The State, Sexuality, and Reproductive Freedom,* rev. ed. (1984; Boston: Northeastern University Press, 1990), 82–83. While middle-class married women still pressed physicians for abortions (often successfully), the new campaign paid little attention to these women or their doctors.

55. C. S. Bacon, "The Midwife Question in America," *JAMA* 29 (November 27, 1897): 1091. The last quotation is in C. S. Bacon, "Failures of Midwives in Asepsis," 247.

56. When New York regulated midwives in 1906, it was not "the first" to do so, as claimed by the New York doctors cited in Joyce Antler and Daniel M. Fox, "The Movement toward a Safe Maternity: Physician Accountability in New York City, 1915–1940," *Bulletin of the History of Medicine* 50 (1976): 569–595; reprint in *Sickness and Health in America: Readings in the History of Medicine and Public Health,* edited by Judith Walzer Leavitt and Ronald L. Numbers (Madison: University of Wisconsin Press, 1978), 379. Litoff suggests that the debates began in about 1910 and, also, that by 1910 the debate had become "fierce" and that it was at its "height . . . between 1910 and 1920." My reading of the medical literature suggests that the latter assessment is correct, but that the debates began in the 1890s. Litoff, *American Midwives,* 64, 137, 138, 140.

57. Bacon, "Failures of Midwives in Asepsis," 247–248.

58. All quotations from Bacon, "The Midwife Question," 1091; see also Kobrin, "The American Midwife Controversy."

59. Holmes et al., "The Midwives of Chicago," 1346.

60. Ibid. On the public-health work of women physicians, see Morantz-Sanchez, *Sympathy and Science*, 296–302. On the public-health activism of organized women, see Jane Addams, *Twenty Years at Hull-House, with Autobiographical Notes* (1910; reprint, New York: The New American Library, 1938); Molly Ladd-Taylor, *Mother-Work: Women, Child Welfare, and the State, 1890–1930* (Urbana: University of Illinois Press, 1994); Judith Walzer Leavitt, *The Healthiest City: Milwaukee and the Politics of Health Reform* (Princeton, N.J.: Princeton University Press, 1982), chap. 6; Suellen M. Hoy, "'Municipal Housekeeping': The Role of Women in Improving Urban Sanitation Practices, 1880–1917," in *Pollution and Reform in American Cities, 1870–1930,* edited by Martin Melosi (Austin: University of Texas Press, 1980), 173–198.

61. On Herbert Stowe, see Entry for Herbert Marion Stowe, *American Medical Directory 1918,* 6th ed. (Chicago: Press of the American Medical Association, 1918), 473. On Alice Hamilton, see Entry for Alice Hamilton by Barbara Sicherman in *Notable American Women: The Modern Period: A Biographical Dictionary,* edited by Barbara Sicherman et al. (Cambridge, Mass.: Belknap Press of Harvard University Press, 1980), 303–306. On Caroline Hedger, see entry for Caroline Hedger, *American Medical Directory 1918,* 448; Mary Riggs Noble, "The Women Doctors of the Children's Bureau," *Medical Woman's Journal* 40 (January 1933): 5–10, cited in Chaff et al, *Women in Medicine.* In 1918, perhaps earlier, Drs. Hedger and Stowe shared an office in downtown Chicago. I am grateful to Lynne Curry for informing me that Hedger worked primarily with the University of Chicago Settlement House.

62. I have calculated the percentage from the figures provided by Crowell. Because of the difficulty of winning convictions for abortion, the New York County Medical Society's attorney pursued midwives suspected of abortion by initiating legal actions against them for "practicing medicine illegally." Seventy-one midwives had been convicted on this charge in five years of work. Crowell, "The Midwives of New York," 44. (Crowell's first name is spelled differently in "The Midwives of New York" and Holmes et al., "The Midwives of Chicago.") J. Milton Mabbott, "The Regulation of Midwives in New York," *AJO* 55 (April 1907): 516–517.

63. Mary Sherwood, "The Midwives of Baltimore: A Report to the Medical and Chirurgical Faculty of Maryland," *JAMA* 52 (June 19, 1909): 2009–2010.

64. Two hundred twenty-three Chicago midwives were investigated. Holmes et al., "The Midwives of Chicago," 1346–1349, quotations, in order, on 1346, 1348, 1347, 1349.

65. Ibid., 1348, 1349.

66. Ibid., 1349.

67. Ibid., 1346.

68. Ibid., 1350.

69. Illinois Medicine and Surgery Act, in Illinois, *All the Laws of Illinois,* 1899, sec. 10, p. 216. This is not to say that physicians had nothing to fear when they got involved in illegal abortion; see chapter 4, this volume.

70. S. Josephine Baker, *Fighting For Life* (New York: Macmillan, 1939), 114–115; Leavitt, *Brought to Bed*, 63, chap. 4. Some physicians thought that the birthing women seen by midwives rightfully belonged to medical students and might be the solution to the poor obstetrical education of physicians. Dr. S. Josephine Baker criticized this idea in "The Function of the Midwife," *WMJ* 23 (September 1913): 197.

71. "Seeks New Nurse Law," *Chicago Record-Herald*, April 25, 1908, p. 16. The hospital ordinance was revised June 1, 1908. *Report of the Department of Health, 1907–1910*, pp. 193–196, Municipal Reference Collection, Chicago Public Library, Chicago, Illinois. On private hospitals, see Morris J. Vogel, *The Invention of the Modern Hospital, Boston, 1870–1930* (Chicago: University of Chicago Press, 1980), 102–103.

72. "Women Press Charges against an Attorney," *Chicago Record-Herald*, September 3, 1910, p. 9; "Boy in 'Hobble' Skirt Spies upon Midwives," *Chicago Record-Herald*, September 17, 1910, p. 18. I have not been able to locate these affidavits.

73. "Boy in 'Hobble' Skirt Spies upon Midwives."

74. Ibid.

75. Historians have discovered only one other instance of turn-of-the-century midwife organization: St. Louis midwives formed the Scientific Association of Midwives; Litoff, *American Midwives*, 39–41.

76. Litoff, *American Midwives*, 106–107, 140; Litoff, *The American Midwife Debate*, 7, 9. Although midwives may have sporadically organized in their own interest, as in Chicago, they did not turn their calling into a profession. On this point, see Borst, *Catching Babies*. James R. Barrett makes a similar critique of historians' assumptions about divisions within the working class and shows how workers of different ethnic groups sometimes organized together in "Unity and Fragmentation: Class, Race, and Ethnicity on Chicago's South Side, 1900–1922," *Journal of Social History* 18 (September 1984): 37–55.

77. Vice Commission of Chicago, *The Social Evil in Chicago. A Study of Existing Conditions with Recommendations by the Vice Commission of Chicago* (1911; reprint, New York: Arno Press, 1970), 225, 223. The Commission investigated midwives in November 1910.

78. Ibid., quotations in order on 226, 225, 223. Judith R. Walkowitz analyzes how Victorians connected prostitution, abortion, and same-sex relationships in "Dangerous Sexualities," in *A History of Women in the West: Emerging Feminism from Revolution to World War*, vol. 4, edited by Genevieve Fraisse and Michelle Perrot (Cambridge, Mass.: Harvard University Press, 1993), 369–398.

79. Grace Abbott, "The Midwife in Chicago," *American Journal of Sociology* 20 (March 1915): 685–686. Dr. Rudolph W. Holmes later commented that the 1896 rules for midwives were "the best system for the control of midwife practice ever devised in this country," but only a few midwives ever registered. The regulations "were never rescinded—they merely fell by the wayside." Rudolph W. Holmes, "Midwife Practice—An Anachronism," *Illinois Medical Journal* 38 (January 1920): 30. On Grace Abbott, see the entry by Jill Ker Conway in *Notable American Women 1607–1950, A Biographical Dictionary*, vol. 1,

edited by Edward T. James (Cambridge, Mass.: Belknap Press of Harvard University Press, 1971), 2–4; Lela B. Costin, *Two Sisters for Social Justice: A Biography of Grace and Edith Abbott* (Urbana: University of Illinois Press, 1983).

80. Abbott, "The Midwife in Chicago," 684–686, 692–694, quotations on 684, 694.

81. Ibid., 689–699, quotation on 699; Mary Elizabeth Fiorenza, "Midwifery and the Law in Illinois and Wisconsin, 1877–1917" (master's thesis, University of Wisconsin, Madison, 1985), 45–46. On medical education in obstetrics, see Virginia G. Drachman, "The Loomis Trial: Social Mores and Obstetrics in the Mid-Nineteenth Century," *Health Care in America,* edited by Susan Reverby and David Rosner (Philadelphia: Temple University Press, 1979), 67–83; reprint, in Leavitt, *Women and Health in America,* 166–174.

82. "Jurors Hold Shavers for Girl Murder," *Chicago Daily Tribune,* May 29, 1915, pp. 1, 4, Abortionists Files, HHFC; "Raid," [1915], n.p., Abortionists Files, HHFC; "End Baby Murder, Cry from Public," *Herald,* May 31, 1915, Abortionists Files, HHFC.

83. Morantz-Sanchez, *Sympathy and Science,* 188–189; Mohr, *Abortion in America,* 161.

84. On the city and sexual danger for women, see Meyerowitz, *Women Adrift;* Peiss, *Cheap Amusements,* chap. 7; Odem, *Delinquent Daughters;* Ellen Carol Dubois and Linda Gordon, "Seeking Ecstasy on the Battlefield: Danger and Pleasure in Nineteenth-Century Feminist Sexual Thought," *Feminist Studies* 9 (spring 1983): 7–25; Walkowitz, "Dangerous Sexualities;" Judith R. Walkowitz, *City of Dreadful Delight: Narratives of Sexual Danger in Late-Victorian London* (Chicago: University of Chicago Press, 1992). On sexuality and the city, see Jean-Christophe Agnew, "Times Square: Secularization and Sacralization," in *Inventing Times Square: Commerce and Culture at the Crossroads of the World,* edited by William R. Taylor (New York: Russell Sage Foundation, 1991), 2–13; Timothy J. Gilfoyle, "Policing of Sexuality," in Taylor, *Inventing Times Square,* 297–314; George Chauncey Jr., "The Policed: Gay Men's Strategies of Everyday Resistance," in Taylor, *Inventing Times Square,* 315–328; Laurence Senelick, "Private Parts in Public Places," in Taylor, *Inventing Times Square,* 329–353.

85. "End Murders by Abortion, Council Order," *Chicago Tribune,* June 2, 1915, Abortionists Files, HHFC; "Jurors Hold Shavers for Girl Murder," Abortionists Files, HHFC.

86. In 1913, for example, of one hundred abortion deaths investigated by the Cook County Coroner, the coroner listed twelve as "criminal" cases, eight "accidental," five "spontaneous" (miscarriages), thirty-three "self-induced," and forty-two "undetermined." Many of the undetermined may have been criminal abortions as well, but the point is that the press coverage of abortion overemphasized the fatalities of criminal abortion by including miscarriages and other abortions. Cook County Coroner, *Biennial Report,* 1918–1919, p. 79, Municipal Reference Collection; Cook County Coroner, *Biennial Report,* 1912–1913, p. 80, Municipal Reference Collection. On the marital status of women who had abortions, see Cook County Coroner, *Biennial Report,* 1918–1919, p. 78; and chapter 1 of this volume.

87. "Coroner Starts War on Wildcat 'Homes,'" *Chicago News,* May 29, 1915, Abortionists Files, HHFC; "Abortion Lairs Facing Clean-Up by Authorities," *Chicago Herald,* May 30, 1915, Abortionists Files, HHFC; "Court Denies Divorce to Woman Aborter," *Chicago Daily Tribune,* June 1, 1915, p. 6, Abortionists Files, HHFC.

88. "Hostetter's [sic] Last Letter to Girl Who Was Quack Victim," n.p., May 28, 1915, Abortionists Files, HHFC; "Jurors Hold Shavers for Girl Murder"; "Body of Slain Girl Robbed, Fiance Claims," *Chicago Post,* May 29, 1915, Abortionists Files, HHFC; "Death Threat to Hostetler," *Chicago Tribune,* June 5, 1915, Abortionists Files, HHFC.

89. "Officials Plan Fight to Curb Abortion Evil," n.p., June 7, 1915, Abortionists Files, HHFC.

90. "Abortion Lairs Facing Clean-Up by Authorities."

91. "Officials Plan Fight to Curb Abortion Evil."

92. "Abortion Lairs Facing Clean-up by Authorities;" "End Baby Murder," *Chicago Herald,* May 31, 1915, Abortionists Files, HHFC.

93. The first mention that I have seen of any group supporting the exposure of abortion in Chicago mentions the city's "women's organizations" only, in "Death of Girl Perils Schools for Abortions," n.p., May 28, 1915, Abortionists Files, HHFC.

94. "End Baby Murder." See also "Alderman to Ask Probe of Quack Homes," *Chicago Tribune,* May 30, 1915, Abortionists Files, HHFC.

95. "Body of Slain Girl Robbed, Fiance Claims."

96. "End Baby Murder."

97. "Letters to 'Tribune' Expose Abortion Crimes," *Chicago Daily Tribune,* June 3, 1915, p. 4, Abortionists Files, HHFC.

98. All quotations in "Abortion Lairs Facing Clean-Up by Authorities."

99. "Crusade against Infant Murders Grows Rapidly," *Chicago Herald,* June 2, 1915, Abortionists Files, HHFC.

100. Ibid.; Chicago City Council, *Proceedings, 1916–1917,* vol. 1, p. 459, Municipal Reference Collection.

101. "Officials Unite to End Practice of Baby Murder," *Chicago Herald,* June 6, 1915, Abortionists Files, HHFC; "End Murders by Abortions."

102. Quotations in "Officials Plan Fight to Curb Abortion Evil," "End Murders by Abortion."

103. "Officials Plan Fight to Curb Abortion Evil;" Abbott's report was summarized in "End Baby Murder;" Fiorenza, "Midwifery and the Law in Illinois and Wisconsin," 45–46.

104. "Practice of Medicine-Act of 1899 Amended," in Illinois, *Laws of Illinois* 1915, p. 504. I am grateful to Elaine Shemoney Evans of the Illinois State Archives for finding this for me. Chicago Department of Police, *Annual Report,* 1878–1916, Municipal Reference Collection. Who fired the gun at Johnson's head and why was never clarified. "Fears Public Opinion in Abortion Cases," *Chicago Sunday Herald,* June 6, 1915, Abortionists Files, HHFC; "Woman Doctor is Convicted," *Chicago News,* March 10, 1916, Abortionists Files, HHFC.

105. Inquest on Edna M. Lamb, February 19, 1917, case no. 43-3-1917, Medical Records Department.

106. Frank Alby in Inquest on Emma Alby, September 11, 1915, case no. 141-10-1915, Medical Records Department. By 1918, Dr. Windmueller was listed as a specialist in laryngology and rhinology. Entry for Charles R. A. Windmueller, *American Medical Directory, 1918,* 479.

107. My thanks to Robert E. Bailey and Elaine Evans at the Illinois State Archives who searched the Chicago City Council files for 1915 and found no reports or investigations on midwives. Chicago Department of Police, *Annual Report,* 1916, Municipal Reference Collection.

108. "'Dr.' Benn Put on Trial as Woman's Slayer," *Chicago Examiner,* March 5, 1918, Abortionists Files, HHFC.

109. Findley, "The Slaughter of the Innocents," 35–36.

110. Ibid., 36.

111. Brickman makes a slightly different but complementary argument about the relationship between the medical profession's attack on midwifery and the Sheppard-Towner Act and public-health efforts in general in her excellent article, "Public Health, Midwives, and Nurses," 66–67, 76–77. On the Sheppard-Towner Act, see J. Stanley Lemons, *The Woman Citizen: Social Feminism in the 1920s* (Urbana: University of Illinois Press, 1973), chap 6; Rosemary Stevens, *American Medicine and the Public Interest* (New Haven: Yale University Press, 1971), 143–144, 200; Ladd-Taylor, *Mother-Work;* Morantz-Sanchez, *Sympathy and Science,* 296–303. On the medical profession and national health insurance, see Ronald L. Numbers, *Almost Persuaded: American Physicians and Compulsory Health Insurance, 1912–1920* (Baltimore: Johns Hopkins Press, 1978).

112. Kobrin and Litoff have divided the people in the midwife debate as either opponents of midwives who favored their abolition or proponents who, as Kobrin described it, took "the public health approach." Kobrin, "The American Midwife Controversy," 320; Litoff, *American Midwives,* chaps. 5, 6. I have found it difficult to determine to which side various doctors and commentators belonged; they often seem to fall in both camps. Individuals' positions could change over time from a negative view of midwives to a more positive view, a change that seems to have been true for female and male physicians most dedicated to public-health work. For example, Dr. S. Josephine Baker's attitude was transformed as she worked to improve maternal and infant health in New York City. S. Josephine Baker, "The Function of the Midwife," 196–197. Nancy Schrom Dye finds a similar change in attitude among dispensary physicians who came to know midwives in New York City in the 1890s. "But," she observes, "obstetricians' professional identity and prestige . . . depended upon the attainment and exercise of unilateral authority. To cooperate with a midwife, or to share responsibility with her, was professionally untenable." "Modern Obstetrics and Working-Class Women: The New York Midwifery Dispensary, 1890–1920," *Journal of Social History* 20 (spring 1987): 554.

113. Lemons, *The Woman Citizen,* 169; Costin, *Two Sisters for Social Justice,* 142; Bonner, *Medicine in Chicago,* 140–141, 218–220, 222; Lynne Elizabeth Curry, "Modern Mothers in the Heartland: Maternal and Child Health Reform in Illinois, 1900–1930" (Ph.D. diss., University of Illinois at Urbana-Champaign, 1995). I am grateful to Lynne Curry for sharing with me the names of physicians who supported the Sheppard-Towner Act.

114. Margaret Sanger, "Why Not Birth Control Clinics in America?" *BCR* 3 (May 1919): 10.

115. Rudolph W. Holmes, chair of the Chicago Medical Society Criminal Abortion Committee, worked with a committee of the Chicago Gynecological Society to oppose birth control clinics and the provision of birth control to the general public. See letter from Rudolph W. Holmes, Joseph L. Haer, and N. Sproat Heaney, "Correspondence. The Regulation of Conception," *Illinois Medical Journal* 43 (March 1923): 193. Dr. Henry W. Cattell of Philadelphia, an antiabortion activist early in the century, testified at a Congressional Hearing in 1931 against a bill granting doctors the right to dispense birth control. Cattell, "Some Medico-Legal Aspects of Abortion," 334–341; Statement of Dr. Henry W. Cattell in U.S. Congress, Senate, *Birth Control Hearings before a Subcommittee of the Committee on the Judiciary* (Washington, D.C.: Government Printing Office: 1931), 59–60. On the relationship between the medical profession and the birth control movement, see Gordon, *Woman's Body, Woman's Right*, 255–269; Kennedy, *Birth Control in America*, 172–217; James Reed, "Doctors, Birth Control, and Social Values, 1830–1970," in Leavitt, *Women and Health*, 124–139.

116. "Birth Controllists and Maternity Legislation," *Illinois Medical Journal* 43 (May 1923): 344; "Birth Control a Corollary of the Sheppard-Towner Bill," *Illinois Medical Journal* 50 (December 1926): 448–449.

117. In 1910, at the peak of the campaign against midwives, midwives still delivered half of the nation's babies, but twenty years later they delivered only 15 percent. The nation's midwives had become concentrated in the South, where most of the midwives and the women they assisted were African American. Louis S. Reed, *Midwives, Chiropodists, and Optometrists: Their Place in Medical Care* (Chicago: University of Chicago Press, 1932), 4–7, 67, table 1A; Kobrin, "The American Midwife Controversy," 318, 324–325; Ladd-Taylor, "'Grannies' and 'Spinsters,'" 269–270.

Chapter 4.   Interrogations and Investigations

1. She had had three children, but one died. Inquest on Carolina Petrovitis, March 21, 1916, case no. 234-3-1916, Medical Records Department. For another physician who closely questioned a woman about abortion, see the Inquest on Matilda Olson, April 30, 1918, case no. 289-4-1918, Medical Records Department.

2. On this point, see Martha Vicinus, "Sexuality and Power: A Review of Current Work in the History of Sexuality," *Feminist Studies* 8 (spring 1982): 133–156. The few histories that examine the control of male heterosexuality include Mary E. Odem, *Delinquent Daughters: Protecting and Policing Adolescent Female Sexuality in the United States, 1885–1920* (Chapel Hill: University of North Carolina Press, 1995); Allan M. Brandt, *No Magic Bullet: A Social History of Venereal Disease in the United States Since 1880*, exp. ed. (New York: Oxford University Press, 1987), 61–64, 66–70; and G. J. Barker-Benfield, *The Horrors of the Half Known Life: Male Attitudes toward Women and Sexuality in Nineteenth Century America* (New York: Harper and Row, 1976). For overviews of

the history of sexuality, see John D'Emilio and Estelle B. Freedman, *Intimate Matters: A History of Sexuality in America* (New York: Harper and Row, 1988); Kathy Peiss and Christina Simmons, eds., with Robert A. Padgug, *Passion and Power: Sexuality in History* (Philadelphia: Temple University Press, 1989).

3. Michael Grossberg argues that the judiciary dominated nineteenth-century family law and claimed patriarchal authority over domestic relations. Michael Grossberg, *Governing the Hearth: Law and the Family in Nineteenth-Century America* (Chapel Hill: University of North Carolina Press, 1985), 289–307. On feminists, see also Carroll Smith-Rosenberg, *Disorderly Conduct: Visions of Gender in Victorian America* (New York: Oxford University Press, 1985), 243–244; Linda Gordon, *Woman's Body, Woman's Right: Birth Control in America,* rev. and updated (1976; reprint, New York: Penguin Books, 1990), chap. 5. Joan Brumberg found that members of the Women's Christian Temperance Union acted as marriage "enforcers" in cases of unmarried pregnant women when they deemed marriage appropriate. Joan Jacobs Brumberg, "'Ruined' Girls: Changing Community Responses to Illegitimacy in Upstate New York, 1890–1920," *Journal of Social History* 18 (winter 1984): 254–257. Linda Gordon finds that feminists had a powerful impact on the welfare state, "particularly its regulatory organizations," at the turn of the century. That influence extended to the state's promotion of male responsibility in cases of pregnant unwed women. Linda Gordon, *Heroes of Their Own Lives: The Politics and History of Family Violence, Boston, 1880–1960* (New York: Viking, 1988), 297. On juvenile courts, see Odem, *Delinquent Daughters.*

4. On the control of medicine, see Paul Starr, *The Social Transformation of American Medicine* (New York: Basic Books, 1982), 102–112, 118, 184–197.

5. H. H. Hawkins in, "Symposium. Criminal Abortion. The Colorado Law on Abortion," *JAMA* 40 (April 18, 1903): 1099; Franz Eschweiler in Wilhelm Becker, "The Medical, Ethical, and Forensic Aspects of Fatal Criminal Abortion," *Wisconsin Medical Journal* 7 (April 1909): 633; James C. Mohr, "Patterns of Abortion and the Response of American Physicians, 1790–1930," in *Women and Health in America: Historical Readings,* edited by Judith Walzer Leavitt (Madison: University of Wisconsin Press, 1984), 121.

6. The Illinois Supreme Court commented on dying declarations in twelve out of the thirty-seven cases concerning an abortion-related death. Dying declarations may have been introduced or discussed in additional cases without having been addressed in the Supreme Court opinions. Furthermore, many dying declarations were collected but never used in court. For examples of Illinois Supreme Court discussion of dying declarations, see *Dunn v. the People,* 172 Ill. 582 (1898), pp. 587–591; *People v. Huff* 339 Ill. 328 (1930), p. 332. For evidence of the importance of dying declarations in other states, see reports of cases in Texas, Wisconsin, and Maryland respectively in "Dying Declarations Obtained in Abortion Case as Condition to Rendering Aid," *JAMA* 52 (April 10, 1909): 1204; "Dying Declarations Made after Refusal of Physician to Treat Abortion Case without History," *JAMA* 60 (June 7, 1913): 1829–1830; "Admissibility of Evidence to Prove Criminal Abortion," *JAMA* 60 (January 4, 1913): 79–80. For nineteenth-century cases, see Grossberg, *Governing the Hearth,* 363 n. 64. On Canada, see Constance B. Backhouse, "Involuntary Motherhood: Abortion, Birth Control, and the Law in Nineteenth Century Canada," *Windsor*

Yearbook of Access to Justice 3 (1983): 61–130; Angus McLaren, "Birth Control and Abortion in Canada, 1870–1920," *Canadian Historical Review* 59, no. 3 (1978): 319–340.

7. The clerk of the Criminal Court of Cook County reported that between 1924 and, I believe, 1934, there were thirty-two prosecutions for murder by abortion and only seven convictions; and out of six prosecutions for abortion, two convictions. [Thomas E. Harris], "A Functional Study of Existing Abortion Laws," *Columbia Law Review* 35 (January 1935): 91 n. 17. Frederick J. Taussig provided the name of the author in *Abortion, Spontaneous and Induced: Medical and Social Aspects* (St. Louis: C. V. Mosby, 1936), 426. In his study of abortion indictments in early twentieth-century Philadelphia, Roger Lane also finds few prosecutions and even fewer convictions. Personal communication from Roger Lane to author, May 31, 1989. Comparable data on the number of arrests and convictions for abortion are not available after the mid-1930s because police annual reports stopped reporting this information in detail.

8. The rise in arrests beginning in 1889 was probably the result of the abortion exposé in the *Chicago Times*, December 12, 1888, through January 6, 1889. On the Comstock raids, see "Fight Race Suicide in Raids All over U.S.," *Chicago* [*News*], November 20, 1912, Abortionists Files, HHFC; "Take Chicagoans in Federal War on Race Suicide," *Chicago Tribune*, November 21, 1912, Abortionists Files, HHFC. The peaks in 1914 to 1917 coincided with local and state investigations of abortion and baby farms, and newspaper coverage of abortion in Chicago. Chicago Department of Health, *Report*, 1911–1918, vol. 1, pp. 1055–1056; Juvenile Protective Association, *Baby Farms in Chicago*, by Arthur Alden Guild ([Chicago], 1917).

9. See, for example, Inquest on Milda Hoffmann, May 29, 1916, case no. 342–5–1916, Medical Records Department; Degma Felicelli, October 11, 1916, case no. 224–10–1916, Medical Records Department.

10. Coroner Peter Hoffman reported sending 185 people to the grand jury for abortion during his fifteen year tenure between 1905 and 1919. I have calculated the average. Cook County Coroner, *Biennial Report*, 1918–1919, Municipal Reference Collection.

11. The following three paragraphs are based on my reading of coroner's inquests and transcripts of criminal abortion trials.

12. William Durfor English, "Evidence—Dying Declaration—Preliminary Questions of Fact—Degree of Proof," *Boston University Law Review* 15 (April 1935): 382.

13. Ibid., 381–382.

14. Quotation from Inquest on Petrovitis. Simon Greenleaf described the dying declaration as "declarations made in extremity, when the party is at the point of death, and when every hope of this world is gone; when every motive to falsehood is silenced, and the mind is induced, by the most powerful considerations, to speak the truth. A situation so solemn and so awful is considered by the law as creating an obligation equal to that which is imposed by a positive oath in a court of justice." Simon Greenleaf, *A Treatise on the Law of Evidence*, vol. 1, 16th ed. (Boston: Little, Brown and Co., 1899), 245. See also John Henry Wigmore, *A Treatise on the System of Evidence in Trials at Common Law, In-*

cluding Statutes and Judicial Decisions of All Jurisdictions of the United States (Boston: Little, Brown and Co., 1904), 1798–1819.

15. "Murder by abortion" was the standard phrase used in the coroner's jury's verdicts and Grand Jury indictments. For example, Inquest on Rosie Kawera, June 15, 1916, case no. 152–5–1916, Medical Records Department; *People v. Dennis* 246 Ill. 559 (1910), pp. 560–561.

16. C. S. Bacon, in "Chicago Medical Society. Regular Meeting, Held Nov. 23, 1904. Symposium on Criminal Abortion," *JAMA* 43 (December 17, 1904): 1889. Roger Lane finds, from his study of indictments in Philadelphia's circuit court, that most abortion cases did not follow the death of a woman, but that women testified as a "result of the damage done." On the nineteenth century, see Roger Lane, *Violent Death in the City: Suicide, Accident, and Murder in Nineteenth-Century Philadelphia* (Cambridge, Mass.: Harvard University Press, 1979), 93; on the early twentieth century, personal communication from Roger Lane to author.

17. Lawrence M. Friedman and Robert V. Percival, *The Roots of Justice: Crime and Punishment in Alameda County, California, 1870–1910* (Chapel Hill: University of North Carolina Press, 1981), 111–116, 310; Sidney L. Harring, *Policing a Class Society: The Experience of American Cities, 1865–1915* (New Brunswick, N.J.: Rutgers University Press, 1983).

In my discussion of the state, I am interested in the broad array of people, institutions, and officials involved in the enforcement of the criminal abortion laws. I do not regard the state as completely unified or consistent in its policies, for certainly there were conflicts between various state agents. The judiciary scrutinized police actions and criticized them, for example, but the differences among the different levels and officers of the state are not my primary focus. For a critical discussion on historians' use of the term *the state,* see Michael Ignatieff, "State, Civil Society, and Total Institution: A Critique of Recent Social Histories of Punishment," in *Legality, Ideology, and the State,* edited by David Sugarman (London: Academic Press, 1983), 183–211.

18. This chapter is based on my examination of forty-four Cook County Coroner's Inquests into abortion deaths between 1907 and 1937, held in the Medical Records Department, Cook County Medical Examiner's Office. Two were found in transcripts of criminal abortion trials.

19. Mohr, "Patterns of Abortion," 122; Paul H. Gebhard et al., *Pregnancy, Birth and Abortion* (New York: Harper and Brothers and Paul B. Hoeber Medical Books, 1958), 194–195, 198. On delay in seeking medical treatment, see James R. Reinberger and Percy B. Russell, "The Conservative Treatment of Abortion," *JAMA* 107 (November 7, 1936): 1530; J. D. Dowling, "Points of Interest in a Survey of Maternal Mortality," *American Journal of Public Health* 27 (August 1937): 804. On the high level of complications and fatalities associated with self-induced abortions, see Regine K. Stix, "A Study of Pregnancy Wastage," *Milbank Memorial Fund Quarterly* 13 (October 1935): 362–363; Raymond E. Watkins, "A Five-Year Study of Abortion," *AJOG* 26 (August 1933), 162.

20. Taussig, *Abortion,* 24; William J. Robinson, *The Law against Abortion: Its Perniciousness Demonstrated and Its Repeal Demanded* (New York: Eugenics Publishing, 1933), 38–39. See also U.S. Dept. of Labor, Children's Bureau, *Ma-*

ternal Mortality in Fifteen States, Bureau publication no. 223 (Washington, D.C.: Government Printing Office, 1934), 103–104. I have not found an incident of families bribing officials, but on the corruption of police and coroners, see Mark H. Haller, "Historical Roots of Police Behavior: Chicago, 1890–1925," *Law and Society Review* 10 (winter 1976), 306–307, 311, 316–317; Julie Johnson, "Coroners, Corruption, and the Politics of Death: Forensic Pathology in the United States," in *Legal Medicine in History,* edited by Michael Clark and Catherine Crawford (Cambridge: Cambridge University Press, 1994), 268–289.

21. I requested the Inquest on Flossie Emerson, who died February 28, 1916, but the Cook County Coroner's Office has no record of her death. Personal communication with Cathy Kurnyta, Director of Medical Records Department, Cook County Medical Examiner's Office. Emerson's abortion-related death was one of the cases for which Dr. Schultz-Knighten was prosecuted, *People v. Schultz-Knighten,* 277 Ill. 238 (1917). I did not find any records from the 1920s or 1930s of black women who had abortions. The paucity of information on the abortion-related deaths of black women may be an artifact of bias in the sources or may reflect the relatively small size of Chicago's African American population. Although World War I migration of African Americans from the South increased Chicago's black population by 148 percent, African Americans still made up only 4 percent of Chicago's population in 1920. Allan H. Spear, *Black Chicago: The Making of a Negro Ghetto* (Chicago: University of Chicago Press, 1967), 140–146, 223. On black women's use of abortion, see Rodrique, "The Black Community and the Birth Control Movement," 140–141.

22. Dr. Anna B. Schultz-Knighten complained that the coroner's physician, Dr. Springer, had "sneered" at her and called her a "nigger." Abstract of Record, p. 117, *People v. Schultz-Knighten,* 277 Ill. 238 (1917), Case Files, no vault no., Supreme Court of Illinois, Record Series 901.

23. Taussig, *Abortion,* 156–158, 185–222.

24. Mortality reached 60 to 70 percent when septicemia or peritonitis had occurred, according to Report of Fred J. Taussig, White House Conference on Child Health and Protection, *Fetal, Newborn, and Maternal Morbidity and Mortality* (New York: D. Appleton-Century, 1933), 466–467. Almuth C. Vandiver, "The Legal Status of Criminal Abortion, with Especial Reference to the Duty and Protection of the Consultant," *AJO* 61 (March 1910): 434–435, quotation on 497.

25. O. B. Will, "The Medico-Legal Status of Abortion," *Illinois Medical Journal* 2 (1900–1901): 506, 508. Edward W. Pinkham, "The Treatment of Septic Abortion, with a Few Remarks on the Ethics of Criminal Abortion," *AJO* 61 (March 1910): 420. Illinois, *All the Laws of Illinois,* 1899, sec. 10, p. 216. In Nebraska and New Jersey, revocation of a physician's license for abortion did not require a criminal conviction. "Procedure before State Board of Health and Revocation of License for Criminal Abortion," *JAMA* 51 (August 29, 1908): 788; "Revocation of License for 'Practice' of Criminal Abortion on Single Occasion," *JAMA* 78 (June 24, 1922): 1988.

26. Inquest on Mary L. Kissell, August 3, 1937, case no. 300–8–1937, Medical Records Department. See also Inquests on Edna M. Lamb, February 19,

1917, case no. 43–3–1917 and Anna P. Fazio, February 14, 1929, case no. 217–2–1929, both held by Medical Records Department.

27. Verdict of Coroner's Jury, Superintendent of Rhodes Avenue Hospital (name illegible) to Coroner Peter M. Hoffman, March 17, 1916 in the Inquest on Annie Marie Dimford, September 30, 1915, case no. 75–11–1915, Medical Records Department. See also Inquest on Ellen Matson, November 19, 1917, case no. 330–11–1917, Medical Records Department; Doctors D. S. J. Meyers and W. W. Richmond commenting on C. J. Aud, "In What Per Cent, Is the Regular Profession Responsible for Criminal Abortions, and What is the Remedy?" *Kentucky Medical Journal* 2 (September 1904): 98, 99.

28. This "agreement" is discussed in the Inquest on Matson. It may have been made in 1915 during the abortion scandal following Anna Johnson's death. See chapter 3, this volume.

29. Dr. Marion S. Swiont in Transcript of *People v. Zwienczak,* 338, Ill. 237 (1929), Case Files, vault no. 44701, Supreme Court of Illinois, Record Series 901.

30. Dr. Coe and others in Vandiver, "Legal Status of Criminal Abortion," 496–501, quotation on 500; "Transactions of the New York Academy of Medicine. Section on Obstetrics and Gynecology. Meeting, of March 23, 1911. Criminal Abortion from the Practitioner's Viewpoint. Paper read by Walter B. Jennings," *AJO* 63 (June 1911): 1094–1096.

31. Meeting of January 9, 1912, Council Minutes, October 1911-June 1912, pp. 53–54, 56–57, Chicago Medical Society Records. The New Orleans Parish Medical Society published a letter to be sent to every physician in New Orleans, which included a model dying declaration. N. F. Thiberge, "Report of Committee on Criminal Abortion," *New Orleans Medical and Surgical Journal* 70 (1917–1918): 802, 807–808.

32. Meeting of January 9, 1912, Council Minutes, p. 57, Chicago Medical Society Records. For examples of dying declarations and judicial discussions on their validity, see *Hagenow v. People,* 188 Ill. 545 (1901), pp. 550–551, 553; *People v. Cheney,* 368 Ill. 131 (1938), pp. 132–135.

33. "Criminal Abortion," *JAMA* 39 (September 20, 1902): 706; Palmer Findley, "The Slaughter of the Innocents," *AJOG* 3 (January 1922): 37.

34. Inquest on Emily Projahn, October 10, 1916, case no. 26–12–1916, Medical Records Department. Abortion convictions appealed to higher courts in Texas and Wisconsin revealed that dying declarations were obtained from women under threats by physicians to refuse medical care. "Dying Declarations Obtained in Abortion Case as Condition to Rendering Aid"; "Dying Declarations Made after Refusal of Physician to Treat Abortion Case without History."

35. John Ross in Inquest on Mathilde C. Kleinschmidt, September 22, 1930, case no. 255–9–30, Medical Records Department.

36. Vandiver, "Legal Status of Criminal Abortion," 435; Furniss commenting on Jennings, "Criminal Abortion from the Practitioner's Viewpoint," 1096.

37. See comments of Louise Hagenow as quoted in *Hagenow v. the People,* 188 Ill. 545 (1901), p. 552.

38. Ernest F. Oakley in discussion of "Legal Aspects of Abortion," *AJOG* 3 (January 1922): 84; "Abortion 'Club' Exposed," *BCR* 4 (November 1936): 5.

See also "Dying Girl Runaway Hides Name of Slayer," *Chicago Examiner,* March 8, 1918, Abortionists Files, HHFC.

39. "End Murders by Abortions," *Chicago Tribune,* June 2, 1915, Abortionists Files, HHFC; Transcript of *People v. Anna Heissler,* 338 Ill. 596 (1930), Case Files, vault no. 44783, Supreme Court of Illinois, Record Series 901.

40. Quotation from an unnamed physician in Hawkins, "Symposium. Criminal Abortion. The Colorado Law on Abortion," 1099. See also Will, "The Medico-Legal Status of Abortion," 508; Simon Marx and George Kosmak in Jennings, "Criminal Abortion from the Practitioner's Viewpoint," 1095–1096.

41. Parkes in Meeting of January 9, 1912, Council Minutes, October 11-June 1912, p. 55, Chicago Medical Society Records; W. Robinson, *The Law against Abortion,* 105–111.

42. Inquest on Lamb; Jennings, "Criminal Abortion from the Practitioner's Viewpoint," 1094.

43. Frank commenting on Aud, "In What Per Cent," 100. See comments of A. C. Morgan and Richard C. Norris in "Society Proceedings. North Branch Philadelphia County Medical Society. Regular Meeting, held April 14, 1904," *JAMA* 42 (May 21, 1904): 1375–1376. Attorneys disagreed about whether or not physicians should act as informers in abortion cases. Allen H. Seaman and Charles R. Brock in "Symposium. Criminal Abortion. The Colorado Law on Abortion," 1097, 1098. Illinois law did not privilege communications between doctors and patients. C. S. Bacon, "The Duty of the Medical Profession in Relation to Criminal Abortion," *Illinois Medical Journal* 7 (January 1905): 22.

44. "Girl's Letters Blame Dr. Mason in Death Case," *Chicago Tribune,* [April] 9, 1916, Abortionists Files, HHFC; "Voice from Grave Calls to Dr. Mason during Trial as His Fiancee's Betrayer," *Denver Post,* April 5, 1916. See also chapter 3, this volume.

45. Quotation from "Dying Girl Runaway Hides Name of Slayer" (emphasis in original). See also "Girl Slain Here Gives Life to Hide Her Tragedy," *Chicago Examiner,* March 5, 1918; "Slain Girl Dies Holding Her Tragedy from Kin," *Chicago Examiner,* March 9, 1918. Both clippings in Abortionists Files, HHFC. All of these stories mention fathers.

46. "Mrs. Ruth Conn," *Chicago Herald,* December 19, 1915, Abortionists Files, HHFC.

47. "Death Arrest Bares List of 1,500 Women," *Chicago Examiner* [1916], Abortionists Files, HHFC.

48. Inquest on Mary Shelley, October 30, 1915, case no. 352–10–1915, Medical Records Department. Bacon, "The Duty of the Medical Profession," 21–22. The Crowell family tried to prevent an investigation into Mamie Ethel Crowell's abortion by lying to physicians and the coroner, Inquest on Crowell, April 16, 1930, case no. 305–4–30, Medical Records Department.

49. For family members who wanted the state to investigate an abortion, see *People v. Hotz,* 261 Ill. 239 (1914). Quotation from "Medical News. A Maryland Abortionist Gets No Pardon," *JAMA* 43 (November 12, 1904): 1476.

50. Edward Flanigan in Inquest on Frances Collins, May 7, 1920, case no. 161–5–20, Medical Records Department.

51. Comments of "Esther E.," *BCR* 4 (September 1920): 15. See also, W. Robinson, *The Law against Abortion*, 106–107.

52. *Hagenow v. People* (1901), p. 551; *People v. Hagenow* 236 Ill. 514 (1908), p. 527; *People v. Heissler* (1930), p. 599. The coroner told Dr. Kruse to "make it a rule" at his hospital to call police in abortion cases so that they could bring the suspect in for identification; Inquest on Lamb.

53. Sgt. O'Connor in Inquest on Petrovitis.

54. Inquest on Petrovitis.

55. Mable Matson in Transcript of *People v. Hobbs,* 297 Ill. 399 (1921), Case Files, vault no. 38773, Supreme Court of Illinois, Record Series 901.

56. Rosie Kronowitz in abstract of *People v. Heisler,* 300 Ill. 98 (1921), p. 38, Case Files, vault no. 39077, Supreme Court of Illinois, Record Series 901.

57. The following account is drawn from the Inquest on Eunice McElroy, November 14, 1928, case no. 486–11–28, Medical Records Department.

58. John Harris in Inquest on Dimford. See also Robert Patrick Crelly in Inquest on Kissell. One man married his lover two days after her abortion; she died three weeks later (see Inquest of Esther Stark, June 12, 1917, case no. 65–6–1917). Quotation in *People v. Rongetti,* 344 Ill. 278 (1931), p. 284.

59. Inquest on Anna Johnson, May 27, 1915, case no. 77790, Medical Records Department.

60. Inquest on Matson.

61. "Death Threat to Hostetler," *Chicago Tribune,* June 5, 1915, Abortionists Files, HHFC. Police and press often called the men in these cases "the sweetheart"; see "Doctor Faces Manslaughter Charge in Girl's Death," *Chicago Tribune,* April 18, 1930, Abortionists Files, HHFC.

62. Inquest on Alma Bromps, April 27, 1931, case no. 35–5–1931, Medical Records Department; *People v. Ney,* 349 Ill. 172 (1932), pp. 173–174. For other lovers who testified against the abortionist, see *Cochran v. The People,* 175 Ill. 28 (1898); *People v. Hobbs,* 297 Ill. 399 (1921).

63. Walter Beisse in Inquest on Rose Siebenmann, April 16, 1920, case no. 266–4–20, Medical Records Department.

64. Charles Morehouse's name is spelled as "Moorehouse" in Transcript of *People v. Hobbs,* 297 Ill. 399 (1921), Case Files, vault no. 38773, Supreme Court of Illinois, Record Series 901; O'Connell in Transcript of *People v. Buettner* 233 Ill. 272 (1908), Case Files, vault no. 30876, ibid. For convictions of boyfriends, see *Dunn v. the People; People v. Patrick,* 277 Ill. 210 (1917). Grace and Edith Abbott found that many foreigners languished in jail because they could not pay their fines; see Lela B. Costin, *Two Sisters for Social Justice: A Biography of Grace and Edith Abbott* (Urbana: University of Illinois Press, 1983), 77.

65. I know of only one case where the husband was charged. Bertis Dougherty pled guilty to abortion and testified as a state witness against the abortionist in *People v. Schneider,* 370 Ill. 612 (1939), pp. 613–614.

66. Juvenile Protective Association of Chicago, *A Study of Bastardy Cases, taken from The Court of Domestic Relations in Chicago,* text by Louise DeKoven Bowen [Chicago, 1914] (History of Women, 1977) microfilm, item 9921, pp. 18, 19, 22.

67. Young men and women understood how the juvenile courts worked

and how statutory rape cases proceeded; young men probably also knew how bastardy and abortion investigations proceeded. Odem, *Delinquent Daughters.*

68. Transcript of *Dunn v. the People,* 172 Ill. 582 (1898), Case Files, vault no. 7876, Supreme Court of Illinois, Record Series 901. On the ways in which women could use the state's regulation for their own ends, see Gordon, *Heroes of Their Own Lives,* 289–299.

69. Abortionists sometimes offered to cover funeral and other expenses as in the unsuccessful cover-up participated in and described by Emil Winter in the Inquest on Margaret B. Winter, November 13, 1916, case no. 274–11–1916, Medical Records Department. In the Winter case the abortionist was a mid-wife. For an unsuccessful attempt to keep abortion quiet by a physician, see Testimony of Walter F. Heidenway and Elizabeth Heidenway in the Inquest on Alma Heidenway, August 21, 1918, case no. 232–8–1918, Medical Records Department.

70. On false death certificates, see *Earll v. the People,* 73 Ill. 329 (1874), p. 336; Rudolph W. Holmes et al., "The Midwives of Chicago," *JAMA* 50 (April 25, 1908), 1348.

71. See Inquest on Fazio; Pinkham, "Treatment of Septic Abortion," 420.

Chapter 5.   Expansion and Specialization

1. "Unemployment," *BCR* 15 (May 1931): 131.

2. Lizabeth Cohen, *Making a New Deal: Industrial Workers in Chicago, 1919–1939* (Cambridge: Cambridge University Press, 1990), 213–249; Alice Kessler-Harris, *Out to Work: A History of Wage-Earning Women in the United States* (Oxford: Oxford University Press, 1982), 250–272.

3. "'Doctor' Jailed after Raid on Abortion Mill," *Chicago Daily Tribune,* November 14, 1932, Abortionists Folders, HHFC; Julian Moynahan to Editor, *New York Times* (hereafter cited as *NYT*), January 15, 1995, p. 16.

4. Carole Joffe and I made similar arguments about the "back-alley butcher" model of abortion history in papers presented on a panel together at the 1990 Berkshire Conference on the History of Women. Hers has since been published; Carole Joffe, "Portraits of Three 'Physicians of Conscience': Abortion before Legalization in the United States," *Journal of the History of Sexuality* 2 (July 1991): 46–67.

5. Lois Rita Helmbold, "Beyond the Family Economy: Black and White Working-Class Women during the Great Depression," *Feminist Studies* 13 (Fall 1987): 640–641; A. J. Rongy, *Abortion: Legal or Illegal?* (New York: Vanguard Press, 1933), 111.

6. Kessler-Harris, *Out to Work,* 256–257; quotations from typed letter from Charleston, IL 61920, April 20, 1985, "Silent No More" Campaign, National Abortion Rights Action League (NARAL), Chicago.

7. The doctor, apparently a chiropractor, performed eight abortions per day. "Abortion 'Club' Exposed," *BCR* 4 (November 1936): 5; "Birth Control 'Club' Revealed in Newark," *NYT,* October 13, 1936, p. 3.

8. Eric M. Matsner, M.D., to Editor, "Differentiation Sought," *NYT,* October 15, 1936, p. 26.

9. Linda Gordon, *Woman's Body, Woman's Right: Birth Control in America,* rev. and updated (1976; reprint, New York: Penguin Books, 1990), chap. 11; John D'Emilio and Estelle B. Freedman, *Intimate Matters: A History of Sexuality in America* (New York: Harper and Row, 1988), 244–248; David M. Kennedy, *Birth Control in America: The Career of Margaret Sanger* (New Haven: Yale University Press, 1970), 246–261, 214–217; James Reed, *From Private Vice to Public Virtue: The Birth Control Movement and American Society Since 1830* (New York: Basic Books, 1978), 239–241.

10. Frederick J. Taussig, *Abortion, Spontaneous and Induced: Medical and Social Aspects* (St. Louis: C. V. Mosby, 1936), quotation on 372, Cincinnati and New York on 363–364. On New Orleans, J. Thornwell Witherspoon, "An Analysis of 200 Cases of Septic Abortion Treated Conservatively," *AJOG* 26 (September 1933): 368. On Minneapolis, Jalmar H. Simons, "Statistical Analysis of One Thousand Abortions," *AJOG* 37 (May 1939): 840; Ransom S. Hooker, *Maternal Mortality in New York City: A Study of All Puerperal Deaths, 1930–1932* (New York: Oxford University Press for the Commonwealth Fund, 1933), 54; Henry J. Sangmeister, "A Survey of Abortion Deaths in Philadelphia from 1931 to 1940 Inclusive," *AJOG* 46 (November 1943): 758.

11. Paul H. Gebhard et al., *Pregnancy, Birth and Abortion* (New York: Harper and Brothers and Paul B. Hoeber Medical Books, 1958). Since much of the data comes from the earlier Kinsey studies on sexuality and this report came out of his institute, hereafter I refer to this book in the text as the Kinsey report or study on abortion.

12. Gebhard et al., *Pregnancy, Birth, and Abortion,* 113–114, 140, table 55.

13. The percentage of first pregnancies aborted in this young generation was no more than 10 percent, but it was more than double the rate of earlier generations of women. Regine K. Stix, "A Study of Pregnancy Wastage," *Milbank Memorial Fund Quarterly* 13 (October 1935): 358, fig. 2, quotation on 359; Gebhard et al., *Pregnancy, Birth, and Abortion,* 97–98.

14. Helmbold, "Beyond the Family Economy," 642–643; Ruth Milkman, "Women's Work and the Economic Crisis: Some Lessons from the Great Depression," *The Review of Radical Political Economics* 8 (spring 1976): 73–91, 95–97; reprint, in *A Heritage of Her Own: Toward a New Social History of American Women,* edited by Nancy F. Cott and Elizabeth H. Pleck (New York: Simon and Schuster, 1979), 507–541.

15. On African Americans and the Kinsey study, see "Why Negro Women are Not in the Kinsey Report," *Ebony* 8 (October 1953): 109–115; quotation from Charles H. Garvin, "The Negro Doctor's Task," *BCR* 16 (November 1932): 270. My thanks to Susan Smith and Leslie Schwalm for giving me the *Ebony* and *BCR* articles respectively. Jessie M. Rodrique, "The Black Community and the Birth Control Movement," in *Passion and Power: Sexuality in History,* edited by Kathy Peiss and Christina Simmons with Robert A. Padgug (Philadelphia: Temple University Press, 1989), 140–141.

16. Peter Marshall Murray and L. B. Winkelstein, "Incomplete Abortion: An Evaluation of Diagnosis and Treatment of 727 Consecutive Cases of Incomplete Abortions," *Harlem Hospital Bulletin* 3 (June 1950): 31, 33, offprint in folder 163, box 76–9, Peter Marshall Murray Papers, used with the permission of the Manuscript Division, Moorland-Spingarn Research Center, Howard

University. I am grateful to Susan Smith for bringing this article to my attention.

17. Endre K. Brunner and Louis Newton, "Abortions in Relation to Viable Births in 10,609 Pregnancies: A Study Based on 4,500 Clinic Histories," *AJOG* 38 (July 1939): 82–83, 88. See also Virginia Clay Hamilton, "Some Sociologic and Psychologic Observations on Abortion," *AJOG* 39 (June 1940): 923, table.

18. John Zell Gaston in George W. Kosmak, "The Responsibility of the Medical Profession in the Movement for 'Birth Control,'" *JAMA* 113 (October 21, 1939): 1559.

19. The Kinsey study did not report directly on women's reproductive practices according to class, but used level of education to signify class status. The study found that, of all the women surveyed who had abortions between the 1920s and 1940s, white married women with a grade school education (therefore presumably lower income) both delivered more babies and had more abortions than did women with greater levels of education (presumably middle or upper class). Women with less education bore more children and did so earlier in life (sixteen to twenty-five years), whereas college educated women tended to abort a greater proportion of pregnancies during these same years while in college and had children later. Gebhard et al., *Pregnancy, Birth, and Abortion,* 114, 120, 109–110, table 54; Brunner and Newton, "Abortions in Relation to Viable Births," 83. Among clients of birth control clinics in New York and Cincinnati in the 1930s, the abortion rate also rose as income rose, although a sample of New York City women found a higher rate of abortion in only "the poorest non-relief group." Regine K. Stix and Dorothy G. Wiehl, "Abortion and the Public Health," *American Journal of Public Health* 28 (May 1938): 624, fig. 2.

20. Hamilton, "Some Sociologic and Psychologic Observations on Abortion," quotations on 922, table on 923; Gebhard et al., *Pregnancy, Birth, and Abortion,* 37, 65–66, 162; Paula Giddings, *When and Where I Enter: The Impact of Black Women on Race and Sex in America* (New York: William Morrow, Bantam Books, 1984), 151–152.

21. Of the unmarried women, the Kinsey survey found that "the Negro college educated women aborted 81 per cent of their pregnancies (essentially the same percentage as for white college women), the high school educated women 25 per cent, and the grade school 19 per cent." The study found too that unwed black women with the least education (and thus from the lowest economic levels) were more likely to give birth and less likely to abort than unwed white women. Gebhard et al., *Pregnancy, Birth, and Abortion,* 162; D'Emilio and Freedman, *Intimate Matters,* 187, 259. Regina G. Kunzel also finds class differences among African-Americans in their use of maternity homes; Kunzel, *Fallen Women, Problem Girls: Unmarried Mothers and the Professionalization of Social Work, 1890–1945* (New Haven: Yale University Press, 1993), 73.

22. Approximately 12 percent of the Catholic women, 13 percent of the Jewish women, and 14 percent of the Protestant women in the Brunner and Newton study had had induced abortions. Brunner and Newton, "Abortions in Relation to Viable Births," 85, 90. A Minneapolis study reached similar conclusions; Simons, "Statistical Analysis of One Thousand Abortions," 840–841. But 35 percent of Stix's informants had had illegal abortions. "A Study of Pregnancy Wastage," 352.

23. The study showed that up to the age of twenty, Catholic, Jewish, and Protestant women all aborted pregnancies at about the same rate, approximately 7 percent. After the age of twenty a major shift occurred. The rate of abortion for Catholic and Jewish women rose only slightly for the twenty-one to twenty-five years of age group, whereas Protestant women's rate of abortion jumped to 20 percent. At the age of thirty-one to thirty-five years, another major shift occurred. The abortion rate for Protestant women dropped dramatically from the highest to zero, whereas the abortion rates for both Jewish and Catholic women increased. Brunner and Newton, "Abortions in Relation to Viable Births," 87, fig. 4.

24. Gebhard et al., *Pregnancy, Birth, and Abortion,* 64–65, 114–118.

25. Ibid., 194–195, 198.

26. *You May Plow Here: The Narrative of Sara Brooks,* edited by Thordis Simonsen (New York: Simon and Schuster, 1986), 176, 177.

27. Stix, "A Study of Pregnancy Wastage," 362–363; complications following abortions are summarized in a table on 362. Raymond E. Watkins, "A Five-Year Study of Abortion," *AJOG* 26 (August 1933): 162. See also a Tennessee study, James R. Reinberger and Percy B. Russell, "The Conservative Treatment of Abortion," *JAMA* 107 (November 7, 1936): 1527.

28. The closing of numerous small hospitals, including maternity hospitals, during the 1930s contributed to the movement of all medical care, including abortion, into public hospitals. Rosemary Stevens, *In Sickness and in Wealth: American Hospitals in the Twentieth Century* (New York: Basic Books, 1989), 141–143, 147–148; Judith Walzer Leavitt, *Brought to Bed: Childbearing in America, 1750–1950* (New York: Oxford University Press, 1986), 171–195.

29. I do not know when this ward first opened. Obstetric staff records beginning in 1938 discuss the number of abortion cases in ward 41. "Staff Conference of the Obstetrics Department," 1938–1958, box 30, "Department of Obstetrics," Medical Director's Office, Cook County Hospital, Cook County Hospital Archives.

30. Dr. Gertrude Engbring in Transcript of *People v. Heissler,* 338 Ill. 596 (1930), Case Files, vault no. 44783, Supreme Court of Illinois, Record Series 901; Augusta Weber, "Confidential Material Compiled for Joint Commission on Accreditation, June 1964," box 5, "Obstetrics Department—Accreditation 1964," Office of the Administrator, Cook County Hospital Archives. An "Abortion Service" was opened at Harlem Hospital in 1935. Murray and Winkelstein, "Incomplete Abortion," 31.

31. The Children's Bureau study was reported on before publication by Fred J. Taussig, "Abortion in Relation to Fetal and Maternal Welfare," *AJOG* 22 (November 1931): 729–738 and *AJOG* 22 (December 1931): 868–878; and Fred J. Taussig, "Abortion in Relation to Fetal and Maternal Welfare," in *Fetal, Newborn, and Maternal Morbidity and Mortality* (New York: D. Appleton-Century by the White House Conference on Child Health and Protection, 1933), 446–472; U.S. Dept. of Labor, Children's Bureau, *Maternal Mortality in Fifteen States,* Bureau publication no. 223 (Washington D.C.: Government Printing Office, 1934), 100–115, 133.

32. Hooker, *Maternal Mortality in New York City,* 51, 54; Taussig, "Abortion in Relation to Fetal and Maternal Welfare" (December 1931), 872.

33. William J. Robinson, *The Law against Abortion: Its Perniciousness Demonstrated and Its Repeal Demanded* (New York: Eugenics Publishing, 1933); A. J. Rongy, *Abortion: Legal or Illegal?* (New York: Vanguard Press, 1933). See also Alan F. Guttmacher, "The Genesis of Liberalized Abortion in New York: A Personal Insight," update by Irwin H. Kaiser, in *Abortion, Medicine, and the Law*, 3d ed., rev., edited by J. Douglas Butler and David F. Walbert (New York: Facts on File Publications, 1986), 231.

34. On Rongy, see "Abraham Rongy, Obstetrician, 71," *NYT*, October 11, 1949. On Robinson, see Gordon, *Woman's Body, Woman's Right*, 173–178; "Dr. W. J. Robinson, Urologist, Is Dead," *NYT*, January 7, 1936, p. 22; entry for William Josephus Robinson in *The National Cyclopaedia of Biography, Being the History of the United States*, vol. 35 (New York: James T. White and Co., 1949), 545–546. For early support for legal abortion, see W. Robinson, *The Law against Abortion*, 26; M. Rabinovitz, "End Results of Criminal Abortion: With Comments on Its Present Status," *New York Medical Journal* 100 (October 24, 1914): 808–811; William J. Robinson, "The Ethics of Abortion," *New York Medical Journal* 100 (October 31, 1914): 897.

35. W. Robinson, *The Law against Abortion*, remark on 26.

36. Rongy, *Abortion*, 39, 90, 146, 200–204, 206–209.

37. "Abraham Rongy, Obstetrician, 71."

38. A. J. Rongy, "Abortion: The $100,000,000 Racket," *American Mercury* 40 (February 1937): 145.

39. Gretta Palmer, "Not to Be Born," *Pictorial Review* 38 (February 1937): 24, 37, 45.

40. B. B. Tolnai, "The Abortion Racket," *Forum* 94 (September 1935): 177.

41. "Book Notices," *JAMA* 102 (January 6, 1934): 71–72.

42. On England, see Barbara Brookes, *Abortion in England, 1900–1967* (London: Croom Helm, 1988); Sheila Rowbotham, *"A New World for Women": Stella Browne, Socialist Feminist* (London: Pluto Press, 1977). On the Soviet Union, see Taussig, *Abortion*, chap. 26. On Germany, see Atina Grossmann, "Abortion and Economic Crisis: The 1931 Campaign against 218 in Germany," *New German Critique* 14 (spring 1978): 119–137; "Demand of the Independent Social Democrats that the Penalties for Abortion Be Removed," *JAMA* 75 (November 6, 1920): 1283; "Attack on the Law Concerning Abortion," *JAMA* 96 (February 14, 1931): 541–542; "The Attitude of Women Physicians toward the Abortion Question," *JAMA* 98 (April 30, 1932): 1580. On Switzerland, see "Bill to Legalize Abortion in Basel," *JAMA* 73 (October 4, 1919): 1095; "Abolishing Penalties for Abortion," *JAMA* 74 (June 12, 1920): 1656. On Vienna, see "Proposed New Legislation Concerning Abortion," *JAMA* 78 (January 21, 1922): 208.

43. Brookes, *Abortion in England*, chap. 4.

44. For examples of coverage of the European movements in medical journals, see note 42. Numerous articles appeared in the *Birth Control Review*. See, for example, Paul Lublinsky, "Birth Control in Soviet Russia," *BCR* 12 (May 1928): 142–143; Margaret Sanger, "Women in Germany," *BCR* 4 (December 1920): 8–9. See also "Sweden Considers a Proposal to Legalize Abortion," *Nation* 140 (March 20, 1935): 318; B. B. Tolnai, "Abortions and the Law," *Nation* 148 (April 15, 1939): 424–427.

45. Tess Slesinger, "Missis Flinders," part 4 of *The Unpossessed; A Novel of the Thirties* (1934; reprint, New York: Feminist Press, 1984). This chapter was first published in 1932 as a short story and "was the first fiction dealing with abortion to appear in a magazine of general circulation," as Janet Sharistanian notes in the afterword to *The Unpossessed,* 377, 385 n. 38. See also Agnes Smedley, *Daughter of Earth* (1929; reprint, New York: Feminist Press, 1973), 197–200, and Meridel Le Sueur, *The Girl* (Minneapolis: West End Press and MEP Publications, 1978), which was written in 1939 but not published until the 1970s. Josephine Herbst wrote autobiographically of abortion in "Unmarried" but did not publish the story. On Herbst, see Elinor Langer, *Josephine Herbst,* An Atlantic Monthly Press Book (Boston: Little, Brown and Co., 1983), 71–72. I am grateful to an anonymous reviewer for alerting me to Langer. That Le Sueur and Langer's stories were left unpublished shows the difficulty for women of publicly discussing this topic.

46. Gordon, *Woman's Body, Woman's Right,* 377–378; Ellen Chesler, *Woman of Valor: Margaret Sanger and the Birth Control Movement in America* (New York: Simon and Schuster, 1992), 300–303.

47. Colorado State Senator George A. Glenn, M.D. to Dr. Sanger, December 26, 1938; Florence Rose to Glenn, January 3, 1939; "A Bill for an Act Relating to the Legalization of Birth Control by Artificial or Natural Methods"; telegram from Rose to Glenn, January 16, 1939; Rose to Glenn, January 16, 1939, all letters in folder 10, box 2, Mary Steichen Calderone Papers, Arthur and Elizabeth Schlesinger Library on the History of Women in America, Radcliffe College, Cambridge, Massachusetts. Calderone Papers used with the permission of the Schlesinger Library. The Colorado State Archives has no material of Senator Glenn's or the Medical Affairs Committee; personal communication from Terry Ketelsen, Colorado State Archivist.

48. Linda Gordon discusses why the birth control movement moved away from the left in *Woman's Body, Woman's Right,* chap. 9, 245–247. See also J. Stanley Lemons, *The Woman Citizen: Social Feminism in the 1920s* (Urbana: University of Illinois Press, 1973), 209–227; Carole R. McCann, *Birth Control Politics in the United States, 1916–1945* (Ithaca: Cornell University Press, 1994), 26–53; Nancy F. Cott, *The Grounding of Modern Feminism* (New Haven: Yale University Press, 1987), 60–61.

49. On the U.S. birth control movement's antiabortion position, see, for example, the response of Mary Knoblauch to letter from Herman Dekker, *BCR* 4 (July 1920): 16; "Here Is an Illogical Situation," *BCR* 14 (March 1930): 73; "The Curse of Abortion," *BCR* 13 (November 1929): 307. On the English movement, see Brookes, *Abortion in England,* 80, 87, 90.

50. Taussig, *Abortion.* On the National Committee on Maternal Health, a committee of doctors that disassociated itself from the radicalism of the birth control movement, see Gordon, *Woman's Body, Woman's Right,* 258–259; Reed, *From Private Vice to Public Virtue,* 168–191.

51. Fred J. Taussig, review of *Abortion: Legal or Illegal?* by A. J. Rongy, *BCR* 17 (June 1933): 153.

52. Taussig, *Abortion,* 443–444.

53. Ibid., 444.

54. Ibid., 443.

55. Norman R. Fielder, "Study of Attitudes, Personality, Social Fitness, Adaptability, Character, and Motivations of Medical Students," *JAMA* 113 (November 25, 1939): 2005.

56. Taussig, *Abortion,* 292–297.

57. Quotations in ibid., 296, 292; see also Gerald B. Webb, "Clinical Aspects of Tuberculosis," in *The Cyclopedia of Medicine,* edited by George Morris, vol. 12 (Philadelphia: F. A. Davis, 1935), 244–268.

58. Taussig, *Abortion,* 296.

59. Ibid., 320–321, 297.

60. Ibid., 277–321.

61. Ibid., 278–279. For a more conservative view, see Hugo Ehrenfest, book review of *Der Kuenstliche Abort. Indikationen und Methoden* (Indications and methods of artificial abortion), 2d ed., by Georg Winter and Hans Naujoks, *AJOG* 25 (March 1933): 463.

62. "Queries and Minor Notes. Abortion or Removal of Pregnant Uterus," *JAMA* 96 (April 4, 1931): 1169.

63. Quotation from Rongy, *Abortion,* 170–171; Guttmacher, "The Genesis of Liberalized Abortion in New York," 229–230.

64. Ed Keemer, *Confessions of a Pro-Life Abortionist* (Detroit: Vinco Press, 1980), 63.

65. Rongy, *Abortion,* 134.

66. On specialization, see Rosemary Stevens, *American Medicine and the Public Interest* (New Haven: Yale University Press, 1971); Charlotte G. Borst, "The Professionalization of Obstetrics: Childbirth Becomes a Medical Specialty," in *Women, Health, and Medicine in America: A Historical Handbook,* edited by Rima D. Apple (New York: Garland Publishing, 1990), 197–216.

67. Lawrence Lader, *Abortion* (Boston: Beacon Press, 1966), 46; Keemer, *Confessions,* 65–68; "Abortaria," *Time* 28 (October 19, 1936): 71.

68. Rongy, *Abortion,* 134–135.

69. Tolnai, "The Abortion Racket," 176.

70. See "Pacific Coast Abortion Ring" File, HHFC; "Abortaria," 70–71. Dr. Robert Douglas Spencer performed abortions for women from all over the East Coast in his office in Ashland, Pennsylvania; see Lader, *Abortion,* 42–47, and Ellen Messer and Kathryn E. May, eds., *Back Rooms: Voices from the Illegal Abortion Era* (New York: St. Martin's Press, 1988), 218–224. On a nonphysician abortionist who practiced for decades in Portland, Oregon, see Ruth Barnett, as told to Doug Baker, *They Weep on My Doorstep* ([Oregon]: Halo Publishers, 1969) and a recent biography of Barnett by Rickie Solinger, *The Abortionist: A Woman against the Law* (New York: Free Press, 1994).

71. This case study is based on patient records and other legal documents discovered in the Transcript of *People v. Martin,* 382 Ill. 192 (1943), Case Files, vault no. 51699, Supreme Court of Illinois, Record Series 901.

72. Gabler went to Dearborn Medical College. In 1921, she gained a second medical license in West Virginia, where she spent part of each year. Perhaps she ran an abortion practice there also. All biographical information on Dr. Josephine Gabler is from the Deceased Physician Master File, AMA.

73. Supplemental Report, Statement of Gordon B. Nash, Assistant State's Attorney, April 23, 1942, in Transcript of *People v. Martin.*

74. A business card of Gabler's introduced into evidence in the Martin trial suggests that the clinic was open every day. The card lists the hours as "8 to 8." Transcript of *People v. Martin*.

75. Supplemental Report, Statement of Gordon B. Nash.

76. Martin estimated that she had worked as a receptionist for Gabler for "about 12 or 15 years." Supplemental Report, Statement of Gordon B. Nash. On Martin's management of the practice, see Ada Martin in the Transcript of *People v. Martin*. On Dr. Millstone's involvement, see "Doctor Bares Abortion Ring, Then Kills Self," *Chicago Daily Tribune*, April 18, 1941, pp. 1–2. Dr. E. D. Howe was also arrested, though it is unclear whether he performed abortions; "Offices of Loop Doctor Raided in Abortion Quiz," *Chicago Sunday Tribune*, May 11, 1941, p. 21.

77. Kristin Luker has assumed that women did not seek illegal abortions from doctors and that doctors did not assist women. Kristin Luker, *Abortion and the Politics of Motherhood* (Berkeley: University of California Press, 1984), 50, 51.

78. Supplemental Report, Statement of Gordon B. Nash; "Millstone's Widow Kills Self in Abortion Probe," *Chicago Daily Tribune*, May 1, 1941, p. 1. Of the eighteen doctors named in the patient records, eleven could be identified. (Sometimes only a last name was included on the record). All eleven were AMA members and eight were specialists of various types. Biographical data found in *American Medical Directory: A Register of Legally Qualified Physicians of the United States*, 16th ed. (Chicago: Press of the AMA, 1940). I am grateful to Rose Holz for collecting this information.

79. Of seventy patient records and seven additional witnesses, the referring individual was identifiable in thirty-eight cases. Eighteen were referred by doctors, or 47 percent. On the process of seeking and finding an abortionist in a later period, see Nancy Howell Lee, *The Search for an Abortionist* (Chicago: University of Chicago Press, 1969).

80. Mrs. Helen B. in Transcript of *People v. Martin*. I have used initials rather than surnames of women who testified in abortion cases and may still be living.

81. Supplemental Report, Statement of Gordon B. Nash. For a referring nurse, see the patient record for Grace E. in Transcript of *People v. Martin*.

82. George Wright, "Tells Bribe behind Killing," *Chicago Daily Tribune*, May 2, 1941, p. 1. The average fee charged for an abortion is my estimate based on records in the transcript of the trial; see the discussion of fees later in this chapter.

83. Stevens, *In Sickness and in Wealth*, 54, 114; Paul Starr, *The Social Transformation of American Medicine* (New York: Basic Books, 1982), 136, 358.

84. Twelve of thirty-eight identifiable referrals found their way to the clinic through friends.

85. While the newspapers covered the Martin story, they reported the deaths of two women due to criminal abortions; "Orders Arrest of Midwife in Woman's Death," *Daily Tribune*, May 7, 1941, p. 17; "Charge Doctor with Murder in Abortion Death," *Daily Tribune*, November 20, 1942, p. 9.

86. Each of the women who testified described the same procedure; this paragraph summarizes their testimony in the Transcript of *People v. Martin*.

87. Quotations from testimony of Helen Z., Gordon Nash, Julia M., Violet S. in Transcript of *People v. Martin*.

88. On standard medical procedures in abortion cases, see Taussig, *Abortion*, 328–340. As one physician noted, "a clean curettage by a skilled abortionist is obviously no more liable to infection than a therapeutic abortion performed in our own operating room"; Virginia Clay Hamilton, "The Clinical and Laboratory Differentiation of Spontaneous and Induced Abortion," *AJOG* 41 (January 1941): 62.

89. A study of working-class New York women found that of the 1,497 women who reported induced abortions, only 33, or 2 percent, were unmarried at the time. Brunner and Newton, "Abortion in Relation to Viable Births," 88.

90. All of the figures are based on my calculations from the seventy patient records included in the Transcript of *People v. Martin*. I have compared the testimony of the witnesses to their medical records. Of twenty-four witnesses, seventeen appeared in the patient records. Fifteen of the records showed the correct information; one patient record had no information on marital status, but she was unmarried; and one woman lied and said she was married when she was not. If other unmarried women lied too, the proportion of unmarried women would be higher.

91. Most of the women with children had one or two. Fourteen had one child, twelve had two, five had three, and one had four. All of these figures are my own calculations from the patient record data.

92. Victoria M. in patient record in Transcript of *People v. Martin*.

93. This is based on comparing the testimony of Helen N., Helen Z., and Helen B. to the information on their patient records in Transcript of *People v. Martin*.

94. Two modal ages, however, were younger, twenty-one and twenty-three years old. Of the women in this sample, 55 percent were under twenty-five; 45 percent were twenty-five or more years old.

95. "Abortion Surveillance: Preliminary Data—United States, 1992," *Morbidity and Mortality Weekly Report: CDC Surveillance Summaries* 43 (December 23, 1994): 930, 932, table 1.

96. Rosalind Petchesky, *Abortion and Woman's Choice: The State, Sexuality, and Reproductive Freedom*, rev. ed. (1984; reprint, Boston: Northeastern University Press, 1990), quotation on 145, and 141–167. Recent abortion data show the trend to delaying childbearing. Teenagers make up a smaller proportion of the women having abortions than in the past: in 1972, 33 percent of the women who had abortions were nineteen years old or less; in 1992, teenagers were only 20 percent of the women having abortions, and women twenty-five or older made up 45 percent of the women having abortions. "Abortion Surveillance," 932, table 1.

97. "Millstone's Widow Kills Self," 12.

98. Based on the information in the patient records under "date" of coming into the office at 190 North State Street and "mstd.," which refers to the last menstrual date, I have calculated at what point in their pregnancies these women came in for abortions. The most frequent length of pregnancy at the time of abortion was two months (thirty cases). Sixty of the women (86 per-

cent) aborted pregnancies that had progressed eight weeks or less. In 1992, 53 percent of abortions were in the first eight weeks. Nearly 90 percent of all abortions are performed in the first twelve weeks of pregnancy. "Abortion Surveillance," 930–933, table 1.

99. I have calculated these figures from the data in the patient records in the Transcript of *People v. Martin*. The Kinsey study was based on 304 cases. Gebhard et al., *Pregnancy, Birth, and Abortion*, 203, table 73.

100. Kessler-Harris, *Out to Work*, 263.

101. A study of births in 1928 found that the most frequent physician fee for delivery of a baby was $50, the fee most frequently charged for abortion at Martin's office. The total cost of an average obstetric case was approximately $200. Richard Arthur Bolt, "The Cost of Obstetric Service to Berkeley Mothers," *JAMA* 94 (May 17, 1930): 1561, 1563.

102. Gordon Nash in Transcript of *People v. Martin*.

103. Patient records for Alice F., Millicent M., Dorothy P., Margaret C., and Marguarita H. and record and testimony of Clara S. in Transcript of *People v. Martin*. One woman's pregnancy was two months, two were three months, and three were four to four and a half months along.

104. Georgina W. in Transcript of *People v. Martin*.

105. Paula F. in Transcript of *People v. Martin*.

106. Ronald L. Numbers, "The Third Party: Health Insurance in America," in *Sickness and Health in America: Readings in the History of Medicine and Public Health*, edited by Judith Walzer Leavitt and Ronald L. Numbers (Madison: University of Wisconsin Press, 1978), 139. Rosemary Stevens discusses how hospital charges varied with the class of the patient and, more recently, the "cost-shifting" in hospital budgets to make up for any "charity care." Stevens, *In Sickness and in Wealth*, 10–11, 112–113, 135, 270.

107. Thirteen of the seventy patient records showed that women owed money for their operations. Transcript of *People v. Martin*.

108. Nine of twenty-four witnesses (37.5 percent) described in Transcript of *People v. Martin* how they suggested or bargained for a lower price. Several of the patient records also show that an initial fee was changed. See the records of Anita P., Bernice M., Pearl G., and Pauline G. in the Transcript.

109. Testimony of Helen N. and Charlotte B. in Transcript of *People v. Martin*.

110. George Wright, "Fires Assistant Prosecutor," *Chicago Daily Tribune*, May 3, 1941, p. 1.

111. As a police officer, Moriarity received a little less than $2,500 per year. Quotations in Wright, "Tells Bribe behind Killing," 1.

112. Letter to Leslie Reagan from Rose S. [pseud.], Maryland, October 3, 1987.

113. Other doctors who appear to have specialized in abortion in Chicago include Dr. William E. Shelton, who may have been involved with Martin ("Dr. William Eugene Shelton," *Daily Tribune*, September 27, 1928; "Loop Physician Held in Abortion Conspiracy Case," *Daily Tribune*, November 21, 1940); Dr. Joseph A. Khamis ("Doctor Accused Second Time as an Abortionist," *Tribune*, August 18, 1942); Dr. Justin L. Mitchell (*People v. Mitchell*, 368 Ill.

399); and Dr. Edward Peyser (*People v. Peyser*, 380 Ill. 404). All newspaper clippings in Abortionists Files, HHFC.

114. Virginia Clay Hamilton, "Abortion," *JAMA* 117 (July 19, 1941): 216.

115. Keemer, *Confessions*, 13, 18, 27, 29, 89–93. I am grateful to Dr. Walter Lear for alerting me to Keemer's autobiography.

116. Ibid., 12, 23–24, 31, 61–65, quotation on 63.

117. Keemer never identified his wife by her full name. My guess is she did abortions as well because he wrote "we were performing more than a dozen [abortions] a month." Ibid., 25–26, 29–31, quotation on 100.

118. Ibid., 65–69, quotations on 65, 68. Feminists also reported that this was a relatively painless method; Jane, "Jane," *Voices*, June-November 1973, typescript, pp. 8–9.

119. "Abortifacient Pastes: The Exploitation and Dangers of Pastes Sold for Producing Therapeutic Abortion," *JAMA* 98 (June 11, 1932): 2155. See also Taussig, *Abortion*, 273, 323–324.

120. Keemer, *Confessions*, 100–101, quotation on 101. On federal efforts to eradicate abortifacients pastes in the late 1930s and early 1940s, see "Two Abortifacients Barred," *JAMA* 113 (October 21, 1939): 1583.

121. Keemer, *Confessions*, 70, 131, 138–142, 144.

122. Lader, *Abortion*, 46; Mary Steichen Calderone, ed., *Abortion in the United States: A Conference Sponsored by the Planned Parenthood Federation of America, Inc. at Arden House and the New York Academy of Medicine* (New York: Harper and Brothers, 1958), 59; Patricia G. Miller, *The Worst of Times* (New York: HarperCollins, 1993), 32–33.

123. On Timanus's practice, see testimony of Bessie E. Nelson and Anne Elizabeth Adams in Transcript, *Adams, Nelson, and Timanus v. State*, 200 Md. 133 (1951), pp. 456–583, Maryland Court of Appeals (transcripts), October 1951 [MSA S434; MdHR 12, 281–24; 1/67/13/34], Maryland State Archives, Annapolis, MD; Lader, *Abortion*, 42–44, 47–48.

124. Lader, *Abortion*, 46.

125. Ibid., 43–47; Joffe, "Portraits of Three 'Physicians of Conscience,'" 46–67; Keemer, *Confessions*, 12–14, 33–34.

126. Bessie E. Nelson in Transcript, *Adams, Nelson, and Timanus v. State*, pp. 485, 488.

Chapter 6.   Raids and Rules

1. Duffy quotation in George Wright, "Tells Bribe behind Killing," *Chicago Daily Tribune*, May 2, 1941, p. 1. This brief summary of events and the quotations of Ada Martin's are drawn from the Transcript of *People v. Martin*, 382 Ill. 192 (1943) Case Files, vault no. 51699, Supreme Court of Illinois, Record Series 901.

2. Testimony of Martin in Transcript of *People v. Martin*.

3. "Seize Physician and Two Nurses in Abortion Raid," *Chicago Tribune*, May 10, 1942, Abortionists Files, HHFC.

4. Wright, "Tells Bribe behind Killing," p. 1.

5. The term *professional abortionist* was widely used. See William J. Robinson, *The Law against Abortion: Its Perniciousness Demonstrated and Its Repeal Demanded* (New York: Eugenics Publishing, 1933), 75; Paul H. Gebhard et al., *Pregnancy, Birth, and Abortion* (New York: Harper and Brothers and Paul B. Hoeber Medical Books, 1958), 198–199.

6. Judith Walzer Leavitt, *Brought to Bed: Childbearing in America, 1750–1950* (New York: Oxford University Press, 1986), 194, 268, 184, graph; Henry J. Olson et al., "The Problem of Abortion," *AJOG* 45 (March 1943): 677; Augusta Webster, "Management of Abortion at the Cook County Hospital," *AJOG* 62 (December 1951): 1327, 1331; W. Nicholson Jones and Eugene H. Howe, "The Role of Antibiotics in the Management of Incomplete Abortions," *AJOG* 67 (April 1954): 825–831; Irvine Loudon, "Maternal Mortality: 1880–1950. Some Regional and International Comparisons," *Social History of Medicine* 1 (August 1988): 196–200.

7. Quotation in *People v. Stanko,* 402 Ill. 558 (1949), p. 560. See also Rolla J. Crick, "Portland 'Abortion Capital' of Northwest," *Portland Oregon Journal* [July 1951], Abortionists Files, HHFC.

8. One "law-breaking midwi[fe]" reportedly said, "There's an abortion boom. . . . I had forty-five patients on Saturday. . . . They come here straight from the factory, in slacks and overalls." Gretta Palmer, "Your Baby or Your Job," *Woman's Home Companion* 70 (October 1943): quotation on 137, 137–138; "Abortionist Convicted," *Time* 43 (March 6, 1944): 62.

9. Alice Kessler-Harris, *Out to Work: A History of Wage-Earning Women in the United States* (Oxford: Oxford University Press, 1982), 273–299.

10. The "feminine mystique" is Betty Friedan's phrase; Betty Friedan, *The Feminine Mystique* (New York: Dell, 1963). Mary P. Ryan shows the emphasis on domesticity in the early 1940s, but suggests that "the partisans of domesticity . . . won cultural hegemony after World War II" in *Womanhood in America: From Colonial Times to the Present* (New York: New Viewpoints, a division of Franklin Watts, 1975), 199; Elaine Tyler May, *Homeward Bound: American Families in the Cold War Era* (New York: Basic Books, 1988); Susan M. Hartmann, *The Home Front and Beyond: American Women in the 1940s* (Boston: Twayne Publishers, 1982); Linda Gordon, *Heroes of Their Own Lives: The Politics and History of Family Violence, Boston, 1880–1960* (New York: Viking, 1988); Linda Gordon, *Woman's Body, Woman's Right: Birth Control in America,* rev. and updated (1976; reprint, New York: Penguin Books, 1990), chap. 12.

11. Anna Kross, "The Abortion Problems Seen in Criminal Courts," in *The Abortion Problem: Proceedings of the Conference Held Under the Auspices of the National Committee on Maternal Health, Inc. at the New York Academy of Medicine, June 19th and 20th, 1942* (Baltimore: Williams and Wilkins, for the National Committee on Maternal Health, 1944), 110, 107; *Ladies Home Journal* quotation as cited in Ryan, *Womanhood in America,* 199, 167–168, 198–209, Rosalind Pollack Petchesky, *Abortion and Woman's Choice: The State, Sexuality, and Reproductive Freedom,* rev. ed. (1984; reprint, Boston: Northeastern University Press, 1990), 106, 111, 114; Paula Giddings, *When and Where I Enter: The Impact of Black Women on Race and Sex in America* (New York: William Morrow and Co., 1984), 250–258.

12. McCarthyism is a convenient label used for the anticommunist hysteria

of the 1940s and 1950s even though Senator Joseph McCarthy himself did not steal the limelight until 1950.

13. Mary Jezer, *The Dark Ages: Life in the United States 1945–1960* (Boston: South End Press, 1982); David Caute, *The Great Fear: The Anti-Communist Purge under Truman and Eisenhower* (New York: Simon and Schuster, 1978); Ellen Schrecker, *The Age of McCarthyism: A Brief History with Documents* (Boston: Bedford Books of St. Martin's Press, 1994); Deborah A. Gerson, "'Is Family Devotion Now Subversive?' Familialism against McCarthyism," in *Not June Cleaver: Women and Gender in Postwar America, 1945–1960,* edited by Joanne Meyerowitz (Philadelphia: Temple University Press, 1994), 151–172.

14. John D'Emilio, *Sexual Politics, Sexual Communities: The Making of a Homosexual Community, 1940–1970* (Chicago: University of Chicago Press, 1983), 41–43, 49–51, 91, quotation on 49. As I find about abortion, George Chauncey finds that prior to this period, the gay male world was much more visible and tolerated than previously realized, *Gay New York: Gender, Urban Culture, and the Making of the Gay Male World, 1890–1940* (New York: Basic Books, 1994).

15. "The Abortion Menace," *Ebony* 6 (January 1951): 24. I am grateful to Susan Smith for bringing this article to my attention.

16. "Sin No More," *Time* 38 (July 28, 1941): 60; "$500,000 Mill," *Time* 50 (September 15 1947): 49–50; "Six Are Arrested in Abortion Raid," *NYT,* July 17, 1941, p. 20; "3 Held in Abortion Case," *NYT,* February 4, 1944, p. 17. The available evidence suggests that Chicago and New York may have led the way in establishing raids as the method for enforcing the abortion laws, but this could be an artifact of the sources.

17. Morton Sontheimer, "Abortion in America Today," *Woman's Home Companion* 82 (October 1955): 96.

18. "Local Doctor Admits Illegal Operations 'To Help Out Needy,'" *Covington Kentucky Post,* February 25, 1952, Abortionists Files, HHFC.

19. Ohio: "One Doctor's Choice," *Time* 67 (March 12, 1956): 46–47; Detroit: "Abortion Raid Nets 2 Medics," *Detroit Free Press,* August 29, 1956; Baltimore: Lawrence Lader, *Abortion* (Boston: Beacon Press, 1966), 42–48; Los Angeles: "Nab 4 in Beach Mansion as Illegal Operation Ring," *Los Angeles, California, Herald and Express,* February 4, 1956; Portland: "Grand Jury Indicts 19," *Portland Oregon Journal,* July 6, 1951, p. 1. Portland and Los Angeles clips are in Abortionists Files, HHFC. No doubt further investigation into the newspapers and records of every state would uncover similar practices elsewhere.

20. As cited in David J. Garrow, *Liberty and Sexuality: The Right to Privacy and the Making of Roe v. Wade* (New York: Macmillan 1994), 279.

21. "Bronx Doctor Indicted on Abortion Rap," *New York Home News,* October 20, 1951; "Woman, 3 Men Seized in Abortion Blackmail," *New York Evening Post,* September 28, 1951, both clips in Abortionists Files, HHFC; Jerome E. Bates and Edward S. Zawadzki, *Criminal Abortion: A Study in Medical Sociology* (Springfield, Ill.: Charles C. Thomas, 1964), 68–70. Ex-patients sometimes tried to blackmail their abortionists, see Rolla J. Crick, "The Abortion Racket," *Portland, Oregon Journal,* July 9, 1951, Abortionists Files, HHFC; Lader, *Abortion,* 48.

22. There were twenty-three cases reviewed dealing with abortions performed between 1940 and 1960.

23. This description of the investigation led by Papanek is based on the testimony of Martin's patients as well as letters from people responding to Papanek's letter in the Transcript of *People v. Martin.*

24. See the humble responses in letters to Papanek, presented as Defendants' exhibits in Transcript of *People v. Martin.*

25. In this particular trial there was no jury.

26. Georgina W., Madeline D., and Evelyn K. in Transcript of *People v. Martin.*

27. Defendant's exhibit 15-a in Transcript of *People v. Martin.*

28. Evelyn K., Helen B., and Stella P. described the state's attorney's office in these words in Transcript of *People v. Martin.*

29. John Harlan Amen, "Some Obstacles to Effective Legal Control of Criminal Abortions," in *The Abortion Problem,* 137; "Abortion Trial Witness Balks; Gets 6 Months," *Chicago Daily Tribune,* November 22, 1949, p. 6; "Convict 2 in Abortion Trial," *Chicago Daily News,* December 1, 1949. Both newspaper clips are in Abortionists Files, HHFC.

The federal government prosecuted abortionists for income tax invasion, which may have been easier than prosecuting for abortion per se. At these trials too the government forced women to speak of their abortions. "Ten Women Tell Abortion Fees at U.S. Tax Trial," *New York Daily News,* October 16, 1952, cited in Bates and Zawadzki, *Criminal Abortion,* 63–64.

30. Compare Evelyn K. and Martha K.; other women also were asked to name their physicians and did so in court. For examples of physicians' names, see the patient records of Helen N., Beatrice S., and Charlotte J. in the Transcript of *People v. Martin.*

31. Transcript of *People v. Martin.*

32. It was particularly important during war, the Court continued, that care be taken against violating people's rights. Furthermore, "These promises are to be construed liberally in favor of the people." *People v. Martin,* 196, 202.

33. The court's opinion in *People v. Martin* referred to both state and U.S. supreme court decisions, pp. 196–203. *People v. Martin* was not the first such case in Illinois, but it was part of a movement coming from the states to apply the U.S. Constitution to criminal procedure in the states. Friedman suggests that the U.S. Supreme Court opinions in the 1950s and 1960s that applied the Bill of Rights to the states and required the states to conform to the same rules of fairness in the criminal process arose from changes developing in the states, but elaborates only slightly on this point. Lawrence M. Friedman, *Crime and Punishment in American History* (New York: Basic Books, 1993), 303.

Applying the fourth amendment of the U.S. Constitution to the states through the fourteenth amendment, which guaranteed due process, is called "incorporation." Applying the fourth amendment to the states meant that state prosecutors, like federal officials, could not use evidence obtained illegally against the defendant at trial. This is called the "exclusionary rule" and is meant to protect all citizens (not criminals as conservatives claim) from abuses by police and other state authorities. The case that applied the exclusionary rule to the states is *Mapp v. Ohio,* 367 U.S. 643 (1961). John E. Nowak, "Criminal

Procedure. Constitutional Aspects," and James B. White, "Search and Seizure," in *Encyclopedia of Crime and Justice*, vol. 2, edited by Sanford H. Kadish (New York: Free Press, 1983), 527–536, 1415–1421; Friedman, *Crime and Punishment in American History*, chap. 14.

34. *People v. Martin*. I have been unable to determine whether the state prosecuted the pair again or dropped the case.

35. Wright, "Tells Bribe behind Killing," 1; George Wright, "Fires Assistant Prosecutor," *Chicago Daily Tribune*, May 3, 1941, p. 1.

36. "Doctor Bares Abortion Ring, Then Kills Self," *Chicago Daily Tribune*, April 18, 1941, p. 1; "Millstone's Widow Kills Self in Abortion Probe," *Chicago Daily Tribune*, May 1, 1941, p. 1; "Offices of Loop Doctor Raided in Abortion Quiz," *Chicago Sunday Tribune*, May 11, 1941, p. 21.

37. Photos in "Doubts Are Cast on Motive Given in Girl Slaying," *Chicago Daily Tribune*, April 30, 1941, p. 9; "Millstone's Widow Kills Self in Abortion Probe," 12.

38. For good examples of critical analysis of this type of journalism, see Judith R. Walkowitz, *City of Dreadful Delight: Narratives of Sexual Danger in Late-Victorian London* (Chicago: University of Chicago Press, 1992); Lisa Duggan, "The Trials of Alice Mitchell: Sensationalism, Sexology, and the Lesbian Subject in Turn-of-the-Century America," *Signs* 18 (summer 1993): 791–814.

39. As Lawrence Friedman has suggested, the notion of a syndicate proved fruitful for the FBI; organized crime gave the FBI reason to expand and conduct far-reaching domestic investigations. Friedman, *Crime and Punishment in American History*, 266–267, 272–273, quotation on 273.

40. Rolla J. Crick, "Portland 'Abortion Capital' of Northwest." Assessing the accuracy of this image is difficult. The press and state authorities regularly described illegal abortion practices as "rings," which could mean merely that several people were involved: an abortionist, often a physician, a nurse, a receptionist, an attorney—people one would expect to find connected to most medical practices—as well as physicians and others who referred patients to the practitioner. To the extent that "the mafia" did take up abortion after the end of Prohibition (which I have often been told but cannot document), this was of course due to the illegality of abortion.

41. For police kicking down doors, see "Seize Physician and Two Nurses in Abortion Raid," *Chicago Tribune*, May 10, 1942, Abortionists Files, HHFC. For quotations and patient record, see Wright, "Tells Bribe behind Killing," 1.

42. "Nab Ex-Doctor and 2 in Loop Abortion Raid," *Chicago Tribune*, September 4, 1947, Abortionists Files, HHFC; "Report 3 True Bills in Abortions," *Chicago Daily News*, August 21, 1951, p. 8, Abortionists Files, HHFC.

43. Compare "Abortion Trial Witness Balks" and "Identifies Doctor in Abortion," *Chicago Daily News*, November 28, 1949, p. 2.

44. Clara L. in the Transcript of *People v. Stanko*, 402 Ill. 558 (1949), Case Files, vault no. 55590, Supreme Court of Illinois, Record Series 901. Other women rounded up by Chicago police gave similar testimony about that day. Stanko was tried twice and the case appealed twice, *People v. Stanko*, 402 Ill. 558 (1949); *People v. Stanko*, 407 Ill. 624 (1951).

45. James P. Hackett in Transcript of *People v. Stanko* (1949).

46. Opening statement by James A. Brown in Transcript of *People v. Stanko* (1949).

47. For a Pennsylvania case, see Patricia G. Miller, *The Worst of Times* (New York: HarperCollins, 1993), 215–216. In a Detroit raid, police picked up sixteen women. "Three of the women," the paper reported, "were taken to Receiving Hospital for treatment." Most likely they were examined there and the state planned to use those examinations for evidence. "Abortion Raid Nets 2 Medics," *Detroit Free Press,* August 29, 1956.

48. *People v. Stanko* (1949), p. 560.

49. Dr. Towne, an obstetrician-gynecologist, was a graduate of Loyola University Medical School in Chicago and an assistant clinical professor there. Dr. Janet Towne in Transcript of *People v. Stanko* (1949); *American Medical Directory,* 18th ed. (Chicago: American Medical Association, 1950), 735. Given her connections, she may have been Catholic and motivated to help the local prosecutor in light of both her religious and her medical beliefs.

50. *People v. Stanko* (1949), p. 559.

51. Clara L. in Transcript of *People v. Stanko* (1949).

52. *People v. Stanko* (1949) and *People v. Stanko* (1951).

53. Affidavits of Helen Stanko, January 14, 1948; questions to Clara L., and closing argument by Edward C. Dufficy in Transcript of *People v. Stanko* (1949).

54. *People v. Stanko* (1949), pp. 558–562; *People v. Stanko* (1951), p. 626.

55. For arrests in Pennsylvania and New Jersey respectively, see Miller, *The Worst of Times,* 215; news clipping, no title, *Union City, New Jersey Dispatch,* July 13, 1951, Abortionists Files, HHFC. For threats, see Sontheimer, "Abortion in America Today," 101.

56. Gordon Nash in Transcript of *People v. Martin.*

57. "State Tax Delay Granted Soldiers," *NYT,* May 9, 1942, p. 6; "Credit Lady Cops in Abortion Drive," *New York World Telegraph,* June 1955, Abortionists Files, HHFC.

58. "Charges Doctors Aid Abortions," *Chicago Daily News,* March 9, 1954. See also "Cops Crack Down on Illegal Surgery," *San Francisco Call Bulletin,* May 1, 1957. Both clips are in Abortionists Files, HHFC.

59. Gerson, "'Is Family Devotion Now Subversive?'"

60. "Abortionist Convicted," *Time,* 43 (March 6, 1944): 60. Ellen Schrecker finds that communist women were stigmatized as bad mothers and consistently associated with sexual deviance. Ellen Schrecker, "The Bride of Stalin: Gender and Anticommunism during the McCarthy Era" (paper delivered to the Berkshire Conference on Women's History, Vassar College, June 11, 1993), 9–13, 15–17.

61. Maxine Davis, "Have Your Baby," *Good Housekeeping* 118 (June 1944): 45; "Soviet Legalizes Abortions Again," *NYT,* December 1, 1955, p. 9.

62. Students at Rutgers University quickly learned that publishing their views on abortion was unacceptable when the Knights of Columbus, Catholic War Veterans, and Catholic Holy Name Societies protested to the state legislature. The students resigned under pressure. "More Quit at Rutgers," *NYT,* December 8, 1950, p. 34; "Rutgers Inquiry Sought," *NYT,* December 13, 1950;

"Rutgers Names Inquiry Board," *NYT,* December 16, 1950, p. 20; "Driscoll Starts Rutgers Inquiry," *NYT,* December 20, 1950.

63. Ellen Schrecker, *The Age of McCarthyism,* 1–94; Caute, *The Great Fear,* 403–486 on the professions; Jezer, *The Dark Ages,* 78–106.

64. J. Stanley Lemons, *The Woman Citizen: Social Feminism in the 1920s* (Urbana: University of Illinois Press, 1973), 171–175; Paul Starr, *The Social Transformation of American Medicine* (New York: Basic Books, 1982), 279–288.

65. "Grand Jury to Scan Brooklyn Abortions," *NYT,* December 11, 1953, p. 26; Sontheimer, "Abortion in America Today," 101. Anti-Semitism was a component of McCarthyism, especially in New York; Caute, *The Great Fear,* 21, 115, 224–225, 434–438.

66. Comments of Dr. Albert E. Catherwood in discussion of H. Close Hesseltine, F. L. Adair, and M. W. Boynton, "Limitation of Human Reproduction. Therapeutic Abortion," AJOG 39 (April 1940): 561. Sterilization will be discussed further in chapter 7, this volume.

67. Remarks in Hesseltine, Adair, and Boynton, "Limitation of Human Reproduction," 561.

68. Harry A. Pearse and Harold A. Ott, "Hospital Control of Sterilization and Therapeutic Abortion," *AJOG* 60 (August 1950): 290.

69. "The Right Thing," *Newsweek* 12 (August 1, 1938): 29; "Great Britain. Test Case," *Time* 32 (August 1, 1938): 17; "Tests Motherhood Law," *NYT,* June 29, 1938, p. 8; "Briton Held in Test on Birth Prevention," *NYT,* July 2, 1938, p. 5; "Aide of King Backs Illegal Operation," *NYT,* July 19, 1938, p. 11; "Foreign Letter. London. The Induction of Abortion in a Case of Rape," *JAMA* 111 (August 20, 1938): 731; Barbara Brookes, *Abortion in England, 1900–1967* (London: Croom Helm, 1988), 40, 133.

70. Hesseltine, Adair, and Boynton, "Limitation of Human Reproduction," 561.

71. Pearse and Ott, "Hospital Control of Sterilization and Therapeutic Abortion," 297, Rudolph W. Holmes comment in discussion on 299.

72. Ibid., 290.

73. Ibid., 291, 293, 294, 296.

74. A study of therapeutic abortion committee members in twenty-six hospitals in San Francisco and Los Angeles learned that the majority agreed that "the committee functions to police the activities of a physician whose procedures might otherwise bring himself and his colleagues into disrepute. . . . And several responses indicated agreement with the view that the committee serves as a curb on the perfectly scrupulous but somewhat 'liberal' obstetrician." Herbert L. Packer and Ralph J. Gampell, "Therapeutic Abortion: A Problem in Law and Medicine," *Stanford Law Review* 11 (May 1959): 429.

75. Charles M. McLane in Mary Steichen Calderone, ed., *Abortion in the United States: A Conference Sponsored by the Planned Parenthood Federation of America, Inc. at Arden House and the New York Academy of Medicine* (New York: Harper and Brothers, 1958), 101–102.

76. On Monmouth Memorial Hospital: comments of Dr. Robert A. MacKenzie in discussion of Walter T. Dannreuther, "Therapeutic Abortion in a General Hospital," *AJOG* 52 (July 1946): 63–64. On California Hospital: Keith

P. Russell, "Therapeutic Abortion in a General Hospital," *AJOG* 62 (August 1951): 435, 437, 438. I have calculated an approximate number of abortions for the five years prior to the formation of the committee from figures provided by Russell. On University of Virginia Hospital: David C. Wilson, "Psychiatric Implications in Abortions," *Virginia Medical Monthly* 79 (August 1952): 448. On Sloan Hospital: Robert E. Hall, "Therapeutic Abortion, Sterilization, and Contraception," *AJOG* 91 (February 15, 1965): 518, 520–521, table 2. On Mt. Sinai Hospital: "Abortion Rates Said Unaffected by Regulations," *Scope Weekly s* (August 31, 1960), no page no., in "Abortion, 1960–1964," Vertical File, American Hospital Association (hereafter cited as AHA), Chicago, Illinois.

77. MacKenzie in Dannreuther, "Therapeutic Abortion in a General Hospital," 64; Alan F. Guttmacher, "Therapeutic Abortion: The Doctor's Dilemma," *Journal of the Mount Sinai Hospital, New York* 21 (May-June 1954): 118.

78. MacKenzie in Dannreuther, "Therapeutic Abortion in a General Hospital," 64.

79. The physician reporting on the hospital's policy believed that "the patients have felt that they have had a fair hearing," but some women must have been annoyed by the repeated prying into their emotional health. Wilson, "Psychiatric Implications in Abortions," 449.

80. S. A. Cosgrove and Patricia A. Carter, "A Consideration of Therapeutic Abortion," *AJOG* 48 (September 1944): 299–304, 305, table 1, quotations on 304, 305. Emphasis in original.

81. Cosgrove and Carter, "A Consideration of Therapeutic Abortion," quotations on 308, 305; "Correspondence. Reply by Dr. Cosgrove," *AJOG* 48 (December 1944): 894.

82. Dr. Nicholson J. Eastman of Johns Hopkins defended the frequency of therapeutic abortion in his hospital, but he first pointed out that the incidence of therapeutic abortion was almost half of what had been reported—an argument that essentially granted the evil of therapeutic abortion. Nicholson J. Eastman, "Correspondence; Therapeutic Abortion," *AJOG* 48 (December 1944): 892–893; and "Reply by Dr. Cosgrove," *AJOG* 48 (December 1944): 893–895. The therapeutic abortion to delivery ratio became a standard way of presenting data and comparing hospitals. See Dannreuther, "Therapeutic Abortion in a General Hospital," 54–65; J. G. Moore and J. H. Randall, "Trends in Therapeutic Abortions. A Review of 137 Cases," *AJOG* 63 (January 1952): 28–29, 31; Roy J. Heffernan and William A. Lynch, "What is the Status of Therapeutic Abortion in Modern Obstetrics?" *AJOG* 66 (August 1953): 337–338; Christopher Tietze in Calderone, *Abortion in the United States,* 85.

83. Comments of Drs. Guttmacher, Rosen, and Lidz, in Calderone, *Abortion in the United States,* 92, 95–96.

84. A Yale medical professor had been attacked as a communist, and Catholic hospitals revoked the admitting privileges of physicians who had spoken in favor of birth control in the Connecticut state legislature. Public support for reproductive control was politically dangerous. Garrow, *Liberty and Sexuality,* 149–150, 113–116, chaps. 1–2.

85. Remarks of Dr. George H. Ryder, Dr. Edward A. Schumann, and Dr. Charles A. Poindexter in Dannreuther, "Therapeutic Abortion in a General

Hospital," 62–64. See also Dr. Raymond Squier, who called for a liberalization of the law, in *The Abortion Problem*, 170–171; and Dr. Sophia J. Kleegman in Calderone, *Abortion in the United States*, 113–116.

86. Bessie E. Nelson in Transcript of *Adams, Nelson, and Timanus v. State* 200 Md. 133 (1951), pp. 474–476, Maryland Court of Appeals (transcripts), October 1951 [MSA S434; MdHR 12,281–24; 1/67/13/34], Maryland State Archives, Annapolis, Maryland. Lawrence Lader also discusses the raid and prosecution of Timanus in *Abortion*, 48–51; Ed Keemer, *Confessions of a Pro-Life Abortionist* (Detroit: Vinco Press, 1980), 163–164.

87. The situation would be different in cases where defendants had no lawyers.

88. Not every lawyer is successful at this, but the best work to keep out extraneous and unanticipated information.

89. A transcript of Keemer's trial and other materials are not available because the records are sealed. Keemer, *Confessions*, 233. My analysis of the Timanus case is based on both the published court opinion, *Adams, Nelson, and Timanus v. State*, 200 Md. 133 (1951), and the trial Transcript.

90. Transcript of *Adams, Nelson, and Timanus v. State*, quotation on p. 217.

91. Ibid., 222.

92. Ibid., 219–221, 255.

93. Ibid., 219, 222.

94. Ibid., 277, 290.

95. Ibid., 576; see also 570, 577.

96. Ibid., 565.

97. Ibid., 579.

98. Nurses referred patients to the Gabler-Martin clinic, but there is no information about them. See Grace E. patient record in Transcript of *People v. Martin;* George Wright, "Tells Bribe behind Killing," 1. For examples of nurses arrested with abortionists, see "Abortion Charges Are Continued Until March 3," *Chicago South End Reporter*, February 17, 1954, Abortionists Files, HHFC; "Credit Lady Cops in Abortion Drive," *New York World Telegraph*, June 1955, Abortionists Files, HHFC. Nurses may appear less often because the state dropped cases against them since many were not actually doing abortions or because nurses did not have the resources to appeal. On the history of nursing, see Barbara Melosh, *"The Physician's Hand": Work Culture and Conflict in American Nursing* (Philadelphia: Temple University Press, 1982); Susan M. Reverby, *Ordered to Care: The Dilemma of American Nursing, 1850–1945* (Cambridge: Cambridge University Press, 1987); Darlene Clark Hine, *Black Women in White: Racial Conflict and Cooperation in the Nursing Profession, 1890–1950* (Bloomington: Indiana University Press, 1989).

99. Transcript of *Adams, Nelson, and Timanus v. State*, pp. 334–335.

100. Testimony of Nancy Lee B., Jerome Goodman, Bessie E. Nelson respectively in ibid., pp. 231–232, 324–332, 463–472; Calderone, *Abortion in the United States*, 63; G. L. Timanus to Alan, March 15, 1962, Alan F. Guttmacher Papers, used with permission of the Countway Library, Harvard University, Boston, Massachusetts. I am grateful to David Garrow for alerting me to the Guttmacher collection.

101. Transcript of *Adams, Nelson, and Timanus v. State,* pp. 376–377.

102. On nineteenth-century doctors in court, see James C. Mohr, *Doctors and the Law: Medical Jurisprudence in Nineteenth-Century America* (New York: Oxford University Press, 1993), 94–108.

103. Christopher Tietze, "Therapeutic Abortions in New York City, 1943–1947," *AJOG* 60 (July 1950): 149, 152; Wilson, "Psychiatric Implications in Abortion," 448. This indication is discussed further in chapter 7, this volume.

104. Timanus in Calderone, *Abortion in the United States,* 62–63; Lader, *Abortion,* 49–51.

105. "Women Tell of Abortions," *The Baltimore Sun,* April 10, 1951. Timanus was not the only one abandoned by his colleagues. When police arrested an Ohio physician-abortionist who had been relied upon by area doctors for years, the medical society kicked him out. "One Doctor's Choice," *Time* 67 (March 12, 1956): 46–47.

106. *Adams, Nelson, and Timanus v. State,* p. 141; Lader, *Abortion,* 51; Transcript of *Adams, Nelson, and Timanus v. State,* p. 2.

107. Most of the description of the investigation and trial comes from Keemer's autobiography. Keemer, *Confessions,* 169–174, quotations on 164, 171.

108. Ibid., 171–172, 178; Isaac Jones, "Physicians Get 2–5 Jail Term," *Detroit Michigan Chronicle,* February 8, 1958, p. 1.

109. "Physicians Issue Final Statement," *Detroit Michigan Chronicle,* February 8, 1958, p. 1. Keemer quotation italicized in original; Keemer, *Confessions,* 176–177.

110. Bill Matney, "Views of the News," *Detroit Michigan Chronicle,* January 18, 1958, p. 1; Garrow, *Liberty and Sexuality,* 361.

111. Gordon, *Woman's Body, Woman's Right,* 217–232. On the birth control movement's work leading up to the U.S. Supreme Court decision in *Griswold v. Connecticut* (1965), which legalized birth control, see Garrow, *Liberty and Sexuality,* 1–269. On the civil rights movement and the NAACP, see Genna Rae McNeil, "Charles Hamilton Houston: Social Engineer for Civil Rights," in *Black Leaders of the Twentieth Century,* edited by John Hope Franklin and August Meier (Urbana: University of Illinois Press, 1982), 221–232; Richard Kluger, *Simple Justice: The History of Brown v. Board of Education and Black America's Struggle for Equality* (New York: Knopf, 1976); Mark V. Tushnet, *Making Civil Rights Law: Thurgood Marshall and the Supreme Court, 1936–1961* (New York: Oxford University Press, 1994); Vicki L. Crawford et al., *Women in the Civil Rights Movement: Trailblazers and Torchbearers, 1941–1965* (Bloomington: Indiana University Press, 1990).

112. On the Timanus case, see "Women Tell of Abortions"; "Dr. Timanus Convicted in Abortion Case," *Baltimore Sun,* April 12, 1951, pp. 38, 26; "Doctor Gets 6 Months for Illegal Operation," *Baltimore Sun,* November 8, 1951. On the Keemer case, see "Conspiracy Charges Aired in Recorder's," *Detroit Michigan Chronicle,* January 18, 1958, p. 1; "Two Medics Guilty in Conspiracy Case," *Detroit Michigan Chronicle,* January 25, 1958, p. 1; "Physicians Get 2–5 Jail Terms," 1, 4.

113. Brookes, *Abortion in England,* 40, 133, 69–70, 79–104, Bourne quotation on 69.

114. Keemer himself returned to practicing abortion, became active in the National Association for the Repeal of Abortion Laws (NARAL), and invited arrest. "4 Arraigned for Illegal Abortions," *Detroit Free Press,* October 28, 1972, p. 3, sec. A.

115. Paul Starr, *The Social Transformation of American Medicine* (New York: Basic Books, 1992), 402–403, 421; Rosemary Stevens, *In Sickness and in Wealth: American Hospitals in the Twentieth Century* (New York: Basic Books, 1989), 341–344. On the power of the medical profession and the struggles between hospitals and physicians earlier in the twentieth century, see Stevens, *In Sickness and in Wealth,* 231, 241–246; Starr, *The Social Transformation of American Medicine,* 161. In scattered instances, a few nineteenth-century hospitals required consultation or staff approval before performing potentially fatal surgery in hospitals. Charles E. Rosenberg, *The Care of Strangers: The Rise of America's Hospital System* (Philadelphia: Basic Books, 1987), 145, 257.

116. Sister M. Patricia, Asa S. Bacon, Fred G. Carter, "The Hospital Administrator: An Analysis of His Duties, Responsibilities, Relationships and Obligations," by the 1934–1935 Study Committee of the American College of Hospital Administrators, p. 13, AHA. See also American Hospital Association, *Manual on Obstetrical Practice in Hospitals* (Chicago: American Hospital Association, 1936), 6, 5, AHA; Malcolm T. MacEachern, *Manual on Obstetric Practice in Hospitals,* American Hospital Association Official Bulletin No. 209 (Chicago: American Hospital Association, 1940), 35, AHA; Joint Commission on Accreditation of Hospitals, *Standards for Hospital Accreditation* (December 1954), AHA. There was no evidence of concern about coercive sterilization practices; the issue of concern was patient control. Some expected that these standards would be applied in biased ways. See Mary Steichen Calderone, M.D. to Howard C. Taylor Jr., M.D., June 4, 1957, folder 15, box 2, Mary Steichen Calderone Papers, Schlesinger Library.

117. Calderone, *Abortion in the United States,* 63.

Chapter 7.   Repercussions

1. Alfred Kinsey in Mary Steichen Calderone, ed., *Abortion in the United States: A Conference Sponsored by the Planned Parenthood Federation of America, Inc. at Arden House and the New York Academy of Medicine* (New York: Harper and Brothers, 1958), 40.

2. Rosalind Pollack Petchesky, *Abortion and Woman's Choice: The State, Sexuality, and Reproductive Freedom,* rev. ed. (1984; Boston: Northeastern University Press, 1990), 100–116. For college participation rates, see Kenneth A. Simon and W. Vance Grant, *Digest of Educational Statistics* (Washington, D.C.: Government Printing Office, 1972), 77, table 103; U.S. Bureau of the Census, *Historical Statistics of the United States, Colonial Times to 1970,* Bicentennial ed., part 1 (Washington D.C.: Government Printing Office, 1975), Series H 602–617, p. 380.

3. Women's labor-force participation transformed in the 1950s and 1960s. More women entered the labor force, remained after marriage, and returned

after childbearing. Alice Kessler-Harris reports, "A third of all women worked in 1950—only half of them full time. By 1975, nearly half worked, more than 70% at full-time jobs." Kessler-Harris, *Out to Work: A History of Wage-Earning Women in the United States* (New York: Oxford University Press, 1982), 300–303; quotation on 301.

4. Julie A. Matthaei, *An Economic History of Women in America: Women's Work, the Sexual Division of Labor, and the Development of Capitalism* (New York: Schocken Books, 1982), 133–136, 224–227; Paula Giddings, *When and Where I Enter: The Impact of Black Women on Race and Sex in America* (New York: William Morrow, 1984), 63, 100–101, 148, 196–197.

5. Rickie Solinger, *Wake Up Little Susie: Single Pregnancy and Race before Roe v. Wade* (New York: Routledge, 1992), 109–110.

6. Solinger, *Wake Up Little Susie*, 103–186; Regina G. Kunzel, "White Neurosis, Black Pathology: Constructing Out-of-Wedlock Pregnancy in the Wartime and Postwar United States," in *Not June Cleaver: Women and Gender in Postwar America, 1945–1960*, edited by Joanne Meyerowitz (Philadelphia: Temple University Press, 1994), 306–308; Morris J. Vogel, "The Rise and Fall of Homes for Unwed Mothers" (paper presented at the Columbia University Seminar on American Civilization, New York, March 18, 1982).

7. Patricia G. Miller, *The Worst of Times* (New York: HarperCollins, 1993), 173; Ellen Messer and Kathryn E. May, *Back Rooms: Voices from the Illegal Abortion Era* (New York: St. Martin's Press, 1988), 31–62.

8. Petchesky, *Abortion and Woman's Choice*, chaps. 3, 7–8.

9. Rose S., [pseud.], to Leslie Reagan, October 3, 1987.

10. Letter to NARAL from "North Suburban" Illinois, August 4, 1985, Illinois File, Silent No More Campaign, NARAL, Washington, D.C. These letters were made available to me without names. Instead, the area or zip code and date, if included, identifies the letters.

11. Dr. Sophia J. Kleegman in Calderone, *Abortion in the United States*, 37, 113. I have calculated the average price for a Chicago abortion in the 1950s from four articles on abortions between 1950 and 1956, Abortionists Files, HHFC. Morton Sontheimer et al., "A Report on Abortion from Nine American Cities," *Woman's Home Companion* 82 (October 1955): 45, 96.

12. Letter to NARAL from Chicago zip code 60640, May 6, 1985, Illinois File, Silent No More Campaign, NARAL, Washington, D.C.

13. John Bartlow Martin, "Abortion," *Saturday Evening Post* 234 (May 20, 1961): 21.

14. "The Abortion Menace," *Ebony* 6 (January 1951): 21–26. The series of photos on p. 24 purporting to show an illegal abortion are probably staged. See also "The Abortion Racket—What Should Be Done?" *Newsweek* 56 (August, 15, 1960): 50; Martin, "Abortion," 19, 21.

15. Two collections of oral histories are Messer and May, *Back Rooms;* Miller, *The Worst of Times*. The National Abortion Rights Action League (NARAL) solicited letters telling of women's abortion histories during its "Silent No More Campaign" in 1985 and kindly allowed me to read their files.

16. Miller, *The Worst of Times*, 34, 245; Letter from Madison, WI to NARAL, April 19, 1985, Silent No More Campaign, Wisconsin File, NARAL,

Washington D.C. See also "3 Are Seized in Midtown Hotel as Members of Abortion Ring," *NYT,* January 26, 1969, p. 44.

17. Letter to NARAL from Chicago zip code 60640, May 6, 1985; Letter to NARAL from Detroit, April 30, 1985, Michigan File, Silent No More Campaign, NARAL, Washington, D.C.

18. Miller finds that black women in this period seemed to talk about and locate abortionists with greater ease than did white women. Miller, *The Worst of Times,* 4–5, 110–114.

19. Letter to NARAL from Milwaukee, April 24, 1985, Wisconsin File; Letter to President Regan [*sic*] from Chicago, zip code 60639, Chicago File; both letters are in Silent No More Campaign, NARAL, Washington, D.C. Miller, *The Worst of Times,* 62.

20. Letter to President Reagan from "Jane Roe," Peoria, IL, zip code 61603, April 17, 1985; Letter to NARAL from Rochelle, IL, zip code 61068, November 25, 1985. Both letters are in Illinois File, Silent No More Campaign, NARAL, Washington, D.C.

21. Miller, *The Worst of Times,* 274–280; Martin, "Abortion," 52; Jerome E. Bates and Edward S. Zawadzki, *Criminal Abortion: A Study in Medical Sociology* (Springfield, Ill.: Charles C. Thomas, 1964), 124.

22. Arthur J. Mandy, "Reflections of a Gynecologist," in *Abortion in America: Medical, Psychiatric, Legal, Anthropological, and Religious Considerations,* edited by Harold Rosen (1954; reprint, Boston: Beacon Press, 1967), 289. See also comments of Dr. Howard C. Taylor Jr. in Calderone, *Abortion in the United States,* 108.

23. For example, see Rickie Solinger, "'A Complete Disaster': Abortion and the Politics of Hospital Abortion Committees, 1950–1970," *Feminist Studies* 19 (summer 1993): 241–259.

24. "Pregnancy and Contracted Pelvis," *JAMA* 38 (February 8, 1902): 433; R. Finley Gayle Jr., "The Psychiatric Consideration of Abortion," *Southern Medicine and Surgery* 91 (April 1929): 251–254.

25. Christopher Tietze, "Therapeutic Abortions in New York City, 1943–1947," *AJOG* 60 (July 1950): 149; Edwin M. Gold et al., "Therapeutic Abortions in New York City: A 20-Year Review," *American Journal of Public Health* (hereafter cited as *AJPH*) 55 (July 1965): 969.

26. Psychiatric indications accounted for 43 percent of all therapeutic abortions. I have calculated this percentage from the data provided in the article. Robert E. Hall, "Therapeutic abortion, sterilization, and contraception," *AJOG* 91 (February 15, 1965): 520–521, table 2.

27. Some of the indications for abortion that had been the most frequent in the 1940s—heart disease, fibroids, toxemia of pregnancy, and tuberculosis— almost completely disappeared as indications by the end of the 1950s. Alan F. Guttmacher, "The Shrinking Non-Psychiatric Indications for Therapeutic Abortion," in Rosen, *Abortion in America,* 12–20; David C. Wilson, "The Abortion Problem in the General Hospital," in Rosen, *Abortion in America,* 191–193; Gold et al., "Therapeutic Abortions in New York City," 969, table 8. On the status of psychiatry, see Gerald N. Grob, *From Asylum to Community: Mental Health Policy in Modern America* (Princeton, N.J.: Princeton University Press, 1991), 273.

28. For example, Miriam C., 1970 letter, box 3, Women's National Abortion Action Coalition Papers, Historical Society of the State of Wisconsin, Madison, Wisconsin.

29. Dr. Alan F. Guttmacher in Calderone, *Abortion in the United States,* 139; Nancy Howell Lee, *The Search for an Abortionist* (Chicago: University of Chicago Press, 1969), 89–90.

30. Oral interview by author with Dr. Jack R. [pseud.], November 1987.

31. Miller, *The Worst of Times,* 37–38.

32. I calculated the proportion of unmarried patients from data presented in table 4, p. 1141 in Kenneth R. Niswander, Morton Klein, and Clyde L. Randall, "Changing Attitudes toward Therapeutic Abortion," *JAMA* 196 (June 27, 1966): 1141–1143, quotation on 1142–1143.

33. Comment of Dr. Lawrence C. Kolb in Calderone, *Abortion in the United States,* 141–142, and see Dr. Robert W. Laidlaw on 138–139.

34. However, Lidz favored liberalization of the law. Theodore Lidz, "Reflections of a Psychiatrist," in Rosen, *Abortion in America,* 277. See also Sidney Bolter, "The Psychiatrist's Role in Therapeutic Abortion: The Unwitting Accomplice," *American Journal of Psychiatry* 119 (October 1962): 313; Harold Rosen, "A Case Study in Social Hypocrisy," in Rosen, *Abortion in America,* 306.

35. Bolter, "The Psychiatrist's Role in Therapeutic Abortion," 314, 312, 314–315. See also Robert B. McGraw, "Legal Aspects of Termination of Pregnancy on Psychiatric Grounds," *New York State Journal of Medicine* 56 (May 15, 1956): 1605–1607.

36. By 1963, 87.5 percent of the therapeutic abortions performed in Buffalo hospitals had been induced for psychiatric indications. Niswander, Klein, and Randall, "Changing Attitudes toward Therapeutic Abortion," 1141.

37. Guttmacher, "The Shrinking Non-Psychiatric Indications for Therapeutic Abortion," 20–21; Gold et al., "Therapeutic Abortions in New York City," 969. For a small debate on this indication, see "Questions and Answers. Pregnancy and Rubella," *JAMA* 166 (February 22, 1958): 991–992.

38. "Abortion: Mercy—or Murder?" *Newsweek* 60 (August 13, 1962): 54; "Abortion Possible for Thalidomide Takers," *Science Newsletter* 82 (August 18, 1962): 99. Not everyone supported abortion for these reasons, but many did; see Sherri Finkbine, as told to Joseph Stocker, "The Baby We Didn't Dare to Have," *Redbook* 120 (January 1963): 102.

39. For helpful discussions of these issues, see Petchesky, *Abortion and Woman's Choice,* 351–354, quotation on 353, emphasis in original; Michael Bérubé, "Life as We Know It," *Harper's* 289 (December 1994): 41–43.

40. Barbara Katz Rothman, *The Tentative Pregnancy: Prenatal Diagnosis and the Future of Motherhood* (New York: Viking Penguin, 1986).

41. Tietze, "Therapeutic Abortions in New York City, 1943–1947"; Gold et al., "Therapeutic Abortions in New York City," 965–966.

42. Gold et al., "Therapeutic Abortions in New York City," 965–966, 971. This article broke down the data into three "ethnic groups": "white," "nonwhite," and "Puerto Rican." I have combined the data for the "nonwhites" and Puerto Ricans so that minority women and majority, white women can be compared in the figures. The decline was 90 percent among Puerto Ricans, 65 percent among "nonwhites," and 40 percent among whites.

43. Hall, "Therapeutic Abortion, Sterilization, and Contraception," 518–519, 522, 524–527, quotation on 519. See also Niswander, Klein, and Randall, "Changing Attitudes toward Therapeutic Abortion," 1143.

44. Gold et al., "Therapeutic Abortions in New York City," 968, table 7. The therapeutic abortion to delivery ratios reported in California hospitals in 1950 ranged from 1:52 deliveries at a private hospital to 1:8,196 deliveries at Los Angeles County Hospital, as reported in Keith P. Russell, "Therapeutic Abortions in California in 1950," *Western Journal of Surgery, Obstetrics, and Gynecology* 60 (October 1952): 497.

45. Calderone, *Abortion in the United States,* 78–80, 90, 100–101, 111; Kristin Luker, *Abortion and the Politics of Motherhood* (Berkeley: University of California Press, 1984), 260–262, table 2; J. G. Moore and J. H. Randall, "Trends in Therapeutic Abortions: A Review of 137 Cases," *AJOG* 63 (January 1952): 35; Hall, "Therapeutic Abortion, Sterilization, and Contraception," 519–522, 527.

46. G. K. Folger in Harry A. Pearse and Harold A. Ott, "Hospital Control of Sterilization and Therapeutic Abortion," *AJOG* 60 (August 1950): 299–300.

47. In 1967, Harold Rosen estimated that five thousand to eight thousand therapeutic abortions were performed every year, but this seems high. Sixty hospitals reported little more than one thousand therapeutic abortions over a several year period to Robert Hall. Rosen, *Abortion in America,* 307; Hall, "Therapeutic Abortion, Sterilization, and Contraception," 524–525, table 6.

48. Hall, "Therapeutic Abortion, Sterilization, and Contraception," 518–519, 522, 526–527.

49. "Illegitimacy Rise Alarms Agencies," *NYT,* August 9, 1959; this article was brought to my attention by a student, Meghan McCloskey. Henry J. Myers, "The Problem of Sterilization: Sociologic, Eugenic, and Individual Considerations," in Rosen, *Abortion in America,* 93; Julius Paul, "The Return of Punitive Sterilization Proposals: Current Attacks on Illegitimacy and the AFDC Program," *Law and Society Review* 3 (August 1968): 77–106; Solinger, *Wake Up Little Susie,* 52–57.

50. See Angela Y. Davis, *Women, Race, and Class* (New York: Random House, 1981), 215–221; Petchesky, *Abortion and Woman's Choice,* 84–89, 159–160, 178–181; Committee for Abortion Rights and Against Sterilization Abuse, *Women under Attack: Victories, Backlash, and the Fight for Reproductive Freedom,* edited by Susan E. Davis (Boston: South End Press, 1988). On the history of the movement for sterilization of mental "defectives," criminals and others, see Linda Gordon, *Woman's Body, Woman's Right: Birth Control in America,* rev. and updated (1976; reprint, New York: Penguin Books, 1990), 307; Mark H. Haller, *Eugenics: Hereditarian Attitudes in American Thought* (New Brunswick: Rutgers University Press, 1963), 130–141.

51. H. Close Hesseltine, F. L. Adair, and M. W. Boynton, "Limitation of Human Reproduction," *AJOG* 39 (April 1940): 551. Robert E. Hall's study of sixty hospitals showed that a third of the women who had therapeutic abortions were sterilized at the same time; "Therapeutic Abortion, Sterilization, and Contraception," 522, table 3.

52. Dr. Laidlaw in Calderone, *Abortion in the United States,* 136.

53. Mandy, "Reflections of a Gynecologist," 289–290.

54. The committee at Florence Crittenton allowed sterilizations on narrow medical grounds and rejected operations primarily justified as desired by the patient. Comments of Albert E. Catherwood in discussion of Hesseltine, Adair and Boynton, "Limitation of Human Reproduction," 561; Pearse and Ott, "Hospital Control of Sterilization and Therapeutic Abortion," 290–296.

55. Miller, *The Worst of Times*, 80–91.

56. Lawrence Lader, *Abortion* (Boston: Beacon Press, 1966), 68–69; Recollection about Chicago Lying-In in Letter to NARAL from Ginny Foxx [pseud.], Haslett, MI, zip code 48840, Michigan File, Silent No More Campaign, NARAL, Washington, D.C.; Sherry Matulis, "Abortion, 1954—Never Again," *Madison, WI Feminist Voices,* September 1989, p. 8.

57. "Vaginal Hemorrhage from Potassium Permanganate Burns," *JAMA* 155 (June 12, 1954): 699.

58. On Los Angeles County Hospital, see Don Harper Mills, "A Medicolegal Analysis of Abortion Statutes," *Southern California Law Review* 31 (February 1958): 182–183, n. 11. On D.C. General Hospital, see Miller, *The Worst of Times,* 72–74, 285–287; "The Abortion Racket."

59. Vital statistics cannot be used to track mortality due to illegal abortions for a variety of reasons; see Christopher Tietze, "Abortion as a Cause of Death," *AJPH* 38 (October 1948): 1434–1437. Abortion-related deaths are presumed to be undercounted because physicians protected their patients (and themselves) by assigning other causes of death on death certificates. These New York City data are the best we have.

60. Gold et al., "Therapeutic Abortions in New York City," 965–966. The percentages of puerperal deaths due to abortion in 1960 to 1962 were 25.2 percent for whites, 49.4 percent for "nonwhites," and 55.6 percent for Puerto Ricans.

61. All of these inequalities continue. Although both infant and maternal mortality have dropped, the racial differences persist. Infant mortality for black children is still twice that of white children and maternal mortality is over three times as high. U.S. Bureau of the Census, *Historical Statistics of the United States, Colonial Times to 1970,* Bicentennial ed., part 1 (Washington D.C.: Government Printing Office, 1975), Series b 136–147, p. 57; U.S. Bureau of the Census, *Statistical Abstract of the United States: 1994* (Washington, D.C.: Government Printing Office, 1994), 91, table 120. On life expectancy, see *Historical Statistics of the United States,* Series B 107–115, pp. 55–56; Wornie L. Reed et al, *Health and Medical Care of African-Americans* (Westport, Conn.: Auburn House, 1993). 1984–1992 data show that more than twice as much money is spent per white American as per black American for health care. See *Statistical Abstract of the U.S.: 1994,* 117, table 164. I am grateful to Rose Holz for collecting these data. For 1987, U.S. infant mortality rates ranked twenty-first in the world, but if those figures are divided by race, white America would rank between twelfth and thirteenth, while black America would rank between twenty-seventh and twenty-eighth; see Christine B. Hale, "Infant Mortality: An American Tragedy," *Black Scholar* 21 (January-February-March 1990): 18, table.

62. Therapeutic abortions in hospitals were extremely safe. Russell S.

Fisher, "Criminal Abortion," in Rosen, *Abortion in America,* 9; Christopher Tietze, "Mortality with Contraception and Induced Abortion," *Studies in Family Planning* 1 (September 1969): 6.

Chapter 8.   Radicalization of Reform

1. Gerald N. Grob, *From Asylum to Community: Mental Health Policy in Modern America* (Princeton, N.J.: Princeton University Press, 1991), 20, 41–43, 274–278.

2. Arthur J. Mandy, "Reflections of a Gynecologist," in *Abortion in America: Medical, Psychiatric, Legal, Anthropological, and Religious Considerations,* edited by Harold Rosen (1954; reprint, Boston: Beacon Press, 1967), 285, 295.

3. Remarks in Mary Steichen Calderone, ed., *Abortion in the United States: A Conference Sponsored by the Planned Parenthood Federation of America, Inc. at Arden House and The New York Academy of Medicine* (New York: Harper and Brothers, 1958), 163, 164, 167.

4. Calderone, *Abortion in the United States,* 6–13.

5. Winfield Best to Mary Calderone, April 19, 1955, folder 3, box 2, Mary Steichen Calderone Papers, Schlesinger Library; Winfield Best to Public Relations Department, February 16, 1955, folder 13, box 2, Calderone Papers.

6. Quotation in Dr. W. Vogt to Dr. Mary Calderone, February 17, 1955, folder 13, box 2, Calderone Papers.

7. Calderone, *Abortion in the United States,* statement on 181–184, quotations on 181, 183.

8. Calderone, *Abortion in the United States,* 193–195.

9. *Proceedings of the American Law Institute,* 1959 (Philadelphia: American Law Institute, 1960), 252–283, quotation on 257–258. On the American Law Institute, see Solon N. Blackmer, "Medical and Legal Foundations for Justifiable Abortions—An Abstract," *Illinois Medical Journal* 121 (January 1962): 59; Herbert F. Goodrich and Paul A. Wolkin, *The Story of the American Law Institute, 1923–1961* (St. Paul: American Law Institute Publishers, 1961), 5–7. The model law was slightly revised in 1962; American Law Institute, *Model Penal Code: Official Draft and Explanatory Notes; Complete Text of Model Penal Code as Adopted at the 1962 Annual Meeting of The American Law Institute at Washington, D.C., May 24, 1962* (Philadelphia: The American Law Institute, 1985), Section 230.3, pp. 165–166.

10. *Proceedings of the American Law Institute,* 258; Leonard Dubin, "The Antiquated Abortion Laws," *Temple Law Quarterly* 34 (winter 1961): 151.

11. *Proceedings of the American Law Institute,* 274–275, 279–281, quotations on 279, 281.

12. Ibid., 259–262, 264.

13. Eugene Quay, "Justifiable Abortion—Medical and Legal Foundations," (in two parts) *Georgetown Law Journal* 49 (winter 1960 and spring 1961): 173–241; 395–443. On the Catholic Church's role in battling birth control, see David M. Kennedy, *Birth Control in America: The Career of Margaret Sanger* (New Haven: Yale University Press, 1970), 96–98, 144–145, 222–223, 232–234;

David J. Garrow, *Liberty and Sexuality: The Right to Privacy and the Making of Roe v. Wade* (New York: Macmillan, 1994), 113–116, 118.

14. "Attorneys Urge Legal Abortions," *AMA News* 3 (July 11, 1960): 8, Vertical Files, AHA; Dubin, "The Antiquated Abortion Laws," 151.

15. Doug Lindgren, "Abortion: State Control or a Woman's Right?" *The Brief* (February 1970): 3. The states that passed reform laws were Colorado, Arkansas, California, Delaware, Georgia, Kansas, Maryland, New Mexico, North Carolina, Oregon, South Carolina, and Virginia. Judith Hole and Ellen Levine, *Rebirth of Feminism* (New York: Quadrangle Books, 1971), 284.

16. Alan F. Guttmacher, "The Law That Doctors Often Break," *Reader's Digest* 76 (January 1960): 51–54.

17. Jerome M. Kummer and Zad Leavy, "Therapeutic Abortion Law Confusion," *JAMA* 195 (January 10, 1966): 143, 144.

18. Maginnis's organization was first named Citizens' Committee for Humane Abortion Laws. Garrow, *Liberty and Sexuality*, 290; Miss. Pat Maginnis to Dr. Alan Guttmacher, March 28, 1962, Correspondence, Guttmacher Papers, Countway Library, Harvard University. Ninia Baehr, *Abortion without Apology: A Radical History for the 1990s* (Boston: South End Press, 1990), 7–18.

19. "Pregnant Women and Self Determination," *Society for Humane Abortion Newsletter* (hereafter cited as *SHA Newsletter*) 1 (August 1965): 1; Kristin Luker, *Abortion and the Politics of Motherhood* (Berkeley: University of California Press, 1984), 95–102.

20. Cartoon by Robert N. Bick in Patricia T. Maginnis, *The Abortees' Songbook*, 1969, Position Papers Part 2 folder, Women's Ephemera Folders (hereafter cited as WEF), Special Collections, Northwestern University Library, Evanston, Illinois. In the 1940s and 1950s, psychiatrists took enlightened views of sexual "deviants" and tried to alleviate the situation for homosexuals, unwed mothers, and sexually unhappy women, but psychiatrists were later considered judgmental, homophobic, and sexist. To its credit, the psychiatric profession heard its clients and revised its views. Allan Bérubé makes this point about homosexuality in *Coming Out under Fire: The History of Gay Men and Women in World War Two* (New York: Free Press, 1990), 149–174. For examples of the psychiatric interpretation of these issues, see Linda Gordon, *Woman's Body, Woman's Right: Birth Control in America*, rev. and updated (1976; reprint, New York: Penguin Books, 1990), 360–361, 366–369; Regina Kunzel, *Fallen Women, Problem Girls: Unmarried Mothers and the Professionalization of Social Work, 1890–1945* (New Haven: Yale University Press, 1993).

21. Quotations from Society for Humane Abortion Statement, *SHA Newsletter* 1 (August 1965), no page no. See also "Abortion vs. Contraception," *SHA Newsletter* 2:1 (February/March 1966); Garrow, *Liberty and Sexuality*, 301, 304. For another early feminist critique of reform, see Alice S. Rossi, "Public Views on Abortion," (February 1966) [reprint] n.p., Abortion—National Association for the Repeal of Abortion Laws folder, WEF.

22. The group had male support, but had originated among women and formulated its arguments from the perspective of women who wanted abortions, not potential providers. For male participants, see "SHA Incorporation," *SHA Newsletter* 2 (April/May 1966).

23. This organization was named the Association to Repeal Abortion Laws (ARAL). Different sources suggest that it started in 1964 or 1966. "Classes in Abortion," flyer, [September 15, 1966], Correspondence, Guttmacher Papers; "Are You Pregnant," flyer, Correspondence, Guttmacher Papers; "Law, Police and Patricia Maginnis," *SHA Newsletter* 3 (January/February 1967): 1; Baehr, *Abortion without Apology*, 10.

24. Report from Juarez, Folder 86 and Evaluations, July 1967, folder 125, box 5, Records of the Society for Humane Abortion and the Association to Repeal Abortion Laws, Schlesinger Library.

25. Interview of Heather Booth by Paula Kamen, September 1, 1992, Paula Kamen Collection, C.D. McCormick Library of Special Collections Department, Northwestern University Library; Lindsey Van Gelder, "The Jane Collective: Seizing Control," *Ms.* (September/October 1991): 83.

26. Different dates are given for the start of the Service. I conclude from the Booth interview that the first collective effort began in 1967 when she contacted Jody Parsons. Interview of Booth, 7; Van Gelder, "The Jane Collective," 83–84; Pauline Bart, "Seizing the Means of Reproduction: An Illegal Feminist Abortion Collective—How and Why it Worked," *Qualitative Sociology* 10 (winter 1987): 339–357.

27. Diane Elze, "Underground Abortion Remembered: Part 2," *Sojourner: The Women's Forum* 13 (May 1988): 12, Abortion—Jane folder, WEF; Bart, "Seizing the Means of Reproduction," 339–357; Interview of Judith Arcana, September 1992, pp. 3–5, Paula Kamen Collection; Jane, "Jane," *Voices*, June-November 1973, typescript, pp. 1–23. Last quotation from "Just Call 'Jane,'" *The Fight For Reproductive Freedom: A Newsletter for Student Activists* 4 (winter 1990): 4. I am grateful to Suzanne Poirier and Bonnie Blustein for giving me copies of the "Jane" typescript and to Anne Champagne for the newsletter.

28. Interview of Arcana, 5; Interview of Anonymous Jane and Husband, September 1992, pp. 1–2, 9, Paula Kamen Collection; Elze, "Underground Abortion Remembered," 12; "Just Call 'Jane,'" 4.

29. Interview of Lorry, November 26, 1992, pp. 2–7, Paula Kamen Collection.

30. "Aborted Women and Silence," *SHA Newsletter* 1 (August 1965): 2; Jane, "Jane," 8.

31. "Law Enforcement," *SHA Newsletter* 1 (August 1965): 2; "Civil Rights are a Part of Good Medical Care," Abortion '68–'73 folder, box 23, Chicago Women's Liberation Union Papers, Chicago Historical Society.

32. Jo Freeman, *The Politics of Women's Liberation: A Case Study of an Emerging Social Movement and its Relation to the Policy Process* (New York: David McKay, 1975); Sara Evans, *Personal Politics: The Roots of Women's Liberation in the Civil Rights Movement and the New Left* (New York: Random House, 1979; Vintage Books, 1980); Paula Giddings, *When and Where I Enter: The Impact of Black Women on Race and Sex in America* (New York: William Morrow, Bantam Books, 1984), 299–324; Hole and Levine, *Rebirth of Feminism*.

33. Women in the United Auto Workers (UAW) got NOW off the ground and the union provided the organization's first funds. Freeman, *The Politics of Women's Liberation*, 50–56, 71–102, 80.

34. Johnnie Tillmon, who "organized the nation's first welfare rights group in the Watts area of Los Angeles in 1963," argued that, "Welfare is a Woman's Issue," reprint in *The First Ms. Reader* (New York: Warner Paperback, 1973), 51–55; Freeman, *The Politics of Women's Liberation*, 73–74; Giddings, *When and Where I Enter*, 312–313; Frances Fox Piven and Richard A. Cloward, *Poor People's Movements: Why They Succeed, How They Fail* (New York: Random House, 1977), 264–280.

35. Women's liberation groups arose in Detroit, Seattle, Gainesville, Boston, New York, and Washington, D.C. Freeman, *The Politics of Women's Liberation*, 50–51, 56–62, 103–111; Evans, *Personal Politics*.

36. *Voices*, August 30, 1971, p. 7, Abortion—Ephemera #2 folder, WEF; *Palante*, March 19, 1971, p. 12, Abortion—Ephemera #4 folder, WEF; Loretta J. Ross, "African-American Women and Abortion, 1800–1970," in *Theorizing Black Feminisms: The Visionary Pragmatism of Black Women*, edited by Stanlie M. James and Abena P. A. Busia (London: Routledge, 1993), 156.

37. John D'Emilio and Estelle B. Freedman, *Intimate Matters: A History of Sexuality in America* (New York: Harper and Row, 1988), 301–325, 350–354; Anne Koedt, "The Myth of the Vaginal Orgasm," *New England Free Press* pamphlet, 1970; Ellen Carol Dubois and Linda Gordon, "Seeking Ecstasy on the Battlefield: Danger and Pleasure in Nineteenth-Century Feminist Sexual Thought," *Feminist Studies* 9 (spring 1983): 7–25.

38. Freeman, *The Politics of Women's Liberation*, 80–81, 153, 171.

39. Gordon, *Woman's Body, Woman's Right*, chap. 5.

40. Hole and Levine, *Rebirth of Feminism*, 296–299; Lucinda Cisler, "Unfinished Business: Birth Control and Women's Liberation," in *Sisterhood is Powerful: An Anthology of Writings from the Women's Liberation Movement*, edited by Robin Morgan (New York: Vintage Books, 1970), 311–312. For a photo of a theatrical skit at a New York City speak-out, see Committee for Abortion Rights and Against Sterilization Abuse, *Women under Attack: Victories, Backlash, and the Fight for Reproductive Freedom*, edited by Susan E. Davis (Boston: South End Press, 1988), 11.

41. Gordon, *Woman's Body, Woman's Right*, 337–345.

42. Ibid., 386–396; Paul R. Ehrlich, *The Population Bomb* (New York: Ballantine Books, 1968); Garrett Hardin, *Exploring New Ethics for Survival: The Voyage of the Spaceship Beagle* (New York: Viking Press, 1968). Barry Commoner, however, criticized this kind of thinking among environmentalists and described Ehrlich and Hardin's horrific plans for coercive sterilization and birth control programs as "political repression" in *The Closing Circle: Nature, Man, and Technology* (1971; reprint, New York: Bantam Books, 1972), 212. I am grateful to Daniel Schneider for these last citations.

43. Hole and Levine, *Rebirth of Feminism*, 285.

44. Mary Smith, "Birth Control and the Negro Woman," *Ebony* 23 (March 1968): 29–30.

45. Michael Kilian, "Kill Welfare Sterilizing Measure," *Chicago Tribune*, May 20, 1971, Birth Control—Sterilization folder, WEF.

46. "Blacks View Limitations on Number in Family as Genocide Effort by U.S.," *Jet* 40 (August 5, 1971): 20–21; Smith, "Birth Control and the Negro Woman," 29.

47. Jessie M. Rodrique, "The Black Community and the Birth Control Movement," in *Passion and Power: Sexuality in History,* edited by Kathy Peiss and Christina Simmons with Robert A. Padgug (Philadelphia: Temple University Press, 1989), 138–154; *D.C. Star,* Aug. 28, 1971, Birth Control—Newspaper Articles folder, WEF.

48. Smith, "Birth Control and the Negro Woman," 29.

49. Ibid., 30–31; Ross, "African-American Women and Abortion," 153–154.

50. Elaine Brown has written of her life in the Black Panther Party and her realization of the party's devaluation of women in *A Taste of Power: A Black Woman's Story* (New York: Pantheon Books, 1992). The Panthers, however, supported abortion and birth control on demand; see Ross, "African-American Women and Abortion," 153–154.

51. Kennedy quotation in Maxine Williams, "Why Black Women Support the Abortion Struggle," [1971], Minority Women (Black) folder, Newspaper Ephemera (Undated Only), WEF; Representative Shirley Chisolm, "Facing the Abortion Question," excerpt from *Unbought and Unbossed* (Boston: Houghton Mifflin, 1970), reprint in *Black Women in White America: A Documentary History,* edited by Gerda Lerner (New York: Vintage Books, 1972), 602–607, quotation on 604; Ross, "African-American Women and Abortion," 154–156.

52. March 8th Movement, "Abortion-Birth Control—A Liberation for Women or Population Control?" in Position Papers folder, box 7, Jenny Knauss Collection, C.D. McCormick Library of Special Collections, Northwestern University Library; Davis, *Women Under Attack,* 28–29; Ross, "African-American Women and Abortion," 156.

53. *NYT,* February 17, 1969, p. 32; "Black MD Hits Abortion Laws," *American Medical News,* October 18, 1971, Abortion—Ephemera #2 folder, WEF.

54. Arlene Carmen and Howard Moody, *Abortion Counseling and Social Change from Illegal Act to Medical Practice: The Story of the Clergy Consultation Service on Abortion* (Valley Forge, Pa.: Judson Press, 1973).

55. Kathy Christensen, speaker at Pro-Choice Rally, January 22, 1985, Madison, Wisconsin.

56. "WONAAC Affiliation Formed at Catholic College," [1972], Abortion—WONAAC #1 folder, WEF. See also Barbara Ferraro and Patricia Hussey with Jane O'Reilly, *No Turning Back: Two Nuns' Battle with the Vatican over Women's Right to Choose* (New York: Ivy Books, 1990).

57. Letterhead, October 12, 1970, Abortion—Total Repeal of Abortion Laws (TRIAL) folder, WEF. The *WONAAC Newsletter* and the *SHA Newsletter,* both held in the Serials Collection at Northwestern University Library, document many organizations and activities.

58. Keith Monroe, "How California's Abortion Law Isn't Working," *The New York Times Magazine,* December 29, 1968, pp. 10–11, 17–20; *People v. Belous,* 80 Cal. Rptr. 354; 458 P. 2d, (1969), pp. 195–196.

59. See R. Bolle to Dr. Guttmacher, February 7, 1966; Alan F. Guttmacher to R. Bolle, February 15, 1966; F. Thomas to Dr. Alan Guttmacher, July 31, 1968; AFG to F. Thomas, September 17, 1968 in Correspondence, Guttmacher Papers; Alan F. Guttmacher, "The Genesis of Liberalized Abortion in New York: A Personal Insight," *Abortion, Medicine, and the Law,* 3d ed., completely

revised, edited by J. Douglas Butler and David F. Walbert (New York: Facts on File Publications, 1986), 229–234.

60. Paul Starr, *The Social Transformation of American Medicine* (New York: Basic Books, 1982); John C. Burnham, "American Medicine's Golden Age: What Happened to It?" *Science* 215 (March 19, 1982): 1474–1479, reprint in *Sickness and Health in America: Readings in the History of Medicine and Public Health*, edited by Judith Walzer Leavitt and Ronald L. Numbers, 2d ed., rev. (Madison: University of Wisconsin Press, 1985), 248–258.

61. "ISMS Symposium on Medical Implications of the Current Abortion Law in Illinois," *Illinois Medical Journal* 131 (May 1967): 666–695.

62. Robert E. Hall, "New York Abortion Law Survey," *AJOG* 93 (December 15, 1965): 1182; "Obstetricians Support Liberal Abortion Policy," *JNMA* 61 (May 1969): 245.

63. On the Group for the Advancement of Psychiatry, see Cisler, "Unfinished Business," 309. On the (African American) Detroit Medical Society, see Edgar B. Keemer, "Update on Abortion in Michigan," *JNMA* 64 (November 1972): 518; also see Era L. Hill and Johan W. Eliot, "Black Physicians' Experience with Abortion Requests and Opinion about Abortion Law Change in Michigan," *JNMA* 64 (January 1972): 52–58. On the American Public Health Association, "APHA Resolutions. 98th Annual Meeting, Oct. 28, 1970. Standards for Abortion Services," *AJPH* 61 (January 1971): 195.

64. "APHA Resolutions," 195.

65. Cisler, "Unfinished Business," 310–311; "Changing Morality: The Two Americas, A Time-Louis Harris Poll," *Time* 93 (June 6, 1969): 27.

66. The case is *Doe v. Scott,* 321 F. Supp. 1385 (1971). My analysis of this legal challenge is based on the original briefs and other materials presented to the federal court, the published opinion, and interviews with the two cooperating attorneys, Sybille Fritzsche and Susan Grossman Alexander. In the text I have used the name that Susan Alexander used at the time, Susan Grossman. I conducted a joint interview with Alexander and Fritzsche, March 8, 1994, Chicago, Illinois, tape in Reagan's possession. This interview is referred to as Alexander and Fritzsche Interview. Additional interviews with Fritzsche, in Chicago on April 6, 1995, and Alexander, by telephone on June 28, 1995, and November 27, 1995, clarified certain points.

67. Roy Lucas came up with a nearly identical plan in 1967, published in 1968; see Garrow, *Liberty and Sexuality,* 338, 351–354, 356–357. *Doe v. Scott* (1971) was started and filed earlier than the Texas and Georgia cases. Alexander and Fritzsche sent copies of their work to Sara Weddington in Texas, Margie Pitts Hames in Georgia, and others; Alexander and Fritzsche Interview. Lawyers around the country shared their strategies, motions, and briefs. See Eva R. Rubin, *Abortion, Politics, and the Courts,* rev. ed. (New York: Greenwood Press, 1987), 54; Sarah Weddington, *A Question of Choice* (New York: G. P. Putnam's Sons, 1992), 25–29. The woman who was "Roe" in *Roe v. Wade* has recently told her life story and of her experience as a subject in the case; see Norma McCorvey, with Andy Meisler, *I Am Roe: My Life, Roe v. Wade, and Freedom of Choice* (New York: HarperCollins, 1994).

68. Alexander in Alexander and Fritzsche Interview.

69. As one of the few women in the legal profession, Fritzsche probably would have identified with the feminists in NOW who focused more on workplace issues and less on domestic arrangements. Fritzsche interview with author, April 6, 1995, Chicago.

70. In 1969–1970, cases were started in Washington, D.C., Colorado, North Carolina, Washington, Iowa, New Jersey, Texas, Georgia, Kentucky, Missouri, Connecticut, Ohio, New Hampshire, South Dakota, Louisiana, Arizona, and perhaps other states as well. Garrow, *Liberty and Sexuality,* 377–378, 381–388, 424–428, 432–433. On physicians' attempts to be arrested, see "Black MD Hits Abortion Laws"; Eileen Shanahan, "Doctor Leads Group's Challenge to Michigan Anti-Abortion Law," *NYT,* October 5, 1971, p. 28; "Defend Dr. Munson, Dr. Koome, Dr. Keemer," *WONAAC Newsletter,* December 1972, p. 7, Northwestern University Library. On Keemer's activism, see Ed Keemer, *Confessions of a Pro-Life Abortionist* (Detroit: Vinco Press, 1980), 215–217, 220–224.

71. Alexander in Alexander and Fritzsche Interview.

72. Martha F. Davis discusses both the activism of poor women themselves and the lawyers inspired to work on their behalf in *Lawyers and the Welfare Rights Movement, 1960–1973* (New Haven: Yale University Press, 1993).

73. "Complaint to Declare the Illinois Abortion Statute Unconstitutional and to Enjoin Its Enforcement," n.d., p. 8, *Doe v. Scott,* 70 C. 395 (Civil Case Files), Northern District of Illinois, Eastern Division (Chicago), Record Group 21, Records of the District Courts of the United States, National Archives—Great Lakes Region, Chicago, Illinois.

74. Sybille Fritzsche, Susan Grossman, and Marshall Patner, "Memorandum of Law of Plaintiffs in Support of Motions for Preliminary Injunction and Summary Judgment and in Opposition to Counterclaim and Motion to Dismiss," pp. 15–16, *Doe v. Scott* (Civil Case Files).

75. Grossman, Transcript of Proceedings, September 29, 1970, p. 36, *Doe v. Scott,* (Civil Case Files).

76. Fritzsche, Grossman, and Patner, "Memorandum of Law of Plaintiffs," 6–13, quotation on 11; *Griswold v. Connecticut* (1965) 381 U.S. 479, phrase at p. 485; Garrow, *Liberty and Sexuality.*

77. Fritzsche, Grossman, and Patner, "Memorandum of Law of Plaintiffs," 7–9. David Garrow argues in *Liberty and Sexuality* that activists in the 1930s began developing the idea of a right to privacy in reference to the use of birth control, which eventually shaped both *Griswold* and *Roe.* Linda Przybyszewski argues that the right to privacy has deeper roots in American history and culture and is part of Americans' long-held fear of government intrusion and abuse. Linda Przybyszewski, "The Right to Privacy: A Historical Perspective," in *Abortion, Medicine, and the Law,* edited by J. Douglas Butler and David F. Walbert, 4th ed. (New York: Facts on File, 1992), 667–692.

78. Alexander and Fritzsche Interview.

79. Alexander and Fritzsche Interview.

80. "Complaint to Declare the Illinois Abortion Statute Unconstitutional and to Enjoin Its Enforcement," 3–5; physician affidavits and vitas in "Plaintiffs' Exhibits," *Doe v. Scott* (Civil Case Files). The lawyers did not contact any-

one at Loyola, the Catholic medical school, knowing it would be futile. Alexander and Fritzsche Interview.

81. David S. Tatel, "Brief of Amici Curiae, Medical School Deans and Others, in Support of Plaintiffs' Motion for Summary Judgment," August 10, 1970, *Doe v. Scott* (Civil Case Files). California lawyers had similarly collected a long list of prestigious medical names in support of the *Belous* case.

82. Brief Amicus Curiae of Committee of Concerned Doctors, August 10, 1970, *Doe v. Scott* (Civil Case Files).

83. In order, quotations by Alexander and Fritzsche in Alexander and Fritzsche Interview.

84. Fritzsche, Grossman, and Patner, "Memorandum of Law of Plaintiffs," 64–71; emphasis added to quotation from Affidavit of David N. Danforth, M.D., pp. 2–3, July 27, 1970, Exhibit D, "Plaintiffs' Exhibits," *Doe v. Scott* (Civil Case Files).

85. Affidavit of Charles Fields, M.D., August 6, 1970, pp. 2–3, Exhibit E, "Plaintiffs' Exhibits," *Doe v. Scott* (Civil Case Files). See also Affidavit of Frederick P. Zuspan, M.D., August 5, 1970, p. 3, *Doe v. Scott* (Civil Case Files).

86. *Doe v. Scott,* p. 1389.

87. Ibid., 1386–1389, 1391.

88. "Abortion Suit Waiting Supreme Court Decision," *The Brief* (March 1971), no page no.; Kenan Heise, "Marvin Rosner, Physician and Local Activist," *Chicago Tribune,* October 17, 1995. I thank Susan Alexander for giving me a copy of this obituary. Alexander and Fritzsche Interview; *Heffernan v. Doe,* appeal filed, 40 *USLW* 3018 (U.S. March 29, 1971) (no. 70–106).

89. Testimony of Mrs. Anne Andich in "Memorandum in Opposition to State's Attorney of Cook County's Petition For a Writ of Mandamus or Prohibition," filed January 26, 1972, p. 6, Transcript of *People ex. rel. Edward v. Hanrahan v. William S. White,* 52 Ill. 2d 71, (March 1972), Case Files, vault no. 68793, Supreme Court of Illinois, Record Series 901; Peter Broeman and Jeannette Meier, "Therapeutic Abortion Practices in Chicago Hospitals—Vagueness, Variation, and Violation of the Law," *Law and Social Order* 4 (1971): 762; Planned Parenthood "Alert," May 1971, folder 1, box 134, accession number 76 116, Chicago Urban League Collection, Department of Special Collections, University of Illinois at Chicago Library.

90. Broeman and Meier, "Therapeutic Abortion Practices in Chicago Hospitals," 757–775. The hypotheticals were first used in a survey of California hospitals by Herbert L. Packer and Ralph J. Gampell, "Therapeutic Abortion: A Problem in Law and Medicine," *Stanford Law Review* 2 (May 1959): 417–445.

91. "Free and Voluntary Abortion Is Every Woman's Right," Abortion, 1968–73 folder, Chicago Women's Liberation Union Papers; Hole and Levine, *Rebirth of Feminism,* 285–291.

92. Letter to Congressman Rostenkowski from Chicago, IL, zip code 60647, [1985], Silent No More Campaign, NARAL, Chicago.

93. Jean Pakter et al., "Two Years Experience in New York City with the Liberalized Abortion Law—Progress and Problems," *AJPH* 63 (June 1973): 524–525.

94. Interview of Spencer Parsons, October 9, 1992, pp. 1, 4, Paula Kamen Collection.

95. Phillip J. O'Connor, "UC Minister to Again Resist Abortion Quiz," *Chicago Daily News,* April 22, 1971, Abortion—Ephemera #3 folder, WEF; Sheila Wolfe, "Agencies Combine Abortion Referrals," *Chicago Tribune,* July 1, 1971, Abortion—Ephemera #2 folder, WEF; Carmen and Moody, *Abortion Counseling and Social Change.*

96. Report of the Executive Director, Planned Parenthood Association, Chicago Area, April 1972, folder 9, box 134, Chicago Urban League Collection; Report of the Executive Director, Planned Parenthood Association, Chicago Area, June 1972, folder 10, box 134, Chicago Urban League Collection.

97. Letter to Senator Dixon from "Jane Roe," March 30, 1985, Chicago, IL, zip code 60615, Silent No More Campaign, NARAL, Chicago.

98. Fritzsche and Grossman knew that many of their opponents, including State's Attorney Hanrahan, were Catholic, but did not consider the opposition to be organized by any church since religious leaders like Rev. Parsons were on their side. Fritzsche in Alexander and Fritzsche Interview.

99. Willard Lassers, "Chicago: Police City," *The Brief* (March-April 1970): 2.

100. O'Connor, "UC Minister to Again Resist Abortion Quiz."

101. *People ex. rel. Edward v. Hanrahan v. William S. White;* "Motion in Opposition to People's Motion for Stay of the Order of the Circuit Court of Cook County, Juvenile Division," January 24, 1972, in Transcript of *People ex. rel. Edward v. Hanrahan v. William S. White.*

102. "Excerpts from Daily News Article, May 4, 1972 by Phil Blake," box 23, Chicago Women's Liberation Union Papers; Arcana Interview, 7, 12; Elze, "Underground Abortion Remembered," 12. On police harassment at peace rallies and so on, see Lassers, "Chicago: Police City."

103. "Is Shirley Wheeler Really Free?" *WONAAC Newsletter,* June 26, 1972, pp. 1, 3; Sherry Smith, "Support Shirley Wheeler," *WONAAC Newsletter,* October 21, 1971, pp. 1–2, 15, Abortion—WONAAC (1972) folder 2, WEF.

104. Keemer, *Confessions,* 224–228.

105. Arcana Interview, 12, 13, 19; Elze, "Underground Abortion Remembered."

106. Keemer, *Confessions,* 233.

107. *Roe v. Wade,* 410 US 113, 35 L Ed 2d 147 (1973); *Doe v. Bolton,* 410 US 179, 35 L Ed 2d 201 (1973).

108. *Roe v. Wade,* quotations on 177, 183.

109. *Doe v. Bolton; People v. Frey,* nos. 43729, 43882, Cons. Illinois S. Ct., (1973); *People v. Bell,* 10 Ill. App. 3d 533 (1973).

110. *Doe v. Bolton,* p. 201.

111. Public-health organizations and welfare recipients submitted an amicus brief that focused on the race and class inequality in access to abortion. Susan Alexander telephone interview, June 28, 1995. See Alan Charles and Susan Alexander, "Abortions for Poor and Nonwhite Women: A Denial of Equal Protection?" *Hastings Law Journal* 23 (November 1971): 147–169.

Epilogue: Post-*Roe*, Post-*Casey*

1. Most hospitals failed to provide abortions: Catholic hospitals did not allow abortions; less than 30 percent of other voluntary hospitals and only 15 percent of municipal hospitals provided abortions by 1974. Harold Speert, *Obstetrics and Gynecology in America: A History* (Chicago: American College of Obstetricians and Gynecologists), 170; Robert E. Hall, "Abortion: Physician and Hospital Attitudes," *AJPH* 61 (March 1971): 517–519.

2. *Chicago Reader*, April 6, 1973, p. 1. However, the problem of limited availability of abortion was foreshadowed by the Chicago Women's Liberation Union's observation that the number of abortion providers was small.

3. Institute of Medicine, *Legalized Abortion and the Public Health* (Washington, D.C.: National Academy of Sciences, May 1975), 79–80.

4. In 1971, the maternal mortality rate (pregnancy associated deaths per 10,000 live births) was 2.9 compared to 5.3 in 1969, the last year abortion was illegal in New York. (During 1970, abortion was illegal part of the year and the new system of legal abortion was being worked out.) I have calculated the decline from figures provided in table 17 in David Harris et al., "Legal Abortion 1970–1971—The New York City Experience," *AJPH* 63 (May 1973): 417; Speert, *Obstetrics and Gynecology in America*, 170; Robert E. Meyer and Paul A. Buescher, "Maternal Mortality Related to Induced Abortion in North Carolina: A Historical Study," *Family Planning Perspectives* 26 (July/August 1994): 179–180; Institute of Medicine, *Legalized Abortion and the Public Health*, 65–68.

5. Irvine Loudon identifies two previous major advances in controlling maternal mortality: the first decline in maternal mortality resulted from the introduction of antiseptic and aseptic procedures in the 1880–1900/1910 period; the "profound fall" in maternal mortality followed the introduction of sulfonamides, and then blood transfusions and penicillin, in the late 1930s and 1940s. Loudon finds that soon after the development of sulfa drugs in 1935–1936, the drugs were quickly manufactured and widely available in England, and maternal mortality soon fell. "Early trials of the sulphonamides showed that they reduced the death rate from puerperal fever by 50 to 60 per cent. . . . The reduction in mortality from puerperal fever in England and Wales from 1936 to 1937 was 35 per cent for total sepsis." However, for a variety of social reasons, the sulfa drugs did not produce as rapid a decline in maternal mortality in the United States as in England. Irvine Loudon, "Maternal Mortality: 1880–1950. Some Regional and International Comparisons," *Social History of Medicine* 1 (August 1988): 183–228, figure A on 186, quotations on 189, 199.

6. Irene Figa-Talamanca et al., "Illegal Abortion: An Attempt to Assess Its Cost to the Health Services and Its Incidence in the Community," *International Journal of Health Services* 16 (1986): 375–376; *Mexico City News*, May 15, 1992, p. 3.

7. In the first two years of legal abortion (1970–1972), "nonwhite" residents had 44.9 percent of the abortions, Puerto Ricans 11.3 percent, and whites, 42.0 percent. Jean Pakter et al., "Two Years Experience in New York City with the Liberalized Abortion Law—Progress and Problems," *AJPH* 63 (June 1973):

528. On mortality rates and abortion use, see Meyer and Buescher, "Maternal Mortality Related to Induced Abortion in North Carolina," 180, table 1; Institute of Medicine, *Legalized Abortion and Public Health*, 3, 34–37.

8. Rosalind Pollack Petchesky, *Abortion and Woman's Choice: The State, Sexuality, and Reproductive Freedom*, rev. ed. (1984; reprint, Boston: Northeastern University Press, 1990), 241–299; Rosalind Pollack Petchesky, "Fetal Images: The Power of Visual Culture in the Politics of Reproduction," *Feminist Studies* 13 (summer 1987): 263–292.

9. Samuel A. Mills, "Abortion and Religious Freedom: The Religious Coalition for Abortion Rights (RCAR) and the Pro-Choice Movement, 1973–1989," *Journal of Church and State* 3 (summer 1991): 569–594; Adele M. Stan, "Frances Kissling: Making the Vatican Sweat," *Ms.* (September/October 1995): 40–43.

10. Stanley K. Henshaw, "Factors Hindering Access to Abortion Services," *Family Planning Perspectives* 27 (March/April 1995): 58–59; Terry Sollom, "State Actions on Reproductive Health Issues in 1994," *Family Planning Perspectives* 27 (March/April 1995): 84; *NYT*, March 11, 1993.

11. Petchesky, *Abortion and Woman's Choice*, chaps. 7–8.

12. Ibid., 205–238.

13. As Linda Gordon points out, all of us receive welfare benefits (in the form of funding for education and highways, unemployment and social security benefits, and so on), but only state aid to mothers of dependent children (through AFDC) is labeled "welfare" and stigmatized. See Linda Gordon, *Pitied but Not Entitled: Single Mothers and the History of Welfare, 1890–1935* (New York: Free Press, 1994).

14. This type of private policing has already begun. In a recent Nebraska case, local antiabortionist activists and state authorities—police, prosecutors, and judge—acted in concert to prevent a young woman from having an abortion and forced her to bear a child. *NYT*, September 25, 1995, p. A8.

15. The only known prosecutions occurred in the 1970s and were political responses to the movement to decriminalize abortion.

16. Patricia Stephenson et al., "Commentary: The Public Health Consequences of Restricted Induced Abortion—Lessons from Romania," *AJPH* 82 (October 1992): 1328–1331.

17. *NYT*, January 31, 1992; *NYT*, November 23, 1987, pp. 1, 12. Barbara Katz Rothman, *Recreating Motherhood: Ideology and Technology in a Patriarchal Society* (New York: W. W. Norton, 1989), 87, 159–168. The American College of Obstetrician-Gynecologists has opposed the use of court orders to force c-sections upon women; "Patient Choice: Maternal-Fetal Conflict," *ACOG Committee Opinion*, no. 55 (October 1987).

18. *Webster v. Reproductive Health Services*, 492 U.S. 490 (1989); *Planned Parenthood v. Casey*, 112 S. Ct. 2791 (1992).

19. The exception for rape exposes the sexual politics of abortion opponents: if the pregnancy resulted from presumably voluntary sexual activity, then it is deserved punishment. Women who are victims, according to this line of thinking, may be permitted to have abortions.

20. Almost all insurance plans cover maternity care, about two-thirds cover

induced abortions, and a minority cover contraceptive services. Alan Guttmacher Institute, *Uneven and Unequal: Insurance Coverage and Reproductive Health Services* (New York: AGI, 1994), 12–19.

21. This is a misnomer; pregnant women are not yet "mothers." Pregnant women looking forward to a child, however, may start relating to the fetus as a child and begin to feel themselves mothers. Barbara Rothman discusses motherhood as a relationship in *Recreating Motherhood*.

22. Sollom, "State Actions on Reproductive Health Issues in 1994," 83; Rachel Benson Gold and Daniel Daley, "Public Funding of Contraceptive, Sterilization, and Abortion Services, Fiscal Year 1990," *Family Planning Perspectives* 23 (September/October 1991): 210.

23. Stanley K. Henshaw and Jennifer Van Vort, "Abortion Services in the United States, 1991 and 1992," *Family Planning Perspectives* 26 (May/June 1994): 103–112.

24. H. Trent MacKay and Andrea Phillips MacKay, "Abortion Training in Obstetrics and Gynecology Residency Programs in the United States, 1991–1992," *Family Planning Perspectives* 27 (May/June 1995): 112–115, quotation on 112.

25. *Webster v. Reproductive Health Services; Planned Parenthood v. Casey.* On *Webster*, see Petchesky, *Abortion and Woman's Choice*, 314–322. In 1994, nine states had instituted waiting periods and twenty-six enforced parental notification or consent laws. Sollom, "State Actions," 84; Frances A. Althaus and Stanley K. Henshaw, "The Effects of Mandatory Delay Laws on Abortion Patients and Providers," *Family Planning Perspectives* 26 (September/October 1994): 228–233.

26. Richard Phelan, President Cook County Board of Commissioners, public lecture, Urbana, Illinois, fall 1992; *Chicago Tribune,* January 28, 1995. My thanks to Rose Holz for giving me this clipping.

27. Linda Gordon reminds radicals to see the backlash as an indicator of how much society has changed in the past thirty years.

28. According to 1993 polls, 83 percent of Americans believe abortion should be legal. Of these, 32 percent think it should be legal "under any circumstances" and 51 percent think it should be legal "only under certain circumstances." Only 13 percent think it should be "illegal in all circumstances." Also interesting is the pro-choice sentiment within the Catholic Church: the majority of Catholics think that a Catholic can have an abortion and still be a "good Catholic" and that the Church should ease its position on abortion. George Gallup Jr., *The Gallup Poll, Public Opinion 1993* (Wilmington, Del.: Scholarly Resources, 1994), 73–74, 145–147.

29. "Vermont Physician Assistants Perform Abortions, Train Residents," *Family Planning Perspectives* 24 (September/October 1992): 225; Melanie Bush, "The Doctor Is Out," *Voice* (June 22, 1993): 18; Katherine McKee and Eleanor Adams, "Nurse Midwives' Attitudes toward Abortion Performance and Related Procedures," *Journal of Nurse-Midwifery* 39 (September/October 1994): 300–311.

30. MacKay and MacKay, "Abortion Training in Obstetrics and Gynecology Residency Programs in the United States, 1991–1992," 112–115.

31. Richard Phelan lecture.

32. Richard U. Hausknecht, "Methotrexate and Misoprostol to Terminate Early Pregnancy," *New England Journal of Medicine* 333 (August 31, 1995): 537–540; Etienne-Emile Baulieu, "Contragestion and Other Clinical Applications of RU 486, an Antiprogesterone at the Receptor, *Science* 245 (September 1989): 1351–1357; James Trussell et al., "Emergency Contraceptive Pills: A Simple Proposal to Reduce Unintended Pregnancies," *Family Planning Perspectives* 24 (November/December 1992): 269–273.

33. Sollom, "State Actions," 84–85.

34. Bylle Y. Avery, "Breathing Life into Ourselves: The Evolution of the National Black Women's Health Project," and Faye Wattleton, "Teenage Pregnancy: A Case for National Action," both in *The Black Women's Health Book: Speaking for Ourselves,* edited by Evelyn C. White (Seattle, Wash.: Seal Press, 1990), 4–10, 107–111. Though African Americans strongly support legal abortion, they are less active in the reproductive rights movement. See Julianne Malveaux, "Black America's Abortion Ambivalence," *Emerge* 4 (February 1993): 33–34. I am grateful to Vanessa Gamble for sharing the last article with me.

Bibliography

Primary Sources

LIBRARY AND ARCHIVAL COLLECTIONS

American Hospital Association Reference Library, Chicago, Illinois.
Joint Commission on Accreditation of Hospitals, *Standards for Hospital Accreditation*, 1953, 1954, 1956, 1960, 1969
Vertical Files
American Medical Association Library and Archives, Chicago, Illinois.
Deceased Physician Master File
Historical Health Fraud Collection
C. D. McCormick Library of Special Collections, Northwestern University Library, Evanston, Illinois.
Jenny Knauss Collection
Paula Kamen Collection
Serials
Women's Ephemera Folders
Chicago Historical Society, Archives and Manuscripts Department, Chicago, Illinois.
Chicago Medical Society Records
Chicago Women's Liberation Union Papers
Cook County Hospital Archives, Chicago, Illinois.
Cook County Hospital Administration Records
Cook County Medical Examiner's Office, Medical Records Department, Chicago, Illinois.
Cook County Coroner's Inquests
Countway Library of Medicine, Harvard University, Boston, Massachusetts.
Alan F. Guttmacher Papers
Horatio R. Storer Papers

Historical Society of the State of Wisconsin, Madison, Wisconsin.
   Women's National Abortion Action Coalition Papers
Illinois State Archives, Springfield, Illinois.
   Supreme Court of Illinois, Case Files, Record Series 901
Illinois State Historical Library, Springfield, Illinois.
   Illinois State Medical Society, Records, 1850–1960
Maryland State Archives, Annapolis, Maryland.
   Maryland Court of Appeals (Transcripts)
Moorland-Spingarn Research Center, Howard University, Washington, D.C.
   E. Franklin Frazier Papers
   Peter Marshall Murray Papers
Municipal Reference Collection, Chicago Public Library, Chicago, Illinois.
   Chicago Bureau of Public Efficiency. *Administration of the Office of Coroner of Cook County, Report,* December 1911
   Chicago City Council. *Proceedings,* 1896–1897, 1908–1909, 1916–1917
   Chicago Department of Health. *Annual Report,* 1899–1930
   ———. *Bulletin,* 1900–1927
   ———. *Committee for the Negro Health Survey,* 1927
   ———. *Handbook of General Orders, Instructions for Field Employees in the Bureau of Medical Inspection,* 1913, 1915
   Chicago Department of Police. *Annual Report,* 1913–1931
   ———. *Report of General Superintendent of Police of the City of Chicago,* 1878–1912
   Chicago Municipal Reference Library. *Coroners of Cook County, 1831–1976*
   Cook County Coroner. *Annual Report,* 1907–1969
   Illinois Department of Public Health. *Annual Report,* 1930–1969
National Abortion and Reproductive Rights Action League, Washington, D.C., and Chicago.
   Silent No More Campaign Files, 1985
National Archives—Great Lakes Region, Chicago, Illinois.
   Civil Case Files, Northern District of Illinois, Eastern Division (Chicago), Record Group 21, Records of the District Courts of the United States
   U.S. District Court, Criminal Docket Book no. 8, U.S. District Court, 1912–1913
Schlesinger Library on the History of Women in America, Radcliffe College, Cambridge, Massachusetts.
   Mary Steichen Calderone Papers
   Records of the Society For Humane Abortion and the Association to Repeal Abortion Laws
University of Illinois at Chicago Library, Department of Special Collections.
   Chicago Urban League Collection
   Jane Addams Collection
University of Illinois at Chicago Library, Reference Section.
   The Chicago Foreign Language Press Survey
William S. Middleton Health Sciences Library, Rare Book Room, University of Wisconsin, Madison.
   Report of the Board of Health of the City of Chicago, 1870–1873

COURT CASES (IN CHRONOLOGICAL ORDER)

United States Supreme Court Cases

Griswold v. Connecticut, 381 U.S. 479 (1965).
Roe v. Wade, 410 U.S. 113 (1973).
Doe v. Bolton, 410 U.S. 179 (1973).
Webster v. Reproductive Health Services, 492 U.S. 490 (1989).
Planned Parenthood v. Casey, 112 S. Ct. 2791 (1992).

Illinois Appellate Court, Illinois Supreme Court, and Other Cases

Holliday v. the People, 9 Ill. 111 (1847).
Yundt v. the People, 65 Ill. 372 (1872).
Earll v. the People, 73 Ill. 329 (1874).
Beasley v. the People, 89 Ill. 571 (1878).
Earll v. the People, 99 Ill. 123 (1881).
Baker v. the People, 105 Ill. 452 (1883).
Scott v. the People, 141 Ill. 195 (1892).
Dunn v. the People, 172 Ill. 582 (1898).
Cochran v. the People, 175 Ill. 28 (1898).
Cook v. the People, 177 Ill. 148 (1898).
Aiken v. the People, 183 Ill. 215 (1899).
Howard v. the People, 185 Ill. 552 (1900).
Hagenow v. the People, 188 Ill. 545 (1901).
Clark v. the People, 224 Ill. 554 (1906).
People v. Buettner, 233 Ill. 272 (1908).
People v. Hagenow, 236 Ill. 514 (1908).
People v. Dennis, 246 Ill. 559 (1910).
People v. Hotz, 261 Ill. 239 (1914).
People v. Patrick, 277 Ill. 210 (1917).
People v. Schultz-Knighten, 277 Ill. 238 (1917).
People v. Hobbs, 297 Ill. 399 (1921).
People v. Heisler, 300 Ill. 98 (1921).
People v. Carrico, 310 Ill. 543 (1924).
People v. Pigatti, 314 Ill. 626 (1924).
People v. Rongetti, 331 Ill. 581 (1928).
People v. Reed, 333 Ill. 397 (1929).
People v. Hagenow, 334 Ill. 341 (1929).
People v. Rongetti, 338 Ill. 56 (1930).
People v. Zwienczak, 338 Ill. 237 (1930).
People v. Heissler, 338 Ill. 596 (1930).
People v. Huff, 339 Ill. 328 (1930).
People v. Stilson, 342 Ill. 158 (1930).
People v. Rongetti, 344 Ill. 107 (1931).

People v. Rongetti, 344 Ill. 278 (1931).

People v. Wyherk, 347 Ill. 28 (1931).

People v. Ney, 349 Ill. 172 (1932).

People v. Kreutzer, 354 Ill. 430 (1933).

People v. Valentino, 354 Ill. 584 (1934).

People v. Gleitsmann, 361 Ill. 165 (1935).

People v. Davis, 362 Ill. 417 (1936).

People v. Braune, 363 Ill. 551 (1936).

People v. Cheney, 368 Ill. 131 (1938).

People v. Mitchell, 368 Ill. 399 (1938).

People v. Holmes, 369 Ill. 624 (1938).

People v. Mann, 370 Ill. 123 (1938).

People v. Schneider, 370 Ill. 612 (1939).

People v. Schyman, 374 Ill. 292 (1940).

People v. Martin, 376 Ill. 569 (1941).

People v. Peyser, 380 Ill. 404 (1942).

People v. Nathanson, 321 Ill. App. 158 (1943).

People v. Nathanson, 382 Ill. 145 (1943).

People v. Martin, 382 Ill. 192 (1943).

People v. Schaffner, 382 Ill. 266 (1943).

People v. Schmoll, 383 Ill. 280 (1943).

People v. Gleitsmann, 384 Ill. 303 (1943).

People v. Pavluk, 386 Ill. 492 (1944).

People v. Thompson, 387 Ill. 134 (1944).

People v. Nathanson, 389 Ill. 311 (1945).

People v. Meyers, 392 Ill. 395 (1946).

People v. Murawski, 394 Ill. 236 (1946).

People v. Gleitsmann, 396 Ill. 499 (1947).

People v. Young, 398 Ill. 117 (1947).

People v. Stanko, 402 Ill. 558 (1949).

People v. Tilley, 406 Ill. 398 (1950).

People v. Stanko, 407 Ill. 624 (1951).

Adams, Nelson, and Timanus v. State, 200 Md. 133 (1951).

People v. Khamis, 411 Ill. 46 (1952).

People v. Tilley, 411 Ill. 473 (1952).

Stalder v. Stone, 412 Ill. 488 (1952).

Castronovo v. Murawsky, 3 Ill. App. 2d 168 (1954).

People v. Ryan, 9 Ill. 2d 467 (1956).

People v. Kalpak, 10 Ill. 2d 411 (1957).

People v. Heidman, 11 Ill. 2d 501 (1957).

People v. Smuk, 12 Ill. 2d 360 (1957).

People v. Sarelli, 34 Ill. App. 2d 380 (1962).

People v. Woods, 24 Ill. 2d 154 (1962).

Iczek v. Iczek, 42 Ill. App. 2d 241 (1963).

People v. Veidt, 28 Ill. 2d 547 (1963).

People v. Gomez, 29 Ill. 2d 432 (1963).

Mateyka v. Smith, 47 Ill. App. 2d 1 (1964).

People v. Johndrow, 71 Ill. App. 2d 75 (1966).
People v. Miller, 82 Ill. App. 2d 304 (1967).
People v. Heidman, 38 Ill. 2d 466 (1967).
People v. Miller, 40 Ill. 2d 154 (1968).
People v. Johndrow, 40 Ill. 2d 288 (1968).
People v. Belous, 80 Cal. Rptr. 354, 458 P. 2d 194 (1969).
People v. Pecora, 107 Ill. App. 2d 283 (1969).
People v. West, 128 Ill. App. 2d 63 (1970).
Doe v. Scott, 321 F. Supp. 1385 (1971).
People v. Stephens, 132 Ill. App. 2d 586 (1971).
People ex rel. Hanrahan v. White, 52 Ill. 2d 70 (1972).
People v. Bell, 10 Ill. App. 3d 533 (1973).
People v. Frey, 54 Ill. 2d 28 (1973).

SELECTED MEDICAL AND HEALTH JOURNALS

American Journal of Obstetrics and Diseases of Women and Children.
     1880–1919. Superseded by *American Journal of Obstetrics and Gynecology.*
     1920–1973.
Birth Control Review. 1917–1940. Reprint, New York: Da Capo, 1970.
Bulletin of the Chicago Medical Society. 1908–1909. Superseded by *The Official
     Bulletin of the Chicago Medical Society.* 1914–1916.
Chicago Medical Journal. 1862–1876. Superseded by *Chicago Medical Journal
     and Examiner.* 1877–1888.
Family Planning Perspectives. 1994–1995.
Illinois State Medical Society. *Transactions.* 1874–1899. Superseded by *Illinois
     Medical Journal.* 1899–1974.
Journal of the American Medical Association. 1883–1973.
Journal of the National Medical Association. 1909–1973.
Milbank Memorial Fund Quarterly. 1935–1960.
Public Health Nurse Quarterly. 1909–1952.
Reports of the American Public Health Association. 1890–1911. Superseded by
     American Journal of Public Health. 1911–1945, 1960–1973.
Transactions of the American Medical Association. 1855–1871.
Woman's Medical Journal. 1893–1934.

NEWSPAPERS

Baltimore Sun, 1951.
Chicago Defender, 1914, 1940–1973.
Chicago Record Herald and Index, 1904–1910.
Chicago Times, 1888–1889.
Chicago Tribune, 1866–1867, 1888–1889, 1940–1941.
Clinton Daily Public, 1867.
Detroit Chronicle, 1958.
Detroit Free Press, 1958, 1972.

New York Times, 1866–1973.
Springfield Illinois State Journal, 1866–1867.
Springfield Illinois State Register, 1866–1867.

ARTICLES, BOOKS, GOVERNMENT DOCUMENTS, AND INTERVIEWS

The Abortion Problem. Proceedings of the Conference Held under the Auspices of the National Committee on Maternal Health. Baltimore: Williams and Wilkins, for the National Committee on Maternal Health, 1944.

"Abortion Surveillance: Preliminary Data—United States, 1992." *Morbidity and Mortality Weekly Report: CDC Surveillance Summaries* 43 (December 23, 1994).

Addams, Jane. *Twenty Years at Hull-House, with Autobiographical Notes.* 1910. Reprint, New York: New American Library, 1938.

Alexander, Susan Grossman. Interview by author. Tape recording. Chicago, March 8, 1994; June 28, 1995. Tape in author's possession.

American College of Physicians Directory, 1929–1930. Edited by Truman Schnabel. Philadelphia: American College of Physicians, 1930.

American Hospital Association. *Manual on Obstetrical Practice in Hospitals.* Chicago: American Hospital Association, 1936.

American Law Institute. *Model Penal Code: Official Draft and Explanatory Notes; Complete Text of Model Penal Code as Adopted at the 1962 Annual Meeting of The American Law Institute at Washington, D.C., May 24, 1962.* Philadelphia: American Law Institute, 1985.

———. *Proceedings of the American Law Institute.* 1959, 1962.

American Medical Directory. Chicago: American Medical Association, 1906, 1914, 1916, 1921, 1942, 1950.

Baker, S. Josephine. *Fighting For Life.* New York: Macmillan, 1939.

Barnett, Ruth. *They Weep on My Doorstep.* [Oregon]: Halo Publishers, 1969.

Bates, Jerome E., and Edward S. Zawadzki. *Criminal Abortion: A Study in Medical Sociology.* Springfield, Ill.: Charles C. Thomas, 1964.

Biographies of Physicians and Surgeons. Edited by F. M. Sperry. Chicago: J. H. Beers and Co., 1904.

Bowen, Louise DeKoven. "The Colored People of Chicago." Chicago: Juvenile Protective Association, 1913.

Breckinridge, Sophonisba P. *Family Welfare Work in a Metropolitan Community, Selected Case Records.* Chicago: University of Chicago Press, 1924.

Bromley, Dorothy Dunbar, and Florence Haxton Britten. *Youth and Sex: A Study of 1300 College Students.* New York: Harper and Brothers, 1938.

Calderone, Mary Steichen, ed. *Abortion in the United States: A Conference Sponsored by the Planned Parenthood Federation of America, Inc. at Arden House and the New York Academy of Medicine.* New York: Harper and Brothers, 1958.

Chicago City Directory. 1889.

Chisolm, Shirley. "Facing the Abortion Question." In *Black Women in White America: A Documentary History,* edited by Gerda Lerner, 602–607. New York: Random House, 1972.

Cisler, Lucinda. "Unfinished Business: Birth Control and Women's Liberation." In *Sisterhood Is Powerful: An Anthology of Writings from the Women's
Liberation Movement,* edited by Robin Morgan, 274–323. New York: Vintage Books, 1970.

Commoner, Barry. *The Closing Circle: Nature, Man, and Technology.* New
York: Knopf, 1971. Reprint, New York: Bantam Books, 1972.

*Connorton's Directory of Physicians, Dentists, and Druggists of Chicago, Includ-
ing Suburbs in Cook County.* Chicago: J. Newton McDonald, 1889.

The Cyclopedia of Medicine. Edited by George Morris. Vol. 12. Philadelphia:
F. A. Davis, 1935.

Davis, Katharine Bement. *Factors in the Sex Life of Twenty-Two Hundred
Women.* 1929. Reprint, New York: Arno Press, 1972.

DeLee, Joseph B. *The Principles and Practice of Obstetrics.* 2d and 4th ed.
Philadelphia: W. B. Saunders, 1916 and 1924.

Ehrlich, Paul R. *The Population Bomb.* New York: Ballantine Books, 1968.

Friedan, Betty. *The Feminine Mystique.* New York: Dell, 1963.

Fritzsche, Sybille. Interview by author. Tape recording. Chicago, March 8,
1994; April 6, 1995. Tape in author's possession.

Gebhard, Paul H., et al. *Pregnancy, Birth, and Abortion.* New York: Harper
and Brothers and Paul B. Hoeber Medical Books, 1958.

Greenleaf, Simon. *A Treatise on the Law of Evidence.* Vol. 1. 16th ed. Boston:
Little, Brown and Co., 1899.

Guttmacher, Alan F. "The Genesis of Liberalized Abortion in New York: A
Personal Insight." Update by Irwin H. Kaiser. In *Abortion, Medicine, and
the Law,* 3d ed., rev., edited by J. Douglas Butler and David F. Walbert,
229–246. New York: Facts on File Publications, 1986.

Hale, Edwin M. *The Great Crime of the Nineteenth Century.* Chicago: C. S.
Halsey, 1867.

Hamilton, Gilbert Van Tassel. *A Research in Marriage.* New York: Albert and
Charles Boni, 1929.

Hardin, Garrett. *Exploring New Ethics for Survival: The Voyage of the Spaceship
Beagle.* New York: Viking Press, 1968.

Hayt, Lillian R., and August H. Groeschel. *Law of Hospital, Physician, and
Patient.* New York: Hospital Textbook, 1952.

Himes, Norman E. *Medical History of Contraception.* Baltimore: Williams and
Wilkins Co., 1936. Reprint, New York: New York University Press, 1963.

Hirst, Barton Cooke. *A Textbook of Obstetrics.* 8th ed. Philadelphia: W. B.
Saunders, 1918.

Hooker, Ransom S. *Maternal Mortality in New York City: A Study of All Puerperal Deaths, 1930–1932.* New York: Commonwealth Fund, by the New York
Academy of Medicine Committee on Public Health Relations, 1933.

Huser, Roger John. *The Crime of Abortion in Canon Law: An Historical Syn-
opsis and Commentary.* Washington, D.C.: Catholic University of America
Press, 1943.

Illinois. *All the Laws of Illinois.* 1899.

———. *Journal of the House of Representatives.* 1867.

———. *Journal of the Senate.* 1867.

———. *Laws of Illinois.* 1899, 1915, 1919, 1961.

————. *Public Laws of Illinois.* 1867, 1872.

————. *Revised Code of Illinois.* 1827.

Illinois State Board of Health. *Annual Report.* 1896–1899, 1903.

Institute of Medicine. *Legalized Abortion and the Public Health, Report of a Study by a Committee of the Institute of Medicine, May 1975.* IOM Publication 75–02. Washington D.C.: National Academy of Science, 1975.

Juvenile Protective Association of Chicago. *Baby Farms in Chicago: An Investigation Made for the Juvenile Protective Association by Arthur Alden Guild.* N.p., 1917.

————. *A Study of Bastardy Cases, Taken from The Court of Domestic Relations in Chicago.* Text by Louise DeKoven Bowen [Chicago, 1914].

Keemer, Ed. *Confessions of a Pro-Life Abortionist.* Detroit: Vinco Press, 1980.

Kelly, Gerald Andrew. *Medico-Moral Problems.* Part 3. St. Louis: Catholic Hospital Association, 1948–1952.

Kopp, Marie E. *Birth Control in Practice: Analysis of Ten Thousand Case Histories of the Birth Control Clinical Research Bureau.* New York: Robert McBride and Co., 1933. Reprint, New York: Arno Press, 1972.

Lader, Lawrence. *Abortion.* Boston: Beacon Press, 1966.

Lee, Nancy Howell. *The Search for an Abortionist.* Chicago: University of Chicago Press, 1969.

Lepawskysy, Albert. *The Judicial System of Metropolitan Chicago.* Chicago: University of Chicago Press, 1932.

Le Sueur, Meridel. *The Girl.* Minneapolis: West End Press and MEP Publications, 1978.

Litoff, Judy Barrett, ed. *The American Midwife Debate: A Sourcebook on Its Modern Origins.* New York: Greenwood Press, 1986.

Logan, Onnie Lee, as told to Katherine Clark. *Motherwit: An Alabama Midwife's Story.* New York: E. P. Dutton, 1989.

MacEachern, Malcolm T. *Manual on Obstetric Practice in Hospitals.* American Hospital Association Official Bulletin, no. 209. Chicago: American Hospital Association, 1940.

McDonald's Illinois State Medical Directory: A Complete List of Physicians in the State. Chicago: J. Newton McDonald, 1891.

Medical and Surgical Register of the United States. Detroit: R. L. Polk, 1886, 1890.

Morgan, Robin, ed. *Sisterhood is Powerful: An Anthology of Writings from the Women's Liberation Movement.* New York: Vintage Books, 1970.

The National Cyclopaedia of Biography, Being the History of the United States. Vol. 35. New York: James T. White and Co., 1949.

R., Dr. Jack [pseud.]. Interview by author. Tape recording. November 1987. Tape in author's possession.

Reed, Louis S. *Midwives, Chiropodists, and Optometrists: Their Place in Medical Care.* Chicago: University of Chicago, 1932.

Robinson, Caroline Hadley. *Seventy Birth Control Clinics: A Survey and Analysis Including the General Effects of Control on Size and Quality of Population.* Baltimore: Williams and Wilkins, 1930.

Robinson, William J. *The Law against Abortion: Its Perniciousness Demon-*

strated and Its Repeal Demanded. New York: Eugenics Publishing Co., 1933.

Rongy, A. J. *Abortion: Legal or Illegal?* New York: Vanguard Press, 1933.

Rosen, Harold, ed. *Therapeutic Abortion: Medical, Psychiatric, Legal, Anthropological, and Religious Considerations in the Prevention of Conception and the Interruption of Pregnancy.* New York: Julian Press, 1954.

S., Rose [pseud.]. Interview by author. Tape recording. November 1987. Tape in author's possession.

Sanger, Margaret. *Motherhood in Bondage.* New York: Brentano's Publishers, 1928.

Schmid, Calvin. *Social Saga of Two Cities: An Ecological and Statistical Study of Social Trends in Minneapolis and St. Paul.* Minneapolis: Minneapolis Council of Social Agencies, 1937.

Simon, Kenneth A., and W. Vance Grant. *Digest of Educational Statistics.* Washington, D.C.: Government Printing Office, 1972.

Storer, Horatio Robinson. *Is It I? A Book for Every Man.* 1868. Reprint as *A Proper Bostonian on Sex and Birth Control,* edited by Charles Rosenberg and Carroll Smith-Rosenberg. New York: Arno Press, 1974.

————. *Why Not? A Book for Every Woman.* 1868. Reprint as *A Proper Bostonian on Sex and Birth Control,* edited by Charles Rosenberg and Carroll Smith-Rosenberg. New York: Arno Press, 1974.

Storer, Horatio Robinson, and Franklin Fiske Heard. *Criminal Abortion: Its Nature, Its Evidence, and Its Law.* Boston: Little, Brown and Co., 1868.

Taussig, Frederick J. *Abortion, Spontaneous and Induced: Medical and Social Aspects.* St. Louis: C. V. Mosby, 1936.

————. *The Prevention and Treatment of Abortion.* St. Louis: C. V. Mosby, 1910.

Tietze, Christopher, et al. *Provisional Estimates of Abortion Need and Services in the Year Following the 1973 Supreme Court Decisions, United States, Each State and Metropolitan Area.* A Report by the Alan Guttmacher Institute, Research and Development Division of Planned Parenthood Federation of America. New York: Planned Parenthood, 1975.

Tillmon, Johnnie. "Welfare is a Woman's Issue." In *The First Ms. Reader,* edited by Francine Klagsbrun, 51–59. New York: Warner Paperback Library, 1973.

Towne, Arthur W. "Young Girl Marriages in Criminal and Juvenile Courts." *Journal of Social Hygiene* 8 (July 1922): 287–290.

U.S. Army. *Index Catalogue of the Library of the Surgeon General's Office.* Washington, D.C.: Government Printing Office, 1880, 1906, 1928.

U.S. Bureau of the Census. *Historical Statistics of the United States, Colonial Times to 1970.* Bicentennial Edition, Part 1. Washington D.C.: Government Printing Office, 1975.

————. *Statistical Abstract of the United States: 1994.* Washington, D.C.: Government Printing Office, 1994.

U.S. Congress. Senate. *Birth Control Hearings before a Subcommittee of the Committee on the Judiciary.* Washington, D.C.: Government Printing Office, 1931.

U.S. Department of Labor. Children's Bureau. *Maternal Mortality in Fifteen States*. Bureau Publication No. 223. Washington D.C.: Government Printing Office, 1934.

Vice Commission of Chicago. *The Social Evil in Chicago. A Study of Existing Conditions with Recommendations*. 1911. Reprint, *The Rise of Urban America*, edited by Richard C. Wade. New York: Arno Press, 1970.

Vincent, Clark E. "Unmarried Fathers and the Mores: 'Sexual Exploiter' as an Ex Post Facto Label." *American Sociological Review* 25 (February 1960): 40–48.

White House Conference on Child Health and Protection. *Fetal, Newborn, and Maternal Morbidity and Mortality*. By Fred J. Taussig. New York: D. Appleton-Century, 1933.

Who's Who in American Medicine, 1925. Edited by Lloyd Thompson. New York: Who's Who Publications, 1925.

Wigmore, John Henry. *A Treatise on the System of Evidence in Trials at Common Law, Including Statutes and Judicial Decisions of All Jurisdictions of the United States*. Boston: Little, Brown and Co., 1904.

Williams, J. Whitridge. *Williams Obstetrics: A Textbook for the Use of Students and Practitioners*. 7th ed. rev. by Henricus J. Stander. New York: D. Appleton-Century, 1936.

You May Plow Here: The Narrative of Sara Brooks. Edited by Thordis Simonsen. New York: Simon and Schuster, 1986.

Secondary Sources

Abelove, Henry. "The Queering of Lesbian/Gay History." *Radical History Review* 62 (Spring 1995): 44–57.

Ackerknecht, Erwin H. *A Short History of Medicine*. 1955. Reprint, Baltimore: Johns Hopkins University Press, 1992.

Alan Guttmacher Institute. *Uneven and Unequal: Insurance Coverage and Reproductive Health Services*. New York: AGI, 1994.

Antler, Joyce, and Daniel M. Fox. "The Movement toward a Safe Maternity: Physician Accountability in New York City, 1915–1940." *Bulletin of the History of Medicine* 50 (1976): 569–595. Reprint in *Sickness and Health in America: Readings in the History of Medicine and Public Health*, edited by Judith Walzer Leavitt and Ronald L. Numbers. Madison: University of Wisconsin Press, 1978.

Apple, Rima D. *Mothers and Medicine: A Social History of Infant Feeding, 1890–1950*. Madison: University of Wisconsin Press, 1987.

———. *Women, Health, and Medicine in America: A Historical Handbook*. New York: Garland Publishing, 1990.

Backhouse, Constance B. "Involuntary Motherhood: Abortion, Birth Control and the Law in Nineteenth Century Canada." *Windsor Yearbook of Access to Justice* 3 (1983): 61–130.

Baehr, Ninia. *Abortion without Apology: A Radical History for the 1990s*. Boston: South End Press, 1990.

Barker-Benfield, G. J. *The Horrors of the Half Known Life: Male Attitudes to-*

ward Women and Sexuality in Nineteenth Century America. New York: Harper and Row, 1976.

Baron, Ava. *Work Engendered: Toward a New History of American Labor.* Ithaca: Cornell University Press, 1991.

Barrett, James R. "Unity and Fragmentation: Class, Race, and Ethnicity on Chicago's South Side, 1900–1922." *Journal of Social History* 18 (September 1984): 37–55.

Bart, Pauline B. "Seizing the Means of Reproduction: An Illegal Feminist Abortion Collective—How and Why it Worked." *Qualitative Sociology* 10 (winter 1987): 339–357.

Basch, Norma. *In the Eyes of the Law: Women, Marriage, and Property in Nineteenth-Century New York.* Ithaca: Cornell University Press, 1982.

Bérubé, Allan. *Coming Out under Fire: The History of Gay Men and Women in World War Two.* New York: Free Press, 1990.

Bérubé, Michael. "Life as We Know It." *Harper's* 289 (December 1994): 41–43.

Bonner, Thomas Neville. *Medicine in Chicago: A Chapter in the Social and Scientific Development of a City, 1850–1950.* Madison, Wis.: American History Research Center, 1957. 2d ed., Urbana: University of Illinois, 1991.

Borst, Charlotte G. *Catching Babies: The Professionalization of Childbirth, 1870–1920.* Cambridge, Mass.: Harvard University Press, 1995.

———. "The Professionalization of Obstetrics: Childbirth Becomes a Medical Specialty." In *Women, Health, and Medicine in America: A Historical Handbook,* edited by Rima D. Apple, 197–216. New York: Garland Publishing, 1990.

Boyer, Paul. *Urban Masses and Moral Order in America, 1820–1920.* Cambridge, Mass.: Harvard University Press, 1978.

Brandt, Allan M. *No Magic Bullet: A Social History of Venereal Disease in the United States Since 1880.* Expanded ed. New York: Oxford University Press, 1987.

Brickman, Jane Pacht. "Public Health, Midwives, and Nurses, 1880–1930." In *Nursing History: New Perspectives, New Possibilities,* edited by Ellen Condliffe Lagemann, 65–88. New York: Teacher's College Press, 1983.

Brieger, Gert H. "American Surgery and the Germ Theory of Disease." *Bulletin of the History of Medicine* 40 (March-April 1966): 135–145.

Brodie, Janet Farrell. *Abortion and Contraception in Nineteenth-Century America.* Ithaca: Cornell University Press, 1994.

Brookes, Barbara. *Abortion in England, 1900–1967.* London: Croom Helm, 1988.

Brown, Elaine. *A Taste of Power: A Black Woman's Story.* New York: Pantheon Books, 1992.

Brumberg, Joan Jacobs. *Fasting Girls: The Emergence of Anorexia Nervosa as a Modern Disease.* Cambridge, Mass.: Harvard University Press, 1988.

———. "'Ruined Girls': Changing Community Responses to Illegitimacy in Upstate New York, 1890–1920." *Journal of Social History* 18 (winter 1984): 247–272.

Burnham, John C. "American Medicine's Golden Age: What Happened to It?" *Science* 215 (March 19, 1982): 1474–1479. Reprint in *Sickness and*

Health in America: Readings in the History of Medicine and Public Health,
2d ed., rev., edited by Judith Walzer Leavitt and Ronald L. Numbers,
248–258. Madison: University of Wisconsin Press, 1985.

Calhoun, Craig. *Habermas and the Public Sphere.* Cambridge, Mass.: MIT
Press, 1992.

Carmen, Arlene, and Howard Moody. *Abortion Counseling and Social Change
from Illegal Act to Medical Practice: The Story of the Clergy Consultation
Service on Abortion.* Valley Forge, Penn.: Judson Press, 1973.

Caute, David. *The Great Fear: The Anti-Communist Purge under Truman and
Eisenhower.* New York: Simon and Schuster, 1978.

Cayleff, Susan E. "Self-Help and the Patent Medicine Business." In *Women,
Health, and Medicine in America: A Historical Handbook,* edited by Rima
D. Apple, 311–336. New York: Garland Publishing, 1990.

Chauncey, George. *Gay New York: Gender, Urban Culture, and the Making of
the Gay Male World, 1890 –1940.* New York: Basic Books, 1994.

Chesler, Ellen. *Woman of Valor: Margaret Sanger and the Birth Control Movement in America.* New York: Simon and Schuster, 1992.

Clark, Anna. *Women's Silence, Men's Violence: Sexual Assault in England,
1770 –1845.* New York: Pandora Press, 1987.

Clark, Michael, and Catherine Crawford, eds. *Legal Medicine in History.*
Cambridge: Cambridge University Press, 1994.

Cohen, Lizabeth. *Making a New Deal: Industrial Workers in Chicago,
1919 –1939.* Cambridge: Cambridge University Press, 1990.

Committee for Abortion Rights and Against Sterilization Abuse. *Women un-
der Attack: Victories, Backlash, and the Fight for Reproductive Freedom.*
South End Press pamphlet no. 7. Edited by Susan E. Davis. Boston: South
End Press, 1988.

Costin, Lela B. *Two Sisters for Social Justice: A Biography of Grace and Edith
Abbott.* Urbana: University of Illinois Press, 1983.

Cott, Nancy F. *The Bonds of Womanhood: "Woman's Sphere" in New England,
1780 –1835.* New Haven: Yale University Press, 1977.

———. "Giving Character to Our Whole Civil Polity: Marriage and the Public Order in the Late Nineteenth Century." In *U.S. History as Women's History: New Feminist Essays,* edited by Linda K. Kerber, Alice Kessler-Harris,
and Kathryn Kish Sklar, 107–121. Chapel Hill: University of North Carolina
Press, 1995.

———. *The Grounding of Modern Feminism.* New Haven: Yale University
Press, 1987.

Cott, Nancy F., and Elizabeth H. Pleck, eds. *A Heritage of Her Own: Toward
a New Social History of American Women.* New York: Simon and Schuster,
1979.

Crawford, Vicki L., et al. *Women in the Civil Rights Movement: Trailblazers
and Torchbearers, 1941 –1965.* Bloomington: Indiana University Press, 1990.

Curry, Lynne Elizabeth. "Modern Mothers in the Heartland: Maternal and
Child Health Reform in Illinois, 1900–1930." Ph.D. diss., University of
Illinois, Urbana-Champaign, 1995.

Davis, Angela Y. *Women, Race, and Class.* New York: Random House, 1981.

Davis, Martha F. *Lawyers and the Welfare Rights Movement, 1960–1973.* New Haven: Yale University Press, 1993.

Dawley, Alan. *Struggles for Justice: Social Responsibility and the Liberal State.* Cambridge, Mass.: Belknap Press of Harvard University Press, 1991.

Dayton, Cornelia Hughes. "Taking the Trade: Abortion and Gender Relations in an Eighteenth-Century New England Village." *William and Mary Quarterly.* 48 (January 1991): 19–49.

Declerq, Eugene R. "The Nature and Style of Practice of Immigrant Midwives in Early Twentieth-Century Massachusetts." *Journal of Social History* 19 (1985): 113–129.

Dedmon, Emmett. *Fabulous Chicago.* New York: Random House, 1953.

Degler, Carl. *At Odds: Women and the Family in America from the Revolution to the Present.* New York: Oxford University Press, 1980.

D'Emilio, John. *Sexual Politics, Sexual Communities: The Making of a Homosexual Minority in the United States, 1940–1970.* Chicago: University of Chicago Press, 1983.

D'Emilio, John, and Estelle B. Freedman. *Intimate Matters: A History of Sexuality in America.* New York: Harper and Row, 1988.

Drachman, Virginia G. *Hospital with a Heart: Women Doctors and the Paradox of Separatism at the New England Hospital, 1862–1969.* Ithaca: Cornell University Press, 1984.

———. "The Loomis Trial: Social Mores and Obstetrics in the Nineteenth Century." In *Childbirth: The Beginning of Motherhood, Proceedings of the Second Motherhood Symposium.* Madison, Wis.: Women's Studies Research Center, 1982. Reprint in *Women and Health in America: Historical Readings,* edited by Judith Walzer Leavitt, 166–174. Madison: University of Wisconsin Press, 1984.

DuBois, Ellen Carol. *Feminism and Suffrage: The Emergence of an Independent Women's Movement in America, 1848–1869.* Ithaca: Cornell University Press, 1978.

DuBois, Ellen Carol, Mari Jo Buhle, Temma Kaplan, Gerda Lerner, and Carroll Smith-Rosenberg. "Politics and Culture in Women's History: A Symposium." *Feminist Studies* 6:1 (1980): 26–62.

DuBois, Ellen Carol, and Linda Gordon. "Seeking Ecstasy on the Battlefield: Danger and Pleasure in Nineteenth-Century Feminist Sexual Thought." *Feminist Studies* 9 (Spring 1983): 7–25.

DuBois, Ellen Carol, and Vicki L. Ruiz, eds. *Unequal Sisters: A Multi-Cultural Reader in U.S. Women's History.* New York: Routledge, 1990.

Duden, Barbara. *Disembodying Women: Perspectives on Pregnancy and the Unborn.* Translated by Lee Hoinacki. Cambridge, Mass.: Harvard University Press, 1993.

Duggan, Lisa. "'Becoming Visible: The Legacy of Stonewall,' New York Public Library, June 18–September 24, 1994." *Radical History Review* 62 (spring 1995): 187–194.

———. "The Trials of Alice Mitchell: Sensationalism, Sexology, and the Lesbian Subject in Turn-of-the-Century America." *Signs* 18 (summer 1993): 791–814.

Dworkin, Andrea, and Catharine A. MacKinnon. *Pornography and Civil Rights: A New Day for Women's Equality.* N.p., 1988.

Dye, Nancy Schrom. "Modern Obstetrics and Working-Class Women: The New York Midwifery Dispensary, 1890–1920." *Journal of Social History* 20 (spring 1987): 549–564.

Ehrenreich, Barbara, and Deirdre English. *For Her Own Good: 150 Years of the Experts' Advice to Women.* Garden City, N.Y.: Anchor Press/Doubleday, 1978.

Engels, Frederick. *The Origin of the Family, Private Property, and the State.* 1884. Reprint, New York: International Publishers, 1972.

Epstein, Barbara Leslie. *The Politics of Domesticity: Women, Evangelism, and Temperance in Nineteenth-Century America.* Middletown, Conn.: Wesleyan University Press, 1981.

Evans, Sara. *Personal Politics: The Roots of Women's Liberation in the Civil Rights Movement and the New Left.* New York: Random House, 1979.

Ewen, Elizabeth. *Immigrant Women in the Land of Dollars: Life and Culture on the Lower East Side, 1890–1925.* New York: Monthly Review Press, 1985.

Ferraro, Barbara, and Patricia Hussey with Jane O'Reilly. *No Turning Back: Two Nuns' Battle with the Vatican over Women's Right to Choose.* New York: Ivy Books, a division of Ballantine Books, 1990.

Fine, Evelyn. "'Belly Ripping Has Become a Mania.' A History of the Cesarean Section Operation in Twentieth Century America." Master's thesis, Department of the History of Science, University of Wisconsin, Madison, 1982.

Fiorenza, Mary Elizabeth. "Midwifery and the Law in Illinois and Wisconsin, 1877 to 1917." Master's thesis, University of Wisconsin, Madison, 1985.

Fissell, Mary E. *Patients, Power, and the Poor in Eighteenth-Century Bristol.* Cambridge: Cambridge University Press, 1991.

Flexner, Eleanor. *Century of Struggle: The Woman's Rights Movement in the United States.* 1959. Rev. ed. Cambridge, Mass.: Belknap Press of Harvard University Press, 1975.

Foucault, Michel. *Discipline and Punish: The Birth of the Prison.* Translated by Alan Sheridan. 1975. Reprint, New York: Vintage Books, 1979.

———. *The History of Sexuality.* Vol. 1. Translated by Robert Hurley. New York: Random House, 1978.

Frankel, Noralee, and Nancy S. Dye, eds. *Gender, Class, Race, and Reform in the Progressive Era.* Lexington: University Press of Kentucky, 1991.

Fraser, Nancy. *Unruly Practice: Power, Discourse, and Gender in Contemporary Social Theory.* Minneapolis: University of Minnesota Press, 1989.

Freedman, Estelle B. *Their Sisters' Keepers: Women's Prison Reform in America, 1830–1930.* Ann Arbor: University of Michigan, 1981.

Freeman, Jo. *The Politics of Women's Liberation: A Case Study of an Emerging Social Movement and its Relation to the Policy Process.* New York: David McKay, 1975.

Friedman, Lawrence M. *Crime and Punishment in American History.* New York: Basic Books, 1993.

Friedman, Lawrence M., and Robert V. Percival. *The Roots of Justice: Crime and Punishment in Alameda County, California, 1870–1910.* Chapel Hill: University of North Carolina Press, 1981.

Gamble, Vanessa Northington. *Making a Place for Ourselves: the Black Hospital Movement, 1920–1945*. New York: Oxford University Press, 1995.

Garrow, David J. *Liberty and Sexuality: The Right to Privacy and the Making of Roe v. Wade*. New York: Maxwell Macmillan International, 1994.

Gerson, Deborah A. "'Is Family Devotion Now Subversive?' Familialism against McCarthyism." In *Not June Cleaver: Women and Gender in Postwar America, 1945–1960*, edited by Joanne Meyerowitz, 151–172. Philadelphia: Temple University Press, 1994.

Gevitz, Norman, ed. *Other Healers: Unorthodox Medicine in America*. Baltimore: Johns Hopkins University Press, 1988.

Giddings, Paula. *When and Where I Enter: The Impact of Black Women on Race and Sex in America*. New York: William Morrow, Bantam Books, 1984.

Gilbert, James. *Perfect Cities: Chicago's Utopias of 1893*. Chicago: University of Chicago Press, 1991.

Ginzberg, Lori D. *Women and the Work of Benevolence: Morality, Politics, and Class in the Nineteenth-Century United States*. New Haven: Yale University Press, 1990.

Goebel, Thomas. "American Medicine and the 'Organizational Synthesis': Chicago Physicians and the Business of Medicine, 1900–1920." *Bulletin of the History of Medicine* 68 (winter 1994): 639–663.

Goodrich, Herbert F., and Paul A. Wolkin. *The Story of the American Law Institute, 1923–1961*. St. Paul, Minn.: American Law Institute Publishers, 1961.

Gordon, Linda. *Heroes of Their Own Lives: The Politics and History of Family Violence, Boston, 1880–1960*. New York: Viking, 1988.

———. *Pitied but Not Entitled: Single Mothers and the History of Welfare, 1890–1935*. New York: Free Press, 1994.

———. *Woman's Body, Woman's Right: Birth Control in America*. New York: Grossman Publishers, 1976. Revised and updated, New York: Penguin Books, 1990.

———, ed. *Women, the State, and Welfare*. Madison: University of Wisconsin Press, 1990.

Green, Norma, Stephen Lacy, and Jean Folkerts. "Chicago Journalists at the Turn of the Century: Bohemians All?" *Journalism Quarterly* 66 (winter 1989): 813–821.

Grob, Gerald N. *From Asylum to Community: Mental Health Policy in Modern America*. Princeton, N.J.: Princeton University Press, 1991.

Grossberg, Michael. *Governing the Hearth: Law and the Family in Nineteenth-Century America*. Chapel Hill: University of North Carolina Press, 1985.

Grossmann, Atina. "Abortion and Economic Crisis: The 1931 Campaign against 218 in Germany." *New German Critique* 14 (spring 1978): 119–137.

Habermas, Jürgen. *The Structural Transformation of the Public Sphere: An Inquiry into a Category of Bourgeois Society*. Translated by Thomas Burger with Frederick Lawrence. Cambridge, Mass.: MIT Press, 1989.

Hale, Christine B. "Infant Mortality: An American Tragedy." *Black Scholar* 21 (January–February–March 1990): 17–26.

Hall, Kermit L. *The Magic Mirror: Law in American History*. New York: Oxford University Press, 1989.

Haller, John S. *American Medicine in Transition, 1840–1910.* Urbana: University of Illinois Press, 1981.

Haller, Mark H. *Eugenics: Hereditarian Attitudes in American Thought.* New Brunswick, N.J.: Rutgers University Press, 1963.

———. "Historical Roots of Police Behavior: Chicago, 1890–1925." *Law and Society Review* 10 (winter 1976): 303–323.

Harring, Sidney L. *Policing a Class Society: The Experience of American Cities, 1865–1915.* New Brunswick, N.J.: Rutgers University Press, 1983.

Hartman, Mary, and Lois W. Banner, eds. *Clio's Consciousness Raised: New Perspectives on the History of Women.* New York: Harper and Row, 1974.

Hartmann, Susan M. *The Home Front and Beyond: American Women in the 1940s.* Boston: Twayne Publishers, 1982.

Hartog, Hendrik. "Pigs and Positivism." *Wisconsin Law Review* 1985, no. 4 (1985): 899–935.

———. "The Public Law of a County Court; Judicial Government in Eighteenth Century Massachusetts," *The American Journal of Legal History* 20 (1976): 282–329.

Hedge, Elaine, and Shelley Fisher Fishkin, eds. *Listening to Silences: New Essays in Feminist Criticism.* New York: Oxford University Press, 1994.

Helmbold, Lois Rita. "Beyond the Family Economy: Black and White Working Class Women during the Great Depression." *Feminist Studies* 13 (fall 1987): 642–643.

Hewitt, Nancy A. "Beyond the Search for Sisterhood: American Women's History in the 1980s." *Social History* 10 (October 1985). Reprint in *Unequal Sisters: A Multi-Cultural Reader in U.S. Women's History,* edited by Ellen Carol DuBois and Vicki L. Ruiz, 1–14. New York: Routledge, 1990.

Hine, Darlene Clark. *Black Women in White: Racial Conflict and Cooperation in the Nursing Profession, 1890–1950.* Bloomington: Indiana University Press, 1989.

Hole, Judith, and Ellen Levine. *Rebirth of Feminism.* New York: Quadrangle Books, 1971.

hooks, bell. *Talking Back: thinking feminist, thinking black.* Boston: South End Press, 1989.

Howe, Louise Kapp. *Moments on Maple Avenue: The Reality of Abortion.* New York: Macmillan, 1984. Reprint, New York: Warner Books, 1986.

Hoy, Suellen M. "'Municipal Housekeeping': The Role of Women in Improving Urban Sanitation Practices, 1880–1917." In *Pollution and Reform in American Cities, 1870–1930,* edited by Martin Melosi, 173–198. Austin: University of Texas Press, 1980.

Hurst, James Willard. *The Growth of American Law: The Law Makers.* Boston: Little, Brown and Co., 1950.

Ignatieff, Michael. "State, Civil Society, and Total Institution: A Critique of Recent Social Histories of Punishment." In *Legality, Ideology and The State,* edited by David Sugarman, 183–211. London: Academic Press, 1983.

James, Stanlie M., and Abena P. A. Busia. *Theorizing Black Feminisms: The Visionary Pragmatism of Black Women.* London: Routledge, 1993.

Jensen, Joan M. "The Death of Rosa: Sexuality in Rural America." *Agricultural History* 67 (fall 1993): 1–12.

Jezer, Mary. *The Dark Ages: Life in the United States, 1945–1960*. Boston: South End Press, 1982.

Joffe, Carole. "Comments on MacKinnon." *Radical America* 18 (March–June 1984): 68–69.

———. "Portraits of Three 'Physicians of Conscience': Abortion before Legalization in the United States." *Journal of the History of Sexuality* 2 (July 1991): 46–67.

Johnson, Julie. "Coroners, Corruption, and the Politics of Death: Forensic Pathology in the United States." In *Legal Medicine in History*, edited by Michael Clark and Catherine Crawford, 268–289. Cambridge: Cambridge University Press, 1994.

Kennedy, David M. *Birth Control in America: The Career of Margaret Sanger*. New Haven: Yale University Press, 1970.

Kerber, Linda K. "A Constitutional Right to Be Treated Like American Ladies: Women and the Obligations of Citizenship." In *U.S. History as Women's History: New Feminist Essays*, edited by Linda K. Kerber, Alice Kessler-Harris, and Kathryn Kish Sklar, 17–35. Chapel Hill: University of North Carolina Press, 1995.

———. "Separate Spheres, Female Worlds, Women's Place: The Rhetoric of Women's History." *Journal of American History* 75 (June 1988): 9–39.

Kerber, Linda K., Alice Kessler-Harris, and Kathryn Kish Sklar, eds. *U.S. History as Women's History: New Feminist Essays*. Chapel Hill: University of North Carolina Press, 1995.

Kessler-Harris, Alice. *Out to Work: A History of Wage-Earning Women in the United States*. New York: Oxford University Press, 1982.

King, Charles R. "The New York Maternal Mortality Study: A Conflict of Professionalization." *Bulletin of the History of Medicine* 65 (winter 1991): 476–502.

Kleinberg, Susan. "Technology and Women's Work: The Lives of Working-Class Women in Pittsburgh, 1870–1900." *Labor History* 17 (winter 1976): 58–72.

Kluger, Richard. *Simple Justice: The History of Brown v. Board of Education and Black America's Struggle for Equality*. New York: Knopf, 1976.

Kobrin, Frances E. "The American Midwife Controversy: A Crisis of Professionalization." *Bulletin of the History of Medicine* 40 (1966). Reprint, in *Women and Health in America: Historical Readings*, edited by Judith Walzer Leavitt, 318–326. Madison: University of Wisconsin Press, 1984.

Konold, Donald E. *A History of American Medical Ethics*. Madison: State Historical Society for the Department of History, University of Wisconsin, 1962.

Kunzel, Regina G. *Fallen Women, Problem Girls: Unmarried Mothers and the Professionalization of Social Work, 1890–1945*. New Haven: Yale University Press, 1993.

———. "White Neurosis, Black Pathology: Constructing Out-of-Wedlock Pregnancy in the Wartime and Postwar United States." In *Not June Cleaver: Women and Gender in Postwar America, 1945–1960*, 304–331, edited by Joanne Meyerowitz. Philadelphia: Temple University Press, 1994.

Ladd-Taylor, Molly. "'Grannies' and 'Spinsters': Midwife Education under the Sheppard-Towner Act." *Journal of Social History* 22 (1988): 255–275.

————. *Mother-Work: Women, Child Welfare, and the State, 1890–1930.* Urbana: University of Illinois Press, 1994.

Lane, Roger. *Policing the City: Boston 1822–1885.* Cambridge, Mass.: Harvard University Press, 1967.

————. *Violent Death in the City: Suicide, Accident, and Murder in Nineteenth-Century Philadelphia.* Cambridge, Mass.: Harvard University Press, 1979.

Leavitt, Judith Walzer. *Brought to Bed: Childbearing in America, 1750–1950.* New York: Oxford University Press, 1986.

————. "The Growth of Medical Authority, Technology, and Morals in Turn-of-the-Century Obstetrics." *Medical Anthropology Quarterly* 1 (September 1987): 230–255.

————. *The Healthiest City: Milwaukee and the Politics of Health Reform.* Princeton, N.J.: Princeton University Press, 1982.

————. "'A Worrying Profession': The Domestic Environment of Medical Practice in Mid-Nineteenth-Century America." *Bulletin of the History of Medicine* 69 (spring 1995): 1–29.

————, ed. *Women and Health in America: Historical Readings.* Madison: University of Wisconsin Press, 1984.

Leavitt, Judith Walzer, and Ronald L. Numbers, eds. *Sickness and Health in America: Readings in the History of Medicine and Public Health.* 2d ed. Madison: University of Wisconsin Press, 1986.

Lemons, J. Stanley. *The Woman Citizen: Social Feminism in the 1920s.* Urbana: University of Illinois Press, 1973.

Lerner, Gerda. *The Grimké Sisters from South Carolina: Rebels against Slavery.* Boston: Houghton Mifflin, 1967.

————, ed. *Black Women in White America: A Documentary History.* New York: Random House, 1972.

————, ed. *The Female Experience: An American Documentary.* Indianapolis: Bobbs-Merrill Educational Publishing, 1977.

Lewis, Jane. *The Politics of Motherhood: Child and Maternal Welfare in England, 1900–1939.* London: Croom Helm, 1980.

Litoff, Judy Barrett. *The American Midwife Debate: A Sourcebook on Its Modern Origins.* New York: Greenwood Press, 1986.

————. *American Midwives: 1860 to the Present.* Westport, Conn.: Greenwood Press, 1978.

————. "Midwives and History." In *Women, Health, and Medicine in America: A Historical Handbook,* edited by Rima D. Apple, 443–458. New York: Garland Publishing, 1990.

Lockwood, Elizabeth Karsen. "The Fallen Woman, the Maternity Home, and the State: A Study of Maternal Health Care for Single Parturients, 1870–1930." Master's thesis, University of Wisconsin, Madison, 1987.

Loudon, Irvine. "Maternal Mortality: 1880–1950. Some Regional and International Comparisons." *Social History of Medicine* 1 (August 1988): 183–228.

Luker, Kristin. *Abortion and the Politics of Motherhood.* Berkeley: University of California Press, 1984.

MacKinnon, Catharine. "The Male Ideology of Privacy: A Feminist Perspective on the Right to Abortion." *Radical America* 17 (July–August 1983): 23–35.

Matthaei, Julie A. *An Economic History of Women in America: Women's Work, the Sexual Division of Labor, and the Development of Capitalism.* New York: Schocken Books, 1982.

May, Elaine Tyler. *Homeward Bound: American Families in the Cold War Era.* New York: Basic Books, 1988.

Mayer, Harold M., and Richard C. Wade, with the assistance of Glen E. Holt. *Chicago: Growth of a Metropolis.* Chicago: University of Chicago Press, 1969.

McCann, Carole R. *Birth Control Politics in the United States, 1916–1945.* Ithaca: Cornell University Press, 1994.

McCorvey, Norma, with Andy Meisler. *I Am Roe: My Life, Roe v. Wade, and Freedom of Choice.* New York: Harper Collins, 1994.

McLaren, Angus. "Birth Control and Abortion in Canada, 1870–1920." *Canadian Historical Review* 59:3 (1978): 319–340.

———. *Reproductive Rituals: The Perception of Fertility in England from the Sixteenth Century to the Nineteenth Century.* London: Methuen, 1984.

McNeil, Genna Rae. "Charles Hamilton Houston: Social Engineer for Civil Rights." In *Black Leaders of the Twentieth Century,* edited by John Hope Franklin and August Meier, 221–232. Urbana: University of Illinois Press, 1982.

Melosh, Barbara. *"The Physician's Hand": Work, Culture, and Conflict in American Nursing.* Philadelphia: Temple University Press, 1982.

Messer, Ellen, and Kathryn E. May. *Back Rooms: Voices from the Illegal Abortion Era.* New York: St. Martin's Press, 1988.

Meyerowitz, Joanne J. "Sexual Geography and Gender Economy: The Furnished Room Districts of Chicago, 1890–1930." *Gender and History* 2 (autumn 1990): 274–296.

———. *Women Adrift: Independent Wage Earners in Chicago, 1880–1930.* Chicago: University of Chicago Press, 1988.

Meyerowitz, Joanne, ed. *Not June Cleaver: Women and Gender in Postwar America, 1945–1960.* Philadelphia: Temple University Press, 1994.

Milkman, Ruth. "Women's Work and the Economic Crisis: Some Lessons from the Great Depression." *The Review of Radical Political Economics* 8 (spring 1976): 73–91, 95–97. Reprint, in *A Heritage of Her Own: Toward a New Social History of American Women,* edited by Nancy F. Cott and Elizabeth H. Pleck, 507–541. New York: Simon and Schuster, 1979.

Miller, Patricia. *The Worst of Times.* New York: Harper Collins, 1993.

Mills, Samuel A. "Abortion and Religious Freedom: The Religious Coalition for Abortion Rights (RCAR) and the Pro-Choice Movement, 1973–1989." *Journal of Church and State* 3 (summer 1991): 569–594.

Mohr, James C. *Abortion in America: The Origins and Evolution of National Policy, 1800–1900.* New York: Oxford University Press, 1978.

———. *Doctors and the Law: Medical Jurisprudence in Nineteenth-Century America.* New York: Oxford University Press, 1993.

———. "Patterns of Abortion and the Response of American Physicians, 1790–1930." In *Women and Health in America: Historical Readings,* edited by Judith Walzer Leavitt, 117–123. Madison: University of Wisconsin Press, 1984.

Monkkonen, Eric H. *The Dangerous Class: Crime and Poverty in Columbus, Ohio, 1860–1885*. Cambridge, Mass.: Harvard University Press, 1975.

———. *Police in Urban America, 1860–1920*. New York: Cambridge University Press, 1981.

Morantz, Regina. "The Lady and Her Physician." In *Clio's Consciousness Raised: New Perspectives on the History of Women*, edited by Mary S. Hartman and Lois Banner, 38–53. New York: Harper and Row, 1974.

Morantz-Sanchez, Regina. *Sympathy and Science: Women Physicians in American Medicine*. New York: Oxford University Press, 1985.

Mott, Frank Luther. *American Journalism: A History of Newspapers in the United States Through 250 Years, 1690–1940*. New York: Macmillan, 1941.

Muncy, Robyn L., *Creating a Female Dominion in American Reform, 1890–1935*. New York: Oxford University Press, 1990.

Noonan, John T., Jr., "An Almost Absolute Value in History." In *The Morality of Abortion: Legal and Historical Perspectives*, edited by John T. Noonan Jr., 1–59. Cambridge, Mass.: Harvard University Press, 1970.

Numbers, Ronald L. *Almost Persuaded: American Physicians and Compulsory Health Insurance, 1912–1920*. Baltimore: Johns Hopkins Press, 1978.

———. "The Fall and Rise of the American Medical Profession." In *Sickness and Health in America: Readings in the History of Medicine and Public Health*, 2d ed., rev., edited by Judith Walzer Leavitt and Ronald L. Numbers, 185–205. Madison: University of Wisconsin Press, 1985.

———. "A Note on Medical Education in Wisconsin." In *Wisconsin Medicine: Historical Perspectives*, edited by Ronald L. Numbers and Judith Walzer Leavitt, 177–184. Madison: University of Wisconsin Press, 1981.

———. "The Third Party: Health Insurance in America." In *Sickness and Health in America: Readings in the History of Medicine and Public Health*, edited by Judith Walzer Leavitt and Ronald L. Numbers, 139–153. Madison: University of Wisconsin Press, 1978.

Numbers, Ronald L., and Darrel W. Amundsen, eds. *Caring and Curing: Health and Medicine in the Western Religious Traditions*. New York: Macmillan, 1986.

O'Brien, Mary. *The Politics of Reproduction*. Boston: Routledge and Kegan Paul, 1981.

Odem, Mary E. *Delinquent Daughters: Protecting and Policing Adolescent Female Sexuality in the United States, 1885–1920*. Chapel Hill: University of North Carolina Press, 1995.

Peiss, Kathy. *Cheap Amusements: Working Women and Leisure in Turn-of-the-Century New York*. Philadelphia: Temple University Press, 1986.

Peiss, Kathy, and Christina Simmons, eds., with Robert A. Padgug. *Passion and Power: Sexuality in History*. Philadelphia: Temple University Press, 1989.

Pernick, Martin S. *A Calculus of Suffering: Pain, Professionalism, and Anesthesia in Nineteenth-Century America*. New York: Columbia University Press, 1985.

Petchesky, Rosalind Pollack. *Abortion and Woman's Choice: The State, Sexuality, and Reproductive Freedom.* New York: Longman, 1984. Rev. ed., Boston: Northeastern University Press, 1990.

———. "Abortion as 'Violence against Women': A Feminist Critique." *Radical America* 18 (March–June 1984): 64–68.

———. "Fetal Images: The Power of Visual Culture in the Politics of Reproduction." *Feminist Studies* 13 (summer 1987): 263–292.

Pierce, Bessie Louise. *The Rise of a Modern City, 1971–1893.* Vol. 3 of *A History of Chicago.* New York: Knopf, 1957.

Piven, Frances Fox, and Richard A. Cloward. *Poor People's Movements: Why They Succeed, How They Fail.* New York: Random House, 1977.

Poovey, Mary. *Uneven Developments: The Ideological Work of Gender in Mid-Victorian England.* Chicago: University of Chicago Press, 1988.

Porter, Roy, ed. *Patients and Practitioners.* Cambridge: Cambridge University Press, 1985.

Przybyszewski, Linda. "The Right to Privacy: A Historical Perspective." In *Abortion, Medicine, and the Law,* 4th ed., edited by J. Douglas Butler and David F. Walbert, 667–692. New York: Facts on File, 1992.

Reed, James. "Doctors, Birth Control, and Social Values, 1830–1970." In *Women and Health in America: Historical Readings,* edited by Judith Walzer Leavitt, 124–139. Madison: University of Wisconsin Press, 1984.

———. *From Private Vice to Public Virtue: The Birth Control Movement and American Society Since 1830.* New York: Basic Books, 1978.

Reverby, Susan. *Ordered to Care: The Dilemma of American Nursing, 1850–1945.* Cambridge: Cambridge University Press, 1987.

Rich, Adrienne. *Of Woman Born: Motherhood as Experience and Institution.* New York: W. W. Norton, 1976.

———. *On Lies, Secrets, and Silence: Selected Prose, 1966–1978.* New York: W. W. Norton, 1979.

Riley, Denise. *"Am I That Name?" Feminism and the Category of "Women" in History.* Minneapolis: University of Minnesota, 1988.

Rodrique, Jessie M. "The Black Community and the Birth Control Movement." In *Passion and Power: Sexuality in History,* edited by Kathy Peiss and Christina Simmons, with Robert A. Padgug, 138–154. Philadelphia: Temple University Press, 1989.

Rosen, George. *The Structure of American Medical Practice, 1875–1941.* Edited by Charles E. Rosenberg. Philadelphia: University of Pennsylvania Press, 1983.

Rosen, Ruth. *The Lost Sisterhood: Prostitution in America, 1900–1918.* Baltimore: Johns Hopkins University Press, 1982.

Rosenberg, Charles E. *The Care of Strangers: The Rise of America's Hospital System.* New York: Basic Books, 1987.

———. *The Cholera Years: The United States in 1832, 1849, and 1866.* Chicago: University of Chicago Press, 1962.

———. "The Therapeutic Revolution: Medicine, Meaning, and Social Change in Nineteenth-Century America." In *The Therapeutic Revolution: Essays in the Social History of American Medicine,* edited by Morris J. Vogel and

Charles E. Rosenberg, 3–26. Philadelphia: Temple University Press, 1970.
———. *The Trial of the Assassin Guiteau: Psychiatry and Law in the Gilded Age.* Chicago: University of Chicago Press, 1968.
Ross, Ellen. *Love and Toil: Motherhood in Outcast London, 1870–1918.* New York: Oxford University Press, 1993.
Ross, Loretta J. "African-American Women and Abortion: 1800–1970." In *Theorizing Black Feminisms: The Visionary Pragmatism of Black Women,* edited by Stanlie M. James and Abena P. A. Busia, 141–159. London: Routledge, 1993.
Rothman, Barbara Katz. *Recreating Motherhood: Ideology and Technology in a Patriarchal Society.* New York: W. W. Norton, 1989.
———. *The Tentative Pregnancy: Prenatal Diagnosis and the Future of Motherhood.* New York: Viking Penguin, 1986.
Rothman, David J. *The Discovery of the Asylum: Social Order and Disorder in the New Republic.* Boston: Little, Brown and Co., 1971.
Rothstein, William G. *American Physicians in the Nineteenth Century: From Sects to Science.* Baltimore: Johns Hopkins University Press, 1972.
Rowbotham, Sheila. *"A New World for Women": Stella Browne—Socialist Feminist.* London: Pluto Press, 1977.
Rubin, Eva R. *Abortion, Politics, and the Courts.* Rev. ed. New York: Greenwood Press, 1987.
Ryan, Mary P. *Womanhood in America: From Colonial Times to the Present.* 2d ed. New York: New Viewpoints, 1979.
———. *Women in Public: Between Banners and Ballots, 1825–1880.* Baltimore: Johns Hopkins University Press, 1990.
Salmon, Marylynne. *Women and the Law of Property in Early America.* Chapel Hill: University of North Carolina Press, 1986.
Schrecker, Ellen. *The Age of McCarthyism: A Brief History with Documents.* Boston: Bedford Books of St. Martin's Press, 1994.
———. "The Bride of Stalin: Gender and Anticommunism during the McCarthy Era." Paper delivered to the Berkshire Conference on Women's History, Vassar College, June 11, 1993.
Schudson, Michael. *Discovering the News: A Social History of American Newspapers.* New York: Basic Books, 1978.
Scott, Joan Walloch. *Gender and the Politics of History.* New York: Columbia University Press, 1988.
Shorter, Edward. *The History of Women's Bodies.* New York: Basic Books, 1982.
Shryock, Richard Harrison. *Medical Licensing in America, 1650–1965.* Baltimore: Johns Hopkins University Press, 1967.
———. *Medicine and Society in America: 1660–1860.* Ithaca: Cornell University Press, 1960.
Silverman, Robert A. *Law and Urban Growth: Civil Litigation in the Boston Trial Courts, 1880–1900.* Princeton: Princeton University Press, 1981.
Simon, Kate. *Bronx Primitive: Portraits in a Childhood.* New York: Harper and Row, 1982.
Smith, Daniel Scott. "Family Limitation, Sexual Control, and Domestic Feminism in Victorian America." *Feminist Studies* 1 (winter–spring 1973): 40–57.
Smith, Susan L. *Sick and Tired of Being Sick and Tired: Black Women's Health*

Activism in America, 1890–1950. Philadelphia: University of Pennsylvania Press, 1995.

Smith-Rosenberg, Carroll. "Beauty, the Beast, and the Militant Woman: A Case Study in Sex Roles and Social Stress in Jacksonian America." *American Quarterly* 23 (1971): 562–584.

———. *Disorderly Conduct: Visions of Gender in Victorian America*. New York: Oxford University Press, 1985.

———. "Female World of Love and Ritual: Relations Between Women in Nineteenth-Century America." *Signs* 1 (1975): 1–29.

Snitow, Ann, Christine Stansell, and Sharon Thompson, eds. *Powers of Desire: The Politics of Sexuality*. New York: Monthly Review Press, 1983.

Solinger, Rickie. *The Abortionist: A Woman Against the Law*. New York: Free Press, 1994.

———. "'A Complete Disaster': Abortion and the Politics of Hospital Abortion Committees, 1950–1970." *Feminist Studies* 19 (summer 1993): 241–259.

———. *Wake Up Little Susie: Single Pregnancy and Race before Roe v. Wade*. New York: Routledge, 1992.

Spear, Allan H. *Black Chicago: The Making of a Negro Ghetto, 1880–1920*. Chicago: University of Chicago Press, 1967.

Speert, Harold. *Obstetrics and Gynecology in America: A History*. Chicago: American College of Obstetricians and Gynecologists, 1980.

Spruill, Julia Cherry. *Women's Life and Work in the Southern Colonies*. Chapel Hill: University of North Carolina Press, 1938. Reprint, New York: W. W. Norton, 1972.

Starr, Paul. *The Social Transformation of Medicine*. New York: Basic Books, 1982.

Stevens, Rosemary. *American Medicine and the Public Interest*. New Haven: Yale University Press, 1971.

———. *In Sickness and in Wealth: American Hospitals in the Twentieth Century*. New York: Basic Books, 1989.

Stowe, Steven M. "Obstetrics and the Work of Doctoring in the Mid-Nineteenth-Century American South." *Bulletin of the History of Medicine* 64 (1990): 540–566.

Susie, Debra Anne. *In the Way of Our Grandmothers: A Cultural View of Twentieth-Century Midwifery in Florida*. Athens: University of Georgia Press, 1988.

Taylor, William R. *Inventing Times Square: Commerce and Culture at the Crossroads of the World*. New York: Russell Sage Foundation, 1991.

Tushnet, Mark V. *Making Civil Rights Law: Thurgood Marshall and the Supreme Court, 1936–1961*. New York: Oxford University Press, 1994.

Ulrich, Laurel Thatcher. *A Midwife's Tale: The Life of Martha Ballard, Based on Her Diary, 1785–1812*. New York: Knopf, 1990.

Vance, Carole S., ed. *Pleasure and Danger: Exploring Female Sexuality*. Boston: Routledge and Kegan Paul, 1984.

Vicinus, Martha. "Sexuality and Power: A Review of Current Work in the History of Sexuality." *Feminist Studies* 8 (spring 1982): 133–156.

Vogel, Morris J. *The Invention of the Modern Hospital: Boston, 1870–1930*. Chicago: University of Chicago Press, 1980.

————. "The Rise and Fall of Homes for Unwed Mothers." Paper presented at the Columbia University Seminar on American Civilization, New York, March 18, 1982.

Vogel, Morris J., and Charles E. Rosenberg, eds. *The Therapeutic Revolution: Essays in the Social History of American Medicine*. Philadelphia: University of Pennsylvania Press, 1979.

Walkowitz, Judith R. *City of Dreadful Delight: Narratives of Sexual Danger in Late-Victorian London*. Chicago: University of Chicago Press, 1992.

————. "Dangerous Sexualities." In *A History of Women in the West: Emerging Feminism from Revolution to World War,* vol. 4, edited by Genevieve Fraisse and Michelle Perrot, 369–398. Cambridge, Mass.: Harvard University Press, 1993.

————. *Prostitution and Victorian Society: Women, Class, and the State*. New York: Cambridge University Press, 1980.

Walsh, Justin E. *To Print the News and Raise Hell! A Biography of Wilbur F. Storey*. Chapel Hill: University of North Carolina Press, 1968.

Walsh, Mary Roth. *"Doctors Wanted: No Women Need Apply": Sexual Barriers in the Medical Profession, 1835–1975*. New Haven: Yale University Press, 1977.

Weddington, Sarah. *A Question of Choice*. New York: G. P. Putnam's Sons, 1992.

Weisberg, D. Kelly. *Property, Family and the Legal Profession*. Vol. 2 of *Women and the Law: A Social Historical Perspective*. Cambridge, Mass.: Schenkman Publishing, 1982.

————. *Women and the Criminal Law*. Vol. 1 of *Women and the Law: A Social Historical Perspective*. Cambridge, Mass.: Schenkman Publishing, 1982.

Wells, Robert V. "Family History and Demographic Transition." *Journal of Social History* 9 (fall 1975): 1–9.

Welter, Barbara. "The Cult of True Womanhood, 1820–1860." *American Quarterly* 18 (summer 1966): 151–174.

Wertz, Richard W., and Dorothy C. Wertz. *Lying-In: A History of Childbirth in America*. New York: Schocken Books, 1979.

Wheeler, Stanton, et al. "Do the 'Haves' Come out Ahead? Winning and Losing in State Supreme Courts, 1870–1970." *Law and Society Review* 21:3 (1987): 403–445.

White, Evelyn C. *The Black Women's Health Book: Speaking for Ourselves*. Seattle, Wash.: Seal Press, 1990.

Wiebe, Robert. *The Search for Order, 1877–1920*. New York: Hill and Wang, 1967.

Williams, Glanville. *The Sanctity of Life and the Criminal Law*. New York: Knopf, 1957.

Wood, Ann Douglas. "'The Fashionable Diseases': Women's Complaints and Their Treatment in Nineteenth-Century America." In *Clio's Consciousness Raised: New Perspectives on the History of Women,* edited by Mary S. Hartman and Lois Banner, 1–22. New York: Harper and Row, 1974.

Wornie, L. Reed, et al. *Health and Medical Care of African-Americans*. Westport, Conn.: Auburn House, 1993.

Yellin, Jean Fagan. *Women and Sisters: The Anti-Slavery Feminists in American Culture*. New Haven: Yale University Press, 1989.

Index

Abbott, Grace, 100–101, 107, 292n79; on immigrants, 303n64; and Sheppard-Towner Act, 110

Abortifacients, 274n106, 274n111; availability of, 9–10, 14; commercial, 43–44; dangers of, 42, 43; government regulation of, 10; herbal, 9, 43, 44; of midwives, 75; paste, 156–57, 314n118; popular knowledge of, 26; use by African American women, 43; use by midwives, 75; use by physician-abortionists, 72

Abortion: advertisements for, 70, 88–89, 225, 262n13, 280n74; availability of, 60–61, 70, 76, 193, 246, 251–52, 339n2; backlashes against, 15, 163, 190, 248, 252; as birth control, 20, 141; case studies of, 17, 268n15, 325n15; censorship of, 140, 172, 309n45, 319n62; in Chicago, 46–59, 71–78, 97–98, 106, 246, 266n3, 339n2; Christian tradition on, 7; in colonial era, 8–9, 42; under common law, 8, 14, 263n32; complications following, 138, 307n27; of defective fetus, 203, 204, 327n38; definition of legality in, 5, 61, 182; on demand, 234, 254; demographics of, 23, 242, *fig. 3, fig. 6;* dissemination of knowledge about, 70; in early nineteenth century, 10, 263n32; in early twentieth century, 14–15, 22; effect of criminalization on, 2; for eugenic reasons, 64, 203–4, 279n59; family support for, 27; female discourse on, 21, 23–24, 44, 229–30;

feminist critique of, 226; feminist networks for, 223, 224, 233, 242; in fiction, 141, 309n45; financial responsibility for, 31; of first pregnancies, 135; frequency of, 23, 134–36, 265n49, 284n110; home remedies for, 43, 44, 209, 274n106; as human right, 254; as infanticide, 13, 85, 248; insurance for, 134, 251, 340n20; location of, 68, 74, 75, 199, 282n83; marriage following, 303n58; media coverage of, 7, 216; medical discourse on, 7–8, 24–25, 61–63, 67, 164; methods of, 72–73, 157, 263n26; motives for, 32–33; parental consent in, 249, 252, 253, 341n25; patient records in, 148–49, 161–62; physicians' fees for, 47, 76, 96, 154, 197, 282n86; physicians' support for, 1, 132, 139, 181, 220; politicization of, 250; popular support for, 6–7, 21–22, 44–45, 81, 116; in postwar era, 164, 190–94, 214–19, 317n22; private policing of, 250, 340n14; public debate on, 104–9, 139–40, 217; public education on, 36; safety of, 76–79, 148, 157, 193, 214, 246–47, 329n62 (*see also* Maternal mortality; Septic infection); as social need, 185, 204; "speak-outs" on, 229–30, 333n40; spontaneous, 284n110, 293n86; standard medical procedures in, 151, 312n88; state surveillance of, 163, 173, 249; trimester system in, 239–40, 244, 252; Victorian view of, 292n78; waiting periods for, 252,

Abortion (*continued*)
341n25; women's demand for, 1, 147,
159, 249, 254, 290n54
Abortion, fatal, 76–79; among African
Americans, 211–12, 222, 232; categories of, 284n110, 293n86; frequency
of, 139, 265n49; as impetus for reform,
222; investigation of, 114, 118; media
coverage of, 102, 114–15; in New York
City, *fig. 5, fig. 6;* peritonitis in, 35,
300n24; in postwar era, 211–12, *fig. 5;*
reductions in, 162; self-induced, 43,
102, 117, 147, 274n111, 293n86, 299n19;
vital statistics in, 329n59. *See also* Dying declarations; Inquests, coroners';
Maternal mortality
Abortion, illegal: arrests for, 109, 116, 117,
120, 129, 164, 298n8; convictions for,
55, 70–71, 118, 291n62, 301n33; court
records on, 255; in exchange for sex,
199; imitation of miscarriage, 72; secrecy in, 21, 45, 48, 151, 193, 196–98;
"underground railroad" for, 233, 242.
See also Abortion clinics; Abortionists; Midwives; Physician-Abortionists
Abortion, instrumental, 42, 43, 72; in
early nineteenth century, 10; by midwives, 75; by physicians, 76, 78–79,
282n89
Abortion, legal, 259n1; in Alaska and
Hawaii, 241; benefits of, 246; under
common law, 8; definition of, 182;
demographics of, 242, 339n7; effect
on maternal mortality, 339n4; effect
on public health, 246–47; equal access to, 244–45, 249, 338n111; following *Doe v. Scott,* 241; in New York,
225, 241–42, 247; opposition to, 248–
54; for poor women, 236, 246; popular support for, 252–53; restrictions
on, 251; safety of, 285n116; social movement for, 140–41; support of black
women for, 342n34; for unmarried
women, 221. *See also* Abortion rights
movement; Therapeutic abortion
Abortion, self-induced, 27, 42–44, 78,
132, 137–38, 281n78; dangers of,
76–77, 209–11; fatalities in, 43, 102,
117, 147, 274n111, 293n86, 299n19;
home remedies for, 43, 44, 209,
274n106; by married women, 312n89;
by poor women, 119, 137–38; in
postwar era, 208–9; by unmarried

women, 312n89; women's knowledge
of, 26–27. *See also* Abortifacients
Abortion, therapeutic. *See* Therapeutic
abortion
Abortion clinics, 10; in Baltimore, 158;
bombing of, 248; of Depression era,
133, 149–67; fees of, 150, 157; feminist,
224–26; harassment at, 253; raids on,
160–61, 164, 167, 181, 243, 316n16,
316n19, 318n41; referrals to, 151, 153,
158, 232–33, 241, 242; following *Roe v.
Wade,* 246. *See also* Gabler-Martin
abortion clinic; "Jane"; Keemer,
Dr. Edgar Bass; Timanus, Dr. George
Loutrell
Abortionists: access to antibiotics, 210;
arrest of, 126, 164, 169; black women's
use of, 326n18; of Chicago, 47, 281n76,
313n113; in *Chicago Times* exposé,
69–70; conviction of, 55, 70–71, 118;
cover-ups by, 130, 304n69; in early
nineteenth century, 10; fatality rates
of, 77; feminists' regulation of, 224;
foreign, 224; kickbacks to physicians,
67; media coverage of, 125; nonphysician, 310n70; of postwar era, 197;
prosecution of, 87–90, 113–31, 298n7,
317n29; raids on, 164, 249; under *Roe
v. Wade,* 252; sexual harassment by,
199, 200, 225; skill of, 78–79; trials of,
107, 153, 154, 155, 160, 169–70; un-
qualified, 199–200, 209. *See also* Midwives; Physician-abortionists
Abortion law: changing patterns in,
14–18; class action suits in, 235; constitutional challenges to, 218, 234–40,
317n33; discrimination in, 244–45; ecumenical resistance to, 241; effect on
abortion safety, 116; enforcement by
state, 1, 81, 107, 114–31, 299n17; exceptions to, 5; of Illinois, 61, 107,
235–40, 261n13, 265n45; implementation of, 3; legal challenges to, 181–92;
model, 143, 220–21, 222; nongovernmental enforcement of, 3, 81–82;
physicians' challenges to, 15; political
resistance to, 241; public policy on,
112; repeal of, 5, 223–24, 233; of states,
64, 252, 261n13, 265n45; test cases in,
181, 189, 190, 191, 237, 335n67, 336n70;
unconstitutionality of, 244; vagueness
of, 61, 148, 238, 241. See also *Doe v.
Scott; Roe v. Wade*

Abortion law reform, 140, 141–42, 216, 217, 219–20; in England, 189–90; feminists on, 331n21; Taussig's proposals for, 142–44. *See also* Abortion rights movement

Abortion Law Reform Association (ALRA), 140, 220

Abortion patients: arrest of, 165, 171, 243, 319n55; blackmail of physicians, 123; blindfolding of, 198, 200, 243; civil rights of, 226; complications of, 138, 307n27; counseling for, 252; delays in seeking treatment, 119, 299n19; follow-up care for, 71, 120–21, 154, 157–58; of Gabler-Martin clinic, 151–52, 310n71; in hospitals, 138–39; interrogation of, 114–15, 118, 126–29, 131, 161, 168, 191–92, 249, 296n1; midwives' identification with, 73–74; physical examination of, 168, 169; police custody of, 47, 168–69, 249; prosecution of, 340n15; as prostitutes, 199; public identification of, 115, 124–26, 167–68, 192; sexual harassment of, 199, 200, 225; sexual histories of, 200; testimony in abortion raid cases, 164–66, 168, 170–71; before therapeutic abortion committees, 321n79; in Timanus trial, 183–87; women's support of, 27, 29–31. *See also* Dying declarations; Inquests, coroners'

Abortion rights movement, 15, 216; African American women in, 253; feminists in, 222–34; groups comprising, 243–44; nonelites in, 223; organizations in, 232–33; professionals' role in, 217, 218–22, 223, 233, 239, 244; psychiatrists in, 218, 223; religious opposition to, 221; right to choose in, 232; students in, 225, 233; white women in, 228. *See also* Abortion, legal; Abortion law reform; Reproductive rights

Abstinence, 36, 38

Academy of Medicine (New York), 139, 140

Adams, Anne, 184–86, 188

Addams, Jane, 95

Adoption, 52–53, 195, 199

Advertising, of abortion, 70, 262n13; in prosecution of abortion, 100, 280n74; suppression of, 88–89

Affiliated Hospitals of the State University of New York at Buffalo, 202

African Americans: in Chicago, 17, 282n93, 300n21; illegitimacy among, 136, 137; nationalist, 231, 232, 334n50; physicians, 82–83, 120, 156, 286n10; population control programs for, 231, 232; support for birth control, 231, 232. *See also* Women, African American

Age: as factor in abortion, 307n23, 312n96; of Gabler-Martin patients, 152; of present-day abortion patients, 152

Aid to Families with Dependent Children (AFDC), 249, 340n13

Aiken, Dr. John W., 69, 280n72

Akron, Ohio, 164

Alaska, 241

Alcohol abuse, 59, 250

Alexander, Susan. *See* Grossman, Susan

American Birth Control League, 132, 133

American Civil Liberties Union, 235, 237, 240

American Law Institute (ALI), 220, 222; model law proposal, 221, 233, 234, 239

American Medical Association: abortionists in, 55, 72; in antiabortion campaigns, 57, 80, 82–83, 89; in birth control movement, 134; Bureau of Investigation, 89; in *Chicago Times* exposé, 60–61; cooperation with state, 4, 89; headquarters of, 57; Historical Health Fraud Collection (HHFC), 255, 256; obstetricians in, 90; opposition to abortion, 10; Section on Obstetrics and Gynecology, 82, 264n6. See also *Journal of the American Medical Association*

American Public Health Association, 234

Amniocentesis, 204

Andrews, J. L., 274n106

Antiabortion campaigns, 11–14, 286n8; activists in, 11, 340n14; antifeminism of, 11, 76; cultural aspects of, 80–81, 85; end of, 111–12; at local level, 81; physicians in, 81, 89–90; as purity campaigns, 85; quickening in, 83, 85; rape in, 340n19; after *Roe v. Wade,* 248–52; against single women, 249; specialists in, 15; strategy of, 81; targeting of women, 81, 83–85; and women's movements, 14

Antibiotics, 162, 210, 246

Anticommunism, 315n12; post–World War I red scare, 142; and repression of abortion, 163–64, 172–73, 180, 181, 319n60

Anti-midwife antiabortion campaign, 90–109; Johnson case in, 101–2, 105, 106, 107–8, 126; physicians in, 290n53; private interest groups in, 91. *See also* Midwives

Anti-Semitism, 320n65

Antiseptic technique, 27, 79, 246, 269n28; in control of maternal mortality, 339n5

Arizona, 336n70

Arkansas, 241; abortion reform in, 331n15

Aseptic technique, 79, 339n5

Ashland Boulevard Hospital (Chicago), 72

Asians: as abortion patients, 207; hostility toward, 11

Association to Repeal Abortion Laws (ARAL), 332n23

Attorneys: Catholic, 221; challenges to abortion law, 218, 234–38, 244, 245, 335n67; courtroom tactics of, 182, 322nn87,88; defense of poor women, 336n72

Auerbach, Dr. Julius, 124

Austria, legalized abortion in, 140

Autonomy: female, 190, 215, 253; of patients, 247; of physicians, 15

Baby farms, 298n8

"Back-alley butchers," 133, 304n4

Bacon, Dr. Charles Sumner, 23, 82, 90, 267n9; on midwives, 94, 95, 96; and Sheppard-Towner Act, 111

Baker, Dr. S. Josephine, 295n112

Ballard, Martha, 31

Baltimore: abortion clinics in, 158; midwives of, 281n81. *See also* Johns Hopkins University; Timanus, Dr. George Loutrell

Bar associations, in abortion rights movement, 222

Barrett, James R., 292n76

Bastardy. *See* Illegitimacy

Bellevue Hospital (New York), 136

Belous, Dr. Leon, 233, 235, 236, 337n81

Benn, Wilhelmina, 73, 74

Bérubé, Michael, 204

Bill of Rights, 166, 317n33

Birth control, 26, 41, 42, 196; abortion as, 36–37, 141; availability of, 117, 134, 196, 229; class as factor in, 40–41; economic reasons for, 35–36; effectiveness of, 229; as genocide, 232; insurance for, 341n20; legalization of, 134, 323n111; physicians' dispensing of,

134, 139, 296n115; popular support for, 111; public debate on, 6–7; racism in, 231; religious publications on, 262n17. *See also names of individual methods*

Birth control clinics, 111; of Chicago, 37; of Depression era, 306n19; opposition to, 296n115; working-class women in, 23

Birth control movement, 6–7, 220; AMA in, 134; criticism of medical profession, 111; English, 140, 142; on family size, 273n94; perspective on abortion, 36–42, 141, 142, 143, 272n76, 309n48; professionals in, 142; and "race suicide," 104; response of organized religion to, 6–7, 262n18; test cases in, 189, 323n111. *See also* Planned Parenthood

Birth Control Review, 37, 41. *See also* Sanger, Margaret

Birth rate: nineteenth-century, 11; rise in, 163

"Black genocide," 231, 232

Black Panther Party, 334n50

Blinn, Dr. Odelia, 57–58, 59

Blood transfusions, 162, 339n5

Bolter, Dr. Sidney, 203

Booth, Heather, 224, 332n26

Borst, Charlotte, 283n97

Boston, 10, 11, 333n35

Bourne, Dr. Aleck, 175, 176; challenge to abortion law, 182, 189–90, 220

Breastfeeding, mandatory, 28, 270n39

Brickman, Jane Pacht, 288n42, 295n111

Brookes, Barbara, 27

Brooks, Sara, 137–48

Brown, Elaine, 334n50

Brown v. Board of Education, 189

Brumberg, Joan Jacobs, 27, 297n3

Buettner, Dr. Adolph, 129

Calderone, Dr. Mary Steichen, 219

California: abortion reform in, 233, 331n15; maternal mortality rates in, 246; Supreme Court, 235. *See also* Los Angeles; San Francisco; Society for Humane Abortion

California Hospital (Los Angeles), 178

Carantzalis, Jennie, 74, 75–76

Carter, Dr. Patricia A., 179, 180

Catherwood, Dr. Albert E., 174

Catheters, 274n106, 274n111; sale of, 44; use by midwives, 75; use by physician-abortionists, 72

Catholic Church: censorship of abortion information, 319n62; on early abortion, 8; on ensoulment, 7; hospitals of, 321n84, 339n1; medical opposition to abortion views of, 62–63; opposition to birth control, 222, 330n13; pro-choice sentiment in, 233, 234, 341n28; on reproductive rights, 7, 180–81, 248; on therapeutic abortion, 62–63

Catholics: abortion rates of, 23, 137, 242, 306n22, 307n23; acceptance of abortion, 7; in ALI, 221–22; of Chicago, 50; hostility toward, and antiabortion campaign, 11; Jesuits, 63

Cattell, Dr. Henry W., 296n115

C. D. McCormick Library of Special Collections (Northwestern University), 256

Censorship, 140, 172, 233, 309n45, 319n62

Cesarean section, 66–67, 145; forced, 250

Chaffee, Dr. John B., 46–47, 48, 50, 51, 52

Chamberlain, Dr. George M., 53

Charity Hospital (New Orleans), 134

Chauncey, George, 316n14

Chicago: abortion clinics in, 149–55, 246; abortion hospitals in, 71–72; abortion in, 16–17, 46–59, 71–78, 266n3; anti-midwife antiabortion campaign in, 91, 92–101; Ashland Boulevard Hospital, 72; Bar Association, 222; birth control clinics in, 37; Board of Health, 88; City Health Department, 94; Clergy Consultation Service on Problem Pregnancies, 241; discourse on women in, 109; frequency of abortion in, 23; health-care system of, 48; as medical center, 57; Medico-Legal Society, 55; Michael Reese Hospital, 240; Michigan Boulevard Sanitarium, 72; newspapers of, 49; Public Library, 256; racial composition of population, 17, 282n93, 300n21; Visiting Nurse Association, 95; Woman's Aid, 105; Woman's City Club, 105; Women's Liberation Union, 225, 232, 339n2; women's organizations, 105–6, 107, 225, 232, 294n93, 339n2. *See also* Cook County coroner; Cook County Hospital; "Jane"; Midwives, of Chicago; Physicians, of Chicago

Chicago City Council, 295n107; in antiabortion debate, 106–7, 108–9; regulation of midwives, 98

Chicago Examiner, 109, 125

Chicago Herald, 106

Chicago Lying-In Hospital: self-induced abortion patients in, 209; therapeutic abortion in, 174, 208

Chicago Medical Society, 106, 107, 117; in *Chicago Times* exposé, 55, 56; Committee on Midwives, 95–97, 100, 101; Criminal Abortion Committee, 82, 83, 84, 88–90, 104; physician-abortionists in, 72; on therapeutic abortion, 62–63

Chicago Midwives' Association, 98

Chicago Times abortion exposé, 46–48, 49–61, 102, 274n2, *plates 1, 3, and 4;* abortionists in, 69–70, 86; American Medical Association in, 60–61; on availability of abortion, 70; defense of immigrants, 50; depiction of women, 58–59; effect on arrests, 298n8; letters to, 55, 277n32; midwives in, 52–53; physicians in, 54–57, 67, 276n29

Chicago Tribune: on abortion raid cases, 167; in antiabortion debate, 123; "Quack Department," 106

Chicago Vice Commission, 99; on midwives, 75, 292n77

Childbearing: of affluent women, 208; attendants during, 285n116; history of, 265n49; at home, 68; in hospitals, 275n5; as medical event, 94, 95; middle-class women's views on, 38, 40; mortality rates in, 39, 77, 162, 285n116; physicians' fees in, 312n101; planned, 230; postponement of, 194, 312n96; refusal of male physicians in, 73, 283n96; social pressure for, 163; state enforcement of, 340n13

Child rearing: responsibility for, 194–95; by unmarried mothers, 29

Children's Bureau, 77; maternal mortality study of, 138–39, 140, 307n31; on pernicious vomiting, 279n56

Chiropractors, abortions by, 304n7

Chisolm, Congresswoman Shirley, 232

Chlevinski, Hattie, 75

Cincinnati, 61, 134–35, 306n19

Cities: abortion in, 17, 60–61, 69; danger to women in, 125, 293n84; fears of, 92, 125; sex reform movements in, 92

Citizen's Committee for Humane Abortion Laws, 331n18. *See also* Society for Humane Abortion

Civil rights, 323n111; abortion as, 44; in abortion raid cases, 166; and legalized abortion, 247–48

Civil Rights Act, 237

Civil rights movement, 189; and abortion reform movements, 217, 224

Clark, Dr. James A., 107

Class: in Chicago, 50; and choice of abortionist, 76; in criminalization of abortion, 11, 13, 15; differences among women, 16, 267n6; as factor in abortion, 16, 58, 135–38, 152, 193, 205, 213–14, 240, 245, 251; in Kinsey study, 306n19; in maternal mortality, 211; and present-day antiabortion movement, 249

Clergy, Protestant: abortion referral services of, 232–33, 241, 242; in *Chicago Times* exposé, 50

Clergy Consultation Service on Problem Pregnancies (Chicago), 241

Cleveland, 207

Clothing, as marker of medical care, 151, 199, 226, *plate 3, plate 4*

Cochrane, Elizabeth, 49

College women, 194, 196–97, 324n2; in Kinsey study, 306n19, 306n21; in loco parentis rules for, 194, 195; therapeutic abortions for, 202

Colonial era: conception in, 8–9; midwife Martha Ballard, 31

Colorado, 116, 141, 331n15, 336n70

Commoner, Barry, 333n42

Common law: abortion under, 8, 14, 88, 263n22; dying declarations in, 118; quickening in, 13

Comstock law, 13; contraceptives in, 134; raids under, 298n8

Conception: as beginning of life, 110; in colonial era, 8–9; during Depression, 135. *See also* Quickening

Condoms, 41, 134, 196

Connecticut, 336n70

Consciousness-raising groups, 228

Contraception. *See* Birth control

Contracted pelvis, 66, 145, 278n55, 279n64

Cook County coroner: on dying declarations, 124; inquests into abortion, 22, 31, 45, 113–31, 256, 273n85, 293n86, 299n18, *fig. 1;* records of maternal mortality, 76, 78. *See also* Inquests, coroners'

Cook County Criminal Court, 298n7

Cook County Hospital: abortion patients in, 43, 209, 240, *fig. 4;* after *Doe v. Scott,* 240; legal abortion in, 246, 253; low-income patients in, 253; septic abortion ward of, 138, 239, 307n29

Cook County Medical Examiner's Office, 256

Coroners, corruption of, 300n20. *See also* Inquests, coroners'

Corruption, police, 155, 167, 300n20

Cosgrove, Dr. Samuel A., 179, 180

Courts: appeal of abortion convictions in, 301n34; control over family law, 297n3; history of, 261n11; juvenile, 303n67; lawyers in, 182; male atmosphere of, 161, 165; records of abortion, 17; reflection of popular morality, 6; scrutiny of police action, 299n17; testimony in, 182. *See also* Illinois Supreme Court; Inquests, coroners'; Juries; U.S. Supreme Court

Craniotomies, 66

Crime, organized: connection with abortion, 167, 318n40; FBI's investigation of, 318n39

Criminal abortion law. *See* Abortion law

Criminal trials, records of abortion in, 17

Crowell, F. Elisabeth, 99; report on midwives, 90, 291n62

Culbertson, Dr. Carey, 87

Curettes, 72, 282n89; *plate 2;* as treatment for miscarriage, 285n113; use by midwives, 75; use by physicians, 75, 78, 79. *See also* Dilation and curettage

Cushing, Dr. G. M., 124

Danforth, Dr. David N., 238, 239

Davis, Martha F., 336n72

D.C. General Hospital, 210

Death certificates, falsification of, 97, 130, 304n70, 329n59

Delaware, abortion reform in, 331n15

DeLee, Dr. Joseph B., 64, 267n7

Depression, Great: abortion activism during, 336n77; abortion during, 14, 132–47, 298n7; fertility rate in, 162; legalized abortion movement during, 141; liberalizing trends of, 173; physician-abortionists during, 148

Detroit: Harper Hospital, 174; raids in, 319n47; therapeutic abortion committees in, 174; women's liberation groups in, 333n35. *See also* Florence Crittendon Hospital; Keemer, Dr. Edgar Bass

Diaphragms, 41, 196

Dilation and curettage (D & C), 72, 78, 156, 225. *See also* Curettes

Discourse: of antiabortionists, 248; feminist, 262n21; radicalization of, 223; on reproductive rights, 223, 254; on sex, 102

Discourse, female: on abortion, 21, 23–24, 44, 229–30; on reproductive rights, 44

Discourse, medical: on abortion, 7–8, 24–25, 61–63, 67, 164

Disease: societal definition of, 278n53; in therapeutic abortion, 278n55

Divorce, 104, 261n8; in abortion decisions, 184

Dixon-Jones, Dr. Mary, 69

Doe v. Bolton, 244, 245, 252

Doe v. Scott, 235–40, 335n66; appeals on, 240; attorneys in, 336n80; filing of, 335n67; judges in, 239; overturn of, 242–43; plaintiffs in, 238–39. *See also* Test cases

Domesticity, of McCarthy era, 315n10

Dorsett, Dr. Walter B., 64, 82, 90

Double standards, sexual, 12, 28; as factor in abortion, 59; feminists on, 230; in prosecution of abortion, 115; in therapeutic abortion committees, 200

Douches, 26, 41, 42, 103

Drugstores. *See* Pharmacies

Dubin, Leonard, 221

Due process rights, 247, 317n33

Duff, Dr. J. Milton, 82

Duffy, Capt. Thomas, 160, 161, 167

Dye, Nancy Schrom, 295n112

Dying declarations: coercion in, 301n34; collection by hospitals, 121; collection by physicians, 119–20, 122, 123–24, 126; in common law, 118; contents of, 126; destruction of, 124; Illinois Supreme Court on, 116, 297n6; legal status of, 298n14, 300n32; marital status in, 128; models of, 122, 301n31; use in court, 297n6. *See also* Inquests, coroners'

Eastman, Dr. Nicholson J., 321n82

Ebony, 197–98, 231, 325n14

Eclectics (physicians), 73, 282n92

Education, in abortion decisions, 195, 306n19, 306n21

Edwards, Dr. E. W., 45, 47, 52, 54

Ehrlich, Paul R., 333n42

Emerson, Flossie, 300n21

England: Abortion Law Reform Association, 140, 220; birth control movement, 140, 142; *Bourne* case in, 175, 176, 220; legalized abortion in, 140–41, 189–90, 236, 308n42; London, as abortion center, 61; maternal mortality in, 339n5; *Pall Mall Gazette* (London), 49, 50; and sex trade, 50

Etheridge, Dr. James H., 55, 56

Ethnicity: in *Chicago Times* exposé, 50; and choice of abortionist, 76; in differences among women, 16; as factor in abortion, 135, 193; in therapeutic abortion, 205, 207, 327n42

Eugenics: in abortion decisions, 64, 203–4, 279n59; and sterilization, 328n50

Europe, legalized abortion in, 140–41, 142, 308n44. *See also* England; Soviet Union

Evidence: in coroners' inquests, 115, 127; illegal, 166, 317n33

Exclusionary rule (evidence), 317n33

Families: in abortion investigations, 125, 126–28, 302nn48,49; contraceptive use in, 40–41; role of medical practice in, 68; size of, 58, 273n94; state intervention in, 115; support for abortion within, 27. *See also* Fathers; Mothers

Families, working-class: birth control for, 36; effect of abortion on, 39–40, 144

Family planning: by working-class women, 35–36, 230. *See also* Birth control

Fatherhood, as expectation, 115, 129

Fathers: attitude toward daughter's abortions, 28, 108; newspaper warnings to, 125; physicians as father figures, 59–60, 84, 234; power over daughters, 237, 248; state as, 115

Federal Bureau of Investigation, 318n39

Fee for service, 49

Fees, abortion: of clinics, 150; compared
    to childbirth, 74, 154, 313n101,
    313n106; at Gabler-Martin clinic,
    154–55, 197, 311n82, 313nn107,108; at
    Keemer clinic, 157; of midwives, 74,
    96, 283n98; negotiation of, 154–55,
    225; physicians', 47, 76, 96, 154, 196,
    197, 282n86; in postwar era, 197,
    325n11; at Timanus clinic, 158
Feminine mystique, 163, 315n10
Feminists: abortion activism of, 217–18,
    223–34, 238, 252; on abortion law
    reform, 331n21; in abortion rights
    movement, 222–34; African Ameri-
    can, 207, 232, 334n50; and birth con-
    trol movement, 141; English, 220;
    on medical profession, 3, 260n6;
    and poor people's movements, 236;
    second-wave, 227, 228–29; smear
    campaigns against, 172; tactics of,
    229; "third-world," 228, 232
Feminists, nineteenth-century, 12; on
    birth control, 36; views on abortion,
    32–33, 35, 36, 76, 278n44; views on
    medicine, 260n6. See also Women's
    movements
Fetus: defects of, 203, 204, 221, 240,
    327n38; images of, 84–85, 287n18;
    medical opinion on, 60, 80; primacy
    over woman, 250; viability of, 245, 248
Fibroids, in therapeutic abortion, 326n27
Fields, Dr. Charles, 238, 239
Findley, Dr. Palmer, 109, 110
Finkbine, Sherri, 203
Fish, Dr. E. F., 67
Fitzbutler, Dr. Henry, 269n38
Florence Crittendon Hospital (Detroit),
    174–75, 176, 177; sterilization at,
    329n54
Folk remedies, for abortion. See Abortifa-
    cients; Abortion, self-induced
Foucault, Michel, 5, 7, 262n21
Frank, Dr. Jacob, 56
Frank, Dr. Louis, 124
Freedmen's Hospital (Washington,
    D.C.), 147
Freedom, sexual, 220; feminists on, 16,
    217, 229; in nineteenth century, 32; in
    sex reform drives, 92. See also Sexuality
Friedan, Betty, 315n10
Friedman, Lawrence, 167, 317n33, 318n39
Friendship, women's, 27, 29–31, 45

Fritzsche, Sybille, 235–38, 239,
    335nn66,67, 336n69; on Cook County
    attorney, 242; on religious opposi-
    tion, 338n98
Furniss, Dr. Henry, 123

Gabler, Dr. Josephine, 148, 149–50, 159,
    311n74; education of, 310n72
Gabler-Martin abortion clinic, 149, 196;
    age of patients, 152; bribes by, 155;
    business records of, 166; fees at,
    154–55, 197, 311n82, 313nn107,108;
    length of pregnancy at, 153–54,
    313n103; patients of, 151–53, 312n90,
    313n99; post-abortion care at, 154;
    procedures of, 151–52, 311n86; race of
    patients, 153; referrals to, 150, 166,
    322n98; secrecy in, 151. See also Mar-
    tin, Ada; People v. Martin
Gallagher, John A., 126
Garrow, David, 336n72
Garvin, Dr. Charles H., 135
Gayle, R. Finley, 279n56
Gay men, 163, 228, 248; marginalization
    of, 266n5; toleration of, 316n14
Gebhard, Paul H., 135
Gender: and anti-midwife campaign, 94;
    as bond between women, 21, 93, 96,
    266n6; in criminalization of abortion,
    11, 115; effect of World War II on, 163;
    and expectations of men, 31, 115, 128,
    129; and expectations of women, 163,
    194; female desire for female atten-
    dants, 57, 76; and honor, 167–68; in
    hospital structure, 213–15; and male
    physicians, 68; moral differences in, 12,
    58–59; and punishment, 5, 115, 131, 171
General practitioners: abortions by, 67,
    79; choice of, 280n66; in history of
    abortion, 4; regulation of, 178; use of
    curette, 285n113
Georgia, 244, 331n15, 336n70
Germany, 140
Germ theory, 269n28. See also Antiseptic
    technique; Aseptic technique
Gleitsman, Dr. Emil, 32
Glenn, Dr. George A., 141
Goldman, Emma, 36, 229
Goodman, Dr. Jerome E., 186, 187
Gordon, Linda, 163, 309n48, 340n13,
    341n27
Grand juries: in abortion cases, 118, 119,

298n10, 299n15; physicians before, 219. *See also* Juries
Greenleaf, Simon, 298n14
Griswold v. Connecticut, 237, 323n111; privacy in, 336n77
Groh, Mary, 74
Grossberg, Michael, 297n3
Grossman, Susan, 235–38, 239, 335nn66,67
Group for the Advancement of Psychiatry, 335n63
Guttmacher, Dr. Alan F., 179, 180, 224; reform efforts of, 222, 233–34; and therapeutic abortion, 201, 219, 233
Gynecologists: in antiabortion campaigns, 82; sterilizations by, 208; support of ALA model law, 234; on therapeutic abortion committees, 175
Gynecology, morality of, 264n38

Habermas, Jürgen, 260n4
Hackett, James P., 168
Hagenow, Dr. Lucy, 77, 284n108
Haisler, Catherine, 75
Hall, Dr. Robert E., 205, 207, 328n51
Hamilton, Dr. Alice, 96
Hamilton, Dr. Virginia Clay, 136
Hanrahan, Edward V., 240, 242–43, 338n98
Hansen, Marie, 29
Hardin, Garrett, 333n42
Harlem Hospital, 135
Harper Hospital (Detroit), 174
Hartmann, Susan, 163
Hawaii, legalization of abortion in, 241
Hawkins, H. H., 116
Health care: of early twentieth century, 48, 110–11; effect of legal abortion on, 246–47; federally funded, 251; feminist-oriented, 223, 225–26; government regulation of, 190; inequalities in, 213, 329n61; and maternal mortality, 213–14; as partnership, 247; state surveillance of, 249. *See also* Hospitals; Public health
Heart disease, in therapeutic abortion, 326n27
Hedger, Dr. Caroline, 96, 111, 291n61
Hellman, Dr. Louis M., 173
Herbs, abortifacient, 9, 43, 44
Herbst, Josephine, 309n45
Hesseltine, Dr. H. Close, 174, 176

Heterosexual relations: abortion in, 18; danger in, 102; dating norms in, 31–33, 271n50; female experience of, 271n59; feminist assumptions on, 32–33, 271n59; power dynamics in, 37–38; regulation of, 115, 296n2; social construction of, 228. *See also* Freedom, sexual; Husbands; Lovers, male; Sexuality
Hoffman, Charles G., 98
Hoffman, Peter, 107, 298n10; on maternity homes, 105
Holmes, Dr. Rudolph W.: in antiabortion campaigns, 84, 88, 89–90; on birth control, 296n115; and midwife regulation, 96, 292n79; on newspapers, 70; report to Chicago Medical Society, 88; on therapeutic abortion, 176
Homeopaths: abortions provided by, 72; as Regulars, 282n92; regulation of, 10; views on abortion, 55, 263n32
Home remedies, for abortion. *See* Abortifacients; Abortion, self-induced
Homosexuality. *See* Gay men; Lesbians
Hospitals: for abortion, 71–72; abortion patients in, 138–39, 146; abortions performed in, 3, 69, 98, 173, 307n28, 339n1; accreditation of, 191; African American, 28, 269n38; births in, 275n5; Catholic, 321n84, 339n1; cooperation with state, 4, 121, 123–24, 162, 173–74, 190, 226, 303n52; fees of, 313n106; government pressure on, 180–81; municipal, 207, 214, 307n38; national standards for, 191; private, 214, 328n44; struggles with physicians, 190, 324n115; therapeutic abortion in, 161–62, 179–80, 329n62; women physicians in, 11. *See also* Septic abortion wards; Therapeutic abortion committees; *names of individual hospitals*
Howe, Dr. E. D., 311n76
Hull-House, 96, 100; investigation of bastardy, 130
Hume, Dr. E. E., 83
Husbands: aid in abortion, 34–35, 272n64; and contraception, 38; control over wives, 35, 41, 59, 237; in coroners' inquests, 129; indictment of, 303n65; notification requirements for, 252
Hyde, Henry, 242, 248

Hyperemesis gravidarum, 63–64, 201, 279n56

Illegitimacy: in ALI model law, 221; comparison by race, 136, 137; prosecution in, 129–30; stigma of, 27–28
Illinois: abortion law reform in, 235–40; abortion laws of, 61, 107, 261n13, 265n45; Bar Association, 222; Medical Practice Act, 107, 116; State Medical Society, 72; state's attorney, 242–43, 317n28; therapeutic abortion in, 13. *See also* Chicago; Cook County; "Jane"
Illinois Board of Health: in antiabortion debate, 106; *Chicago Times* on, 50; physicians' cooperation with, 88; regulation of midwives, 97, 98
Illinois Supreme Court: abortion rulings of, 61, 244; appeals to, 255–56; on dying declarations, 116, 297n6; overturn of *People v. Martin,* 166; in Stanko case, 170, 171; on therapeutic abortion, 242–43. See also *Doe v. Scott*
Immigrants: abortions for, 68; in antiabortion campaigns, 13; to Chicago, 17; in *Chicago Times,* 50; in coroners' inquests, 119; and criminalization of abortion, 11; midwives among, 73, 81, 91–92, 147; neighborhoods of, 31, 270n48; physicians among, 139; preferences in childbearing, 73, 283nn96–97; sense of community among, 31; use of midwives, 73, 76
Immigrants' Protection League, 100
Incest, abortion following, 220–21, 251
Indiana, 149
Infant health, national policy on, 110, 111
Infanticide: abortion as, 13, 85; in *Chicago Times* exposé, 50–51
Infant mortality, 250; African American, 213
Inquests, coroners', 22, 31, 45, 114, 256, 299n18; evidence in, 115, 127; husbands in, 129; interrogation in, 126–29, 131, 182; legal purpose of, 119; physicians' cooperation in, 120–25, 131; specialists' testimony in, 88; unmarried men in, 115, 128–30; unmarried women in, 128–30. *See also* Cook County coroner; Dying declarations
Insurance: for abortion, 134, 340n20; national health, 172, 295n111
Iowa, 61, 336n70

Irregulars (medical providers), 11, 48; of Chicago, 57, 276n29, 282n92; practice of abortion, 263n32

"Jane" (abortion provider), 223, 224–27, 240, 242; founders of, 237; origins of, 224, 332n26; political support for, 243–44; raid on, 243
Japan, 224
Jarrett, Dr. Elizabeth, 94
Jay, Dr. Milton, 53
Jewish law on abortion, 7
Jewish women, 23, 37, 137, 173, 306n22, 307n23; reproductive rights of, 7
Joffe, Carole, 304n4
Johns Hopkins University (Baltimore), 158, 179–80, 187, 218, 321n82
Johnson, Dr. Joseph Taber, 25, 80, 82
Joint Commission on Accreditation of Hospitals (JCAH), 191
Journalism: investigative, 47, 48–49; sensational, 318n38
Journal of the American Medical Association (JAMA): abortion debate in, 67, 140; anti-midwife campaign in, 97; *Bourne* case in, 175; on *Chicago Times* exposé, 57, 60; on dying declarations, 122; Leunbach method in, 157; on maternity homes, 28; on therapeutic abortion, 64, 65–66, 146. *See also* American Medical Association
Juries: acquittal of abortionists, 6; coroners', 118, 119, 299n15. *See also* Grand juries; Inquests, coroners'

Kahn, Dr. Maurice, 113, 120, 122
Kansas, 331n15
Keemer, Dr. Edgar Bass: abortion clinic of, 156–58; autobiography of, 323n107; convictions of, 244; education of, 156; fees of, 157; in NARAL, 232, 243, 324n114; post-abortion care by, 157–58; raids on, 181, 243; in Socialist Workers Party, 189; trial of, 182, 188–89, 322n89; wife of, 156, 314n117
Kennedy, Florynce, 232
Kentucky, 336n70; Louisville National Medical College, 28, 269n38
Kessler-Harris, Alice, 325n3
Khamis, Dr. Joseph A., 313n113
Kinnally, Nate, 168
Kinsey, Dr. Alfred, 193
Kinsey Institute for Sex Research, 305n11;

study of abortion, 135, 136, 154, 305n15, 306n19, 306n21, 313n99
Klinetop, Dr. Charles, 72
Knights of Columbus, 319n62
Kobrin, Francis E., 295n112
Kruse, Dr. Henry, 124, 303n52
Kuder, Josephine, 150; arrest of, 160; trial of, 154, 155, 160
Kummer, Jerome M., 222
Kunzel, Regina, 29

Lader, Lawrence, 322n86
Lane, Roger, 299n16
Latina women: as feminists, 232; and sterilization abuse, 232. *See also* Mexicans; Puerto Ricans
Law, American: ambiguity in, 262n15; history of, 261n10
The Law against Abortion (Robinson), 139
Leavitt, Judith Walzer, 38, 280n69
Leavy, Zad, 222
Left, political: on "the woman question," 228; women's movements and, 142, 309n48. *See also* Socialist movements
Legal Aid, 236
Lesbians, 163, 228, 248, 249; marginalization of, 266n5
Le Sueur, Meridel, 309n45
Leunbach's Paste, 156–57, 314n118
Lewis, Dr. Denslow, 69
Lidz, Dr. Theodore, 180, 203, 327n34
Life expectancy, 213, 329n59
Litoff, Judy Barrett, 290n53, 290n56, 295n112
Livingston, Dr. Margaret, 280n74
Living wills, 247
Lobdell, Dr. Effie L., 105
London. *See* England
Long, Dr. John Hermon, 186–87
Los Angeles, 164; California Hospital, 178; County Hospital, 210
Lotz, Dr. George, 87
Loudon, Irvine, 284n111, 339n5
Louisiana, 336n70
Louisville National Medical College, 28, 269n38
Lovers, male: as aid in abortion, 31, 270n50; arrest of, 129; conviction of, 129, 303n64; in coroners' inquests, 128–30, 303n58, 303nn61,62
Loyola Medical School, 319n45, 337n80
Lucas, Roy, 335n67
Luker, Kristin, 311n77

MacKenzie, Dr. Robert A., 178–79
Maginnis, Patricia, 223, 224, 331n18
Male-dominated spaces, 126, 127, 161, 165, 194, 229
Mandy, Dr. Arthur J., 218
Mann, Sophie, 75
Marbury, William, 221
Margaret Hague Maternity Hospital (New Jersey), 179, 180
Marquette University School of Medicine, 63
Marriage, 261n8; as alternative to abortion, 84, 115, 133; in coroners' investigations, 128; enforcement of, 297n3; interracial, 237; power relations in, 37–38, 59; state intervention in, 115, 129–31
Martin, Ada, 149, 151, 311n76; arrest of, 160; conviction of, 166. *See also* Gabler-Martin abortion clinic; *People v. Martin*
Maryland, 331n15; Court of Appeals, 188
Massachusetts: Medical Society, 87, 120; midwives of, 281n81
Maternal health, national policy on, 110–11
Maternal mortality, 39, 77, 284nn109,110, 285n116; after legalized abortion, 246–47; blame of midwives for, 91, 95; decline in, 339n5; under legal abortion, 339n4; public opinion on, 190–91; race as factor in, 211–12, 329nn60,61; resulting from abortion, 43, 138–39, 140, 340n7, *fig.* 7
Maternity homes, 28–29, 107, 195, 306n21; investigation of, 105–6
May, Elaine Tyler, 163
McCarthyism, 163, 172–73, 192, 315n12; anti-Semitism in, 320n65; effect on therapeutic abortion, 180, 192
McGoorty, John P., 104
Medical practice: ambiguities in, 145–46; locations of, 48, 68; monitoring of, 219
Medical practice acts, of Illinois, 107, 116
Medical profession, 1; on abortion law reform, 143, 234; admission of women to, 11–12; antiabortion policies of, 4, 48, 55–56, 82; business aspects of, 48–49, 84–85; in *Chicago Times* exposé, 50; claims to moral superiority, 57, 82, 85, 234, 277n39; class identity of, 208; competition in, 67; conservatism of, 172; control of reproductive rights, 3, 208, 214; cooperation with

Medical profession (*continued*)
state, 3, 81, 88–90, 115–16, 120–25, 131, 226, 249, 260n5; disagreement within, 4, 5, 48, 64, 247; discourse on abortion, 7–8, 24–25, 61–63, 67, 164; eighteenth-century, 9; elimination of abortionists from, 81; exemption from abortion debate, 100, 105, 108; feminists on, 3, 260n6; and national health insurance, 172, 295n111; power in, 324n115; rejection of male authority in, 226; self-regulation of, 88, 97; social authority of, 13–14; state control of, 11, 116; support of abortion reform, 216, 234, 244

Medical schools: in antiabortion campaigns, 87, 90; Catholic, 337n80; of Chicago, 57; cooperation with state, 4; women in, 4

Medical societies: African American, 234; physician-abortionists in, 61, 72, 81. *See also* American Medical Association; Chicago Medical Society; National Medical Association

Medical students: abortion training for, 252; acceptance of abortion, 143; in *Chicago Times* exposé, 55–56; obstetrical training of, 92, 97, 101, 292n70, 293n81

Medico-Legal Society (Chicago), 55

Men: and alcohol abuse, 59; control over women, 35, 44, 237, 245, 253; as legislators, 13; penalties for abortion, 115; sexual domination of women, 12. *See also* Gay men; Gender; Heterosexual relations; Husbands; Lovers, male; Male-dominated spaces

Menstruation: 19, 38; restoration of, 8–9, 13, 20, 24, 51; government surveillance of, 126, 127, 128, 250

Mental illness, therapeutic abortion for, 183, 184, 187, 201–3, 207, 241, 326n26, 327n36

Mercereau, Dr. C. W., 71

Mexicans: hostility toward, 11; use of abortion, 136

Mexico, 224, 233

Meyerowitz, Joanne, 32, 270n41

Michael Reese Hospital (Chicago), 240

Michigan Boulevard Sanitarium (Chicago), 72

Midwifery schools, 57, 101; proposed, 107

Midwives: abortion charges against, 288n42; abortions provided by, 70–71, 74–75, 96, 281nn76,81; African American, 73, 137–48; alliances with physicians, 96, 290n53; arrangement of adoption, 52–53; blackmailing of, 98; boarding of abortion patients, 74–75; check-ups by, 74, 283n100; clientele of, 76; convictions of, 291n62; disappearance of, 111, 147, 281n80, 296n117; of early nineteenth century, 10; fees of, 74, 96, 283n98; feminist historians of, 91; frequency of abortions by, 71; history of, 288n42, 290n53; identification with patients, 73–74, 76; immigrant, 73, 81, 91–92, 147; licensing of, 93; location of practice, 48; mistreatment by officials, 98–99; national distribution of, 283n105; of New York, 90, 96, 281n81, 291n62; obstetric practices of, 95; organizations of, 98, 292n76; physicians' defense of, 96, 290n53; prosecution of, 88; public debate on, 104–5; refusal of abortion, 52–53, 276n21; regulation of, 94–95, 97, 107, 109, 290n56, 292n79; safety records of, 77–79, 91, 95–96, 100, 284n111; surveillance of, 98–100; techniques of, 75–76; training of, 57, 100–101, 107. *See also* Antimidwife antiabortion campaign

Midwives, of Chicago, 47, 281nn76,81; Anti-Graft Association, 98; campaign against, 92–101; clients of, 73; regulation of, 97–98; self-defense of, 98–99; in *Times* exposé, 52–53; in vice investigation, 99

Miller, Dr. G.-P., 122–23

Miller, Dr. Truman W., 25

Miller, Patricia, 326n18

Millstone, Dr. Henry James, 149, 311n76

Milwaukee, 78

Minneapolis, 78, 134

Miscarriage: abortion disguised as, 72; coroners' investigation of, 270n61, 273n85; fatal, 284n110, 293n86; mortality in, 77, 102, 117, surveillance of, 250; suspicion of, 123

Mississippi, 241

Missouri, 336n70

Mitchell, Dr. Justin L., 29, 72, 313n113

Mohr, James C., 10, 268n15, 286n8

Monmouth Memorial Hospital (New Jersey), 178, 320n76

Montana, 253

Morality: gender differences in, 12, 58–59; physicians' superiority in, 57, 82, 234, 277n39; women's superiority in, 12, 264n39

Morality, popular: acceptance of abortion, 6–7, 21–22, 44–45, 81, 112, 116, 244

Moriarity, Daniel, 155, 313n111

Mortality. See Infant mortality; Maternal mortality

Motherhood: as expectation, 163, 195; immigrant, 91; and pregnancy, 273n86; "voluntary," 12, 229, 264n39

Mothers: and children, 39–40; and housework, 40; support for unmarried daughters, 27–28; threats to life of, 251, 341n21; use of abortion, 38, 273n85

Mothers, unmarried: charities for, 28–29; child rearing by, 29; male responsibility for, 297n3; mothers' support for daughters, 27–28; New Right on, 196; psychiatrists' views on, 331n20; sterilization of, 207. See also Women, unmarried

Mt. Sinai Hospital, 179, 180

NARAL. See National Abortion Rights Action League; National Association for the Repeal of Abortion Laws

National Abortion Rights Action League (1973–1993), 325n15

National Association for the Repeal of Abortion Laws (1969–1973), 232, 243, 324n114

National Committee on Maternal Health, 142, 143, 309n50

National Council of Jewish Women, 173

National health insurance, 172, 295n111

National Medical Association, 83

National Organization for Women (NOW), 227–28; UAW women in, 332n33; welfare work of, 253

National Welfare Rights Organization, 228

Nelson, Bessie E., 188

New Hampshire, 336n70

New Jersey, 178, 179, 319n55, 336n70

New Journalism, 47, 49

Newmayer, Babetta, 74

New Mexico, 331n15

New Orleans: Charity Hospital, 134; Parish Medical Society, 301n31

New Right, 196, 229; attacks on abortion rights, 248–49, 253

Newspapers: abortion advertisements in, 70, 88–89, 225, 226, 262n13, 280n74; abortion raids in, 167, 192; African American, 135; anti-midwife antiabortion campaign in, 92, 108, 109; coverage of abortion, 7, 23, 25, 49, 104–6, 114–15, 121, 125, 130, 132–33, 185, 216, 268n15, 298n8; Johnson case in, 102, 104, 105, 125; messages to doctors, 172; messages to men, 130; messages to women, 102, 108, 125, 130, 168; use of illustrations, 50–51; use by prosecutors, 168, 172. See also Chicago Times

New York, 10; abortion use in, 134–35, 306n19; abortion investigations in, 119, 136, 287n29; abortion raids in, 164, 316n16, 316n19; Bellevue Hospital, 136; Harlem Hospital, 135; legal abortion in, 225, 241–42, 247, 339n4; maternal mortality in, 139, 211, 213, fig. 5, fig. 6; midwives of, 90, 96, 281n81, 290n56, 291n62; public health in, 295n112; Sloane Hospital, 205, 207; speak-outs in, 333n40; therapeutic abortion in, 204, 205, fig. 2, fig. 3; women's liberation groups in, 333n35

New York Academy of Medicine, 139, 140

New York County Medical Society, 291n61

New York Public Library, 140

New York Times, 134, 268n15; Bourne case in, 175

New York World, 49

North Carolina, 246, 331n15, 336n70

Nurses, 68, 185, 253, 322n98

Oakley, Ernest F., 123

Obstetricians: in AMA, 90; in antiabortion campaigns, 82; campaign against midwives, 90–94, 108; influence on public policy, 105; professional identity of, 295n112; regulation of general practitioners, 178; regulation of midwives, 94–95, 109; support of ALI model law, 234; and therapeutic abortion committees, 173, 175. See also Gynecologists; Midwives

Obstetrics: medical training in, 92, 97, 101, 292n70, 293n81; morality of, 11–12, 264nn37,38

O'Callaghan, Rev. Peter J., 62–63

O'Connor, Sgt. William E., 113, 126

Ohio, 336n70

Oregon, abortion reform in, 331n15

Orphans, 39; orphanages, 132
Ott, Dr. Harold A., 176
Our Bodies, Ourselves (Boston Women's
Health Collective), 226

Packwood, Sen. Robert, 231
Pall Mall Gazette, 49, 50
Papanek, Samuel, 165, 317nn23,24
Parental notification or consent require-
ments, 249, 252, 253, 341n25
Paris, infanticide in, 50, 51
Parkes, Dr. Charles H., 122, 124
Parsons, Jody, 237, 332n26
Parsons, Rev. E. Spencer, 241, 242, 338n98
Paternity cases, 129–30
Patients, 9; decision-making of, 65–67,
223, 224, 247; influence on politics,
217; state surveillance of, 247–48, 249.
See also Abortion patients; Physician-
patient relationship
Patients' rights, 247–48, 250–51
Pearse, Dr. Harry A., 176
Pelvis, contracted, 66, 145, 278n55, 279n64
Pemmer, Elizabeth, 52–53
Penicillin, 162, 339n5
Pennsylvania, 319n55
People ex rel. Hanrahan v. White, 242–43
People v. Belous, 235, 236, 337n81
People v. Martin, 153, 154, 155, 160, 312n90,
314n1; press coverage of, 311n85; refer-
ring physicians in, 166, 317n30; sui-
cides in, 167; testimony in, 317n23;
verdict in, 317n33. *See also* Martin,
Ada; Gabler-Martin abortion clinic
Peritonitis, 35, 300n24
Petchesky, Rosalind, 153, 194, 204
Peyser, Dr. Edward, 314n113
Pharmaceutical colleges, 57
Pharmacies: condoms in, 134; sale of
abortifacients, 44
Pharmacists, 100, 291n69
Philadelphia, 10; abortion in, 61, 134–35;
abortion indictments in, 298n7, 299n16;
abortion investigations in, 119, 287n29;
County Medical Society, 88
Philbrick, Dr. Inez, 61
Physician-abortionists, 50, 313n113;
African American, 156; assassination
of, 248; caricature of, 86, *plate 4;* case
studies of, 133; Chicago Medical Soci-
ety's control of, 95; in *Chicago Times*
exposé, 54–57, 276n29; of Depression

era, 148; expulsion from medical societies, 87, 120, 323n105; expulsion from
profession, 81, 97, 110, 120; following
Roe v. Wade, 246; hospitals of, 71–72;
in medical societies, 61, 72; methods
of, 72–73; motives of, 158–59; prosecution of, 181–92; as prostitutes, 85;
raids on, 181, 233; referrals to, 46, 54,
67, 148–50, 158, 311n79; role in reproductive rights, 47, 48; safety records
of, 77–79, 284n111; sex of, 76; as specialists, 147, 159; training for, 147–48,
252; use of abortifacients, 72; women
among, 73. *See also* Abortionists; Gabler, Dr. Josephine; Keemer, Dr. Edgar
Bass; Midwives; Timanus, Dr. George
Loutrell
Physician-patient relationship, 4, 67–68,
254, 260n7; antiabortion counseling
in, 83–84; communication in, 48,
67–69, 176, 178, 201; confidentiality
in, 124–25, 302n43; denial of patient
autonomy, 208, 215, 220, 234; distrust
in, 64, 179, 190, 248; effect of abortion laws on, 131, 226; equality in,
247; freedom of speech in, 238; negotiation in, 62, 244; patients' views ignored in, 208, 252; women's power in,
67. *See also* Patients
Physicians: alliances with midwives, 96;
antiabortion, 83–84, 89–90, 109; arrest of, 120, 171, 236, 336n70; attitude
toward inquests, 121; challenges to
abortion laws, 15; collection of dying
declarations, 119–20, 122, 123–24,
126; cooperation in inquests, 120–
25, 131; cooperation with state, 88,
288n32, 302n43; cover-up of abortion,
304n69; dispensing of contraceptives,
134, 139, 296n115; in *Doe v. Scott,*
238–39; Eclectic, 73, 282n92; economic concerns of, 67, 85–86; elite,
53, 54–55; enforcement of abortion
laws, 3, 115; exemption from abortion
debate, 100, 105, 108; fear of prosecution, 122–24, 174, 175; fees for abortion, 47, 76, 96, 154, 197, 282n86;
frequency of abortions by, 70–71;
hygienic practices of, 79, 265n46;
influence of private sphere on, 4; interrogation of abortion patients,
296n1; kickbacks from abortionists,

67; legal protection for, 174–76; loss of license, 120, 172, 300n25; observation of abortion complications, 146–47, 210, 217, 222, 239; obstetrical training of, 92, 97, 101, 292n70, 293n81; post-abortion treatment by, 120–21; prosecution of, 233; public-health work of, 295n112; on quickening, 12; radical, 132, 139, 146, 173, 217; reasons for performing abortion, 67–68; red-baiting of, 180, 321n84; referrals by, 148–50, 171, 233, 311n79; reformers among, 217; refusal of treatment, 122–23; review committees of, 223; rights to privacy and to practice, 238, 244; rural, 69, 280n69; safety records of, 91, 284n111; self-regulation of, 3; state regulation of, 116; struggles with hospitals, 190, 324n115; support for abortion, 1, 15, 132, 139, 181, 220; sympathy with midwives, 107, 290n52; testimony in abortion trials, 186–87, 188; and therapeutic abortion committees, 178–79, 190–91, 218; threats of prosecution, 120–21, 171–72; training of midwives, 101. *See also* Irregulars; Medical profession; Regulars

Physicians, African American, 82–83, 156, 286n10; female, 300n21; prosecution of, 120

Physicians, of Chicago: abortionists among, 53, 70, 72, 313n113; in *Chicago Times* exposé, 54–57, 67, 276n29; cooperation with Board of Health, 88; Regulars among, 55, 56, 276n29

Physicians, female, 149, 264n37; on abortion, 57–58; abortions performed by, 73, 76; African American, 300n21; hostility to, 11–12; public-health work of, 96, 291n60, 295n112

Physicians, nineteenth-century, 10–11; autonomy of, 15; ignorance of contraceptives, 41; opposition to abortion, 13, 82; referrals by, 46, 54, 67, 148–50; use of placebos, 26; on women's attitudes, 25

Pierce, Mrs. (nurse), 46–47, 48

Pill (contraceptive), 229

Planned Parenthood, 173; advocacy of birth control, 220; conference on abortion (1955), 219–20, 221; and population control, 230–31; referral service of, 241; welfare work of, 253

Planned Parenthood v. Casey, 251, 252

Police: arrests in abortion cases, 109, 116, 117, 120, 129, 164, 298n8; corruption, 155, 167, 300n20; custody of abortion patients, 168–69, 249; interrogation of abortion patients, 114, 118, 126, 249; raids on abortion clinics, 160–62, 164–68, 170–71, 181, 243, 249, 316nn16,19, 318n41; self-protection in abortion cases, 126; as voyeur, *plate 6*

Political movements, and abortion rights, 14, 15, 180, 228

Poor people's movements, 236, 336n72

Population control, 230; as political repression, 333n42; for poor women, 231; support for legal abortion, 231, 233

Pornography, 270n59

Portland, Ore., 138, 164

Powell, Roberta, 153

Pregnancy: in common law, 8; dangerous, 41; as developmental process, 60; ectopic, 266n7; fear of, 38–39, 40; first, 135, 305n13; history of, 265n49; medical advances in, 144–45, 162; medical profession's control of, 12, 83–84; as menstrual problem, 8–9, 23; and motherhood, 273n86; as punishment for sex, 249, 340n19; of students, 195; toxemia of, 326n27; tuberculosis during, 143–44, 145, 146; women's friendship in, 30–31; in the workplace, 194

Privacy: in birth control, 336n77; in medical treatment, 49, 124–25, 238, 302n43; in reproductive rights, 254; state intervention in, 131; in Supreme and Federal Court decisions, 237, 239, 244; violation of bodily integrity, 168–71

Private sphere: abortion in, 21; in anti-abortion debate, 106; influence on physicians, 4, 67–68; nineteenth-century, 2; and public debate, 2–3, 229–30; reproductive rights in, 254

Professional abortionists. *See* Physician-abortionists

Progressive Era, 289n43; abortion in, 81, 102, 110; sexual discourse in, 102; social movements in, 81, 91

Pronatalism, 163, 195

Prosecutors: in abortion fatalities, 116–18;

Prosecutors (*continued*)
  in abortion raid cases, 164, 165, 187;
  investigation of physicians, 173
Prostitution, 59, 264n39; campaigns
  against, 12, 92; as metaphor, 85; related to abortion, 99–100, 292n78
Protestants: abortion practices of, 50, 137,
  306n22; attitude toward abortion,
  6–7; birth rate of, 11
Protest movements, 228
Przybyszewski, Linda, 336n77
Psychiatrists: in abortion rights movement, 218, 223, 234, 335n63; on sexual
  deviance, 331n20
Public discussion, of abortion, 142,
  172–73, 219, 229, 230, 233. *See also*
  Speak-outs
Public health, 295n111; effect of legal
  abortion on, 246–47; in midwife debate, 295n112; reformers in, 138. *See
  also* Health care
Public-health officers, 106, 248; on access
  to abortion, 338n111; on maternal mortality, 214; in Planned Parenthood
  conference, 219; reformers among, 217
Public opinion: acceptance of abortion,
  6–7, 21–22, 44–45, 81, 112, 234,
  252–53, 321n84, 341n28; formation of,
  2; on maternal mortality, 190–91
Public policy, 1; in enforcement of abortion laws, 112; exclusion of women,
  107; implementation of, 3, 16; on maternal health, 110–11; medical societies' role in, 106; on midwives, 101;
  obstetricians' influence on, 105; on
  reproduction, 81, 110, 214, 218, 244
Public sphere: abortion discourse in,
  141, 229–30; antiabortion debate in,
  106, 217; debate in, 2, 3; nineteenth-
  century, 2; reproductive rights in,
  254; scholarship on, 260n4
Puerto Ricans: abortion rates of, 327n42,
  fig. 6; fatal abortions among, 222, 232,
  329n60; therapeutic abortion for, 205
Punishment, 5, 114–15, 131; pregnancy as,
  249, 340n19; for unmarried women,
  221, 249. *See also* Abortion, illegal

Quay, Eugene, 221
Queer Theory, 226n5
Quickening: abortion after, 8; in antiabortion campaigns, 83, 85; colonial
  concept of, 8, 9; in common law, 13;

in nineteenth-century law, 10; nineteenth-century perception of, 25, 51,
  80; persistence of belief in, 109–10;
  Storer on, 12–13

Race: in criminalization of abortion, 11,
  15; differences among women, 16; as
  factor in abortion, 16, 135–38, 193,
  213–14, 251, *fig. 6;* in infant mortality, 213, 329n61; in Keemer trial, 188;
  in maternal mortality, 211, 213, 232,
  329nn60,61, *fig. 6;* and therapeutic
  abortion, 205, 206, *fig. 3;* and welfare, 249. *See also* African Americans;
  Puerto Ricans; Whites
"Race suicide," 92, 102, 104
Racism, 11, 208, 213
Raids: on abortion clinics, 160–62,
  164–68, 181, 243, 249, 316n16, 316n19;
  newspaper coverage of, 192; testimony on, 164–66, 168, 170–71; use of
  force in, 167, 318n41
Rape: abortion following, 33–34, 65, 175,
  199, 221, 251, 340n19; in hypothetical
  abortion requests, 240; marital, 59;
  pregnancy following, 64; statutory,
  92, 304n67; of unmarried women, 33,
  270n61
Reed, Dr. Charles B., 82, 83
Reformers: in anti-midwife campaign, 96;
  on maternal health, 111; medical, 217;
  in public health, 138; views on abortion, 99–100
Regulars (physicians), 10–11, 48, 263n32;
  abortions performed by, 72, 282n92;
  in *Chicago Times* exposé, 55, 56,
  276n29; consolidation of, 282n92
"Relief babies," 134
Religion, organized: in abortion rights
  movement, 221, 244; fundamentalism
  in, 248; leadership in abortion issues,
  13; response to birth control movement, 6–7, 262n18; teaching on abortion, 6, 7, 262nn17,18,19
Religious belief, and abortion rates, 23,
  137, 242
Reproduction: centrality to society,
  266n50; economic factors in, 133;
  medical profession's control over policy, 3, 208, 214; public policy on, 110,
  214; shame in regulation of, 5, 28, 125,
  126–28, 171, 200
Reproductive rights, 18, 204, 253–54; af-

ter *Roe v. Wade,* 245; under ALI model law, 221; in backlash against abortion, 252; birth control movement in, 111; Catholic Church on, 7, 180–81, 248; in challenges to abortion law, 237; in Chicago abortion trade, 48; choice in, 133; in coroners' inquests, 45; in *Doe v. Scott,* 239–40; feminist interest in, 190, 224; history of, 6, 7, 8; Jewish tradition of, 7; mass movements for, 217; in McCarthy era, 164; nineteenth-century, 229; and patients' rights, 247–48, 251; and population control programs, 231; in postwar era, 194; in private sphere, 254; in public policy, 110; public support for, 321n84; resentment against, 102, 104; of teenagers, 248, 253; in therapeutic abortion, 66, 67, 146, 279n64; of unmarried women, 108; without physician's approval, 220; women's discourse on, 44; and women's goals, 195

Restell, Madam, 10

Right to decide. *See* Reproductive rights

Right to die, 247

Ripczynski, Veronica, 75

Robinson, Dr. William J., *The Law against Abortion,* 139; as "A.B.C.," 45, 268n22

Rockefeller, Nelson, 234

Roe v. Wade, 198, 244, 245; attacks on, 249, 251; coalitions supporting, 248; right to privacy in, 244

Rolick, Marie, 98–99

Romania, 250

Rongetti, Dr. Amante, 72, 128

Rongy, Dr. A.-J., *Abortion: Legal or Illegal,* 139–40; on fatal abortion, 146–47

Root, Dr. Eliza H., 92–93

Rosen, Dr. Harold, 328n47

Rosner, Dr. Marvin, 240

Ross, Ellen, 38, 270n49

Royston, Dr. G. D., 43

Rubella, 203, 240

Rural areas, abortion in, 17, 43, 69

Ryan, Mary P., 163, 315n10

Ryder, Dr. George H., 181

Saint Louis, Mo., 61

San Francisco, 61, 89, 226

Sanger, Margaret, 36, 141, 229; letters to, 37, 38, 40, 41, 132

Schmid, Calvin, 274n111

Schoenian, Mme. M., 52, 73

Scholtes, Mrs., 74

Schreckcr, Ellen, 319n60

Schultz-Knighten, Dr. Anna B., 300nn21–22

Scott, Joan Wallach, 262n21

Search and seizure, illegal, 166, 248

Septic abortion wards, 138, 210, 214, 239, 307n29; closure of, 246; reopening of, 249

Septic infection: among poor women, 134; fatal, 147, 242, 300n24; in legal abortion, 284n110; physician-induced, 79, 265n46, 285n113; women's knowledge of, 27

"The Service" (abortion provider). *See* "Jane"

Settlement houses, 107

Sexism: in abortion system, 194; of men, 228, 231, 232, 334n50; in present-day antiabortion movement, 249

Sex trade, British, 50

Sexual harassment, by abortionists, 199, 200, 225

Sexual immorality: in abortion raid cases, 167; in anti-midwife campaign, 92; male, 59

Sexuality: history of, 297n2; social history of, 7, 8; Victorian view of, 292n78. *See also* Freedom, sexual; Heterosexual relations

Sexuality, female: autonomy in, 253; in birth control movement, 36, 229; as dangerous to women, 108; feminist thought on, 270n59; maternity in, 163; reformers' views on, 100; regulation of, 3, 269n36; in second wave feminism, 228–29; social concern over, 91, 92, 108; as threat, 102, 109

Sexuality, male: immorality in, 59; regulation of, 115, 296n2

Sexual norms: in abortion reform movements, 221; in antiabortion campaigns, 12; deviation from, 163; psychiatrists' views on, 331n20; state regulation of, 115, 130–31; violation of, 5

Shame, 36, 125, 126–28, 230; in regulation of reproductive behavior, 5, 28, 36, 171, 200, 230

Shaver, Clarence, 104

Shaver, Dr. Eva, 101, 105; newspaper coverage of, 104; office of, *plate 5;* trial of, 107

Shelton, Dr. William E., 313n113
Sheppard-Towner Act, 81, 110, 172; abolition of, 111; and attacks on midwifery, 291n111
Shorter, Edward, 284n111
Silence: in McCarthy era, 192; as metaphor for subordination, 20, 21, 266nn4,5
Silva, Dr., 56
Simon, Kate, 68
Slaves, abortifacients of, 9
Slippery elm, 43, 44, 274nn106,111
Sloane Hospital (New York), 205, 207
Socialist movements: and birth control, 141; and legal abortion, 142, 218, 233. *See also* Left, political
Socialized medicine, 172
Society for Humane Abortion (SHA, California), 223, 224, 227; male support of, 331n22; newsletter of, 257; underground arm of, 224
South, midwives in, 296n117
South Carolina, 331n15
South Dakota, 336n70
Soviet Union, 139, 140, 141, 172, 180, 285n114, 308n42
"Speaking," liberatory aspects of, 20, 21, 266nn4,5
Speak-outs, 20, 229–30, 333n40
Specialists, 285n1; antiabortion campaigns of, 15; in coroners' inquests, 88; in history of abortion, 4; physician-abortionists as, 147, 159, 310n66; on use of curette, 285n113. *See also* Gynecologists; Obstetricians
Speculums, 75
Spencer, Dr. Robert Douglas, 310n70
Springer, Dr., 300n21
Squier, Dr. Raymond, 322n85
Stackable, Dr. W. H., 104, 105
Stahl, Dr. Frank A., 42
Stanko, Helen, 168; trials of, 169–70, 171, 318n44
Stanley, Dr., 56
State: cooperation of hospitals with, 4, 121, 123–24, 162, 173–74, 190, 226, 303n52; enforcement of abortion law, 1, 81, 107, 114–31, 299n17; enforcement of childbearing, 340n13; intervention in marriage, 115, 129–31; medical profession's cooperation with, 3, 81, 88–90, 115–16, 120–25, 131, 226, 249, 260n5; surveillance of

abortion, 163, 173, 249; surveillance of health care, 249
States: abortion laws of, 64, 252, 261n13, 265n45; abortion reform in, 331n15; test cases in, 335n67, 336n70
State v. Martin, 166
Stead, W. T., 49–50
Sterilization, 320n66; coercive, 207, 208, 232, 324n116, 333n42; for eugenic reasons, 328n50; of low-income patients, 207, 231; medical grounds for, 329n54; during therapeutic abortion, 328n51; therapeutic abortion committees' oversight of, 177
Stevens, Rosemary, 313n106
Stevenson, Dr. Sarah Hackett, 58, 290n52; in anti-midwife campaign, 93–94
Stix, Dr. Regine K., 23
Storer, Dr. Horatio R., 20, 82; on quickening, 11–12
Storer, Dr. Humphreys, 82
Stowe, Dr. Herbert M., 96, 291n61
Students, in abortion rights movement, 225. *See also* Medical students
Styskal, Cecilia, 75
Suicide: in *People v. Martin,* 167; "race," 102, 104; in therapeutic abortion decisions, 201–2, 241; of unmarried women, 185
Sulfonamides, 339n5
Supreme Court. *See* U.S. Supreme Court
Sweden, 224
Switzerland, 140, 308n42

Tampa, Fla., 198
Taussig, Dr. Frederick J.: on frequency of abortion, 23, 134, 139; on infection, 285n113; organization of lectures, 84; reform proposals of, 142–44, 145, 179; on tuberculosis, 146
Teachers, 158
Technology, medical, 247; and liberalization of abortion, 216
Teenagers: abortions by, 312n96; reproductive rights of, 248, 253
Temperance movements, 12, 264n39
Test cases: in abortion law, 181, 189, 190, 191, 237, 335n67, 336n70; in birth control movement, 189, 323n111. See also *Doe v. Scott*
Texas, 336n70
Thalidomide, 203

Therapeutic abortion: under ALI model law, 233; Catholic Church on, 7; during Depression, 143; for economic reasons, 146, 181; effect of McCarthyism on, 180; effect of police raids on, 161–62; in England, 141; ethnicity in, 207, 327n42; for eugenic reasons, 64–65, 203–4; in exchange for sterilization, 208; fatalities in, 284n110; following *Doe v. Scott,* 240; frequency of, 328n47; in hospitals, 161–62; hypothetical cases in, 240–41, 337n90; before Illinois Supreme Court, 242–43; lack of standards for, 218; Leunbach method in, 157; medical consensus on, 5, 262n14; medical discourse on, 67; medical indications for, 63–64, 143–46, 176, 177, 278n55, 326n27; moral protection for, 176–77; of nineteenth century, 13; for poor women, 144, 205; of postwar era, 173, 200–202, 214; psychiatric indications for, 183, 184, 187, 201–3, 207, 241, 326n26, 327n36; by race, 205, 206, *fig. 3;* ratio to live births, 179–80, 321n82, 328n44, *fig. 2;* reductions in, 191, 204, *fig. 2, fig. 3;* reform of, 219–22; restrictiveness of, 235; for rubella, 203, 240; safety of, 214, 329n62; social indications for, 62, 64–65, 132, 143–44, 181, 203; state statutes on, 64; sterilization during, 328n51; in Timanus trial, 186–88; women's right to decision in, 66, 67, 146, 279n64. *See also* Abortion, legal

Therapeutic abortion committees, 173–79; control of physicians, 178–79, 190–91, 218; and decline in abortions, 204; dismantling of, 246; following *Doe v. Scott,* 240; institutionalization of, 214; membership of, 320n74; origins of, 174; in postwar era, 214; procedures of, 177, 178–79; psychiatrists' challenges to, 218; review process of, 186; and sterilization, 177; unconstitutionality of, 244; women before, 179, 200, 321n79. *See also* Hospitals

Thiery, Mary E., 53

Thurston, Dr., 56

Timanus, Dr. George Loutrell, 148, 158–59; abandonment by colleagues, 187, 323n105; imprisonment of, 188;

on medical profession, 191; professional ethics of, 187; raid on, 181, 322n86; referrals to, 183, 186

Timanus trial, 323n112; court opinion on, 322n89; defense in, 187; physicians' testimony in, 186–87; prosecution in, 322n86; therapeutic abortion in, 186–88; transcript of, 183

Time magazine, 172

Towne, Dr. Janet, 168, 169, 319n49

Trade unions, 227, 233

Tuberculosis, as indication for abortion, 63, 143–44, 145, 146, 240, 326n27

Underworld: commercial abortion in, 52–53, 57, 99, 106, 149; in popular press, 167; sexual, 50

United Auto Workers (UAW), 332n33

United Charities, 236

United States: abortion statutes in, 10; Constitution, 317n33; nature of state in, 3

University of Chicago Settlement House, 291n61

University of Virginia Hospital, 179

University of Wisconsin in Madison, 196

Unmarried mothers. *See* Mothers, unmarried

U.S. Children's Bureau. *See* Children's Bureau

U.S. Supreme Court: abortion cases before, 16, 216, 235, 244–45, 323n111; in *Doe v. Scott,* 240; on economic discrimination, 244–45; on "potential life," 252; on right to privacy, 237, 244; on search and seizure, 166

Uterine perforation, 79, *plate 2*

Uterine sounds, 72, 282n89; use by midwives, 75

Vandiver, Almuth, 120, 123

Vermont, 253

Virginia: abortion reform in, 331n15; University of Virginia Hospital, 179

Visiting Nurse Association (Chicago), 95

Void-for-vagueness doctrine, 239

Vomiting, as indication for abortion, 63–64, 201, 279n56

Walkowitz, Judith R., 50, 292n78

Warner, Dr. A. S., 19, 266n1

Washington, D.C.: Freedmen's Hospital,

Washington, D.C. (*continued*)
147; General Hospital, 210; Obstetrical and Gynecological Society, 80; test cases in, 336n70; women's liberation groups in, 333n35
Washington University Dispensary (St. Louis), 70
Wayman, John, 122
Webster v. Reproductive Health Services, 251, 252
Weiss, Dr. E. A., 64
Welfare, 134, 249, 253, 340n13; and access to abortion, 338n111; attacks on, 249; feminist influence on, 297n3; National Welfare Rights Organization, 228; sterilization of recipients, 231
Wetherhill, Dr. H. G., 82
Wheeler, Shirley, 243
Whites: ethnic groups, 16; legislators, 13; racial fears of, 11, 50; reformers, 91. *See also* Women, white
Wife beating, 41
Will, Dr. O. B., 120
Windmueller, Dr. Charles R. A., 108, 295n106
Winter, Margaret, 39
Wisconsin, 61, 149
Withdrawal, 41, 196
Womanhood: "bonds" of, 266n6; of midwives, 76
Woman's City Club (Chicago), 105
Women: admission to medical profession, 11–12; arrest of, for abortion, 243; attitude toward abortion, 25–26; Catholic, 233, 268n12; class divisions among, 94; communist, 172, 319n60; community obligation among, 31, 270n49; demand for abortions, 1, 147, 159, 249, 254, 290n54; and discourse on abortion, 8, 21, 23–24, 44, 109, 220; discrimination against, 228; empowerment of, 226, 253; in history of crime, 5, 261n8; influence on physicians, 6; Jewish, 7, 137, 173, 306nn22,23; medical lectures for, 84–85; moral character of, 58–59; moral superiority of, 12, 264n39; nonprofessional, 222; perceptions of abortion, 23–24; property rights of, 261n8; Protestant, 10, 23, 50, 137, 306n22; reasons for abortion, 42; silence of, 20–21, 266nn4,5; status in American society, 245; subordination of, 20, 21,

217; targeting in antiabortion campaigns, 81, 83–85; before therapeutic abortion committees, 179, 200, 321n79; in workforce, 163, 194, 324n3; in World War II, 162–63; writers, 141, 309n45. *See also* Abortion patients
Women, affluent: abortion practices of, 53, 54, 58, 69, 236; childbearing of, 208; choice of physicians, 137; during Depression, 135; investigation of, 119; legalized abortion for, 251; in physician-patient relationship, 67; support of legal abortion, 342n34
Women, African American, 2; abortion records of, 300n21; in abortion rights movement, 232, 253; in black power movement, 334n50; childrearing by, 194; in coroners' inquests, 119–20; education levels of, 306n21; effect of illegal abortion on, 193; fatal abortions of, 211–12, 222, 232; feminists among, 232; at Gabler-Martin clinic, 153; history of, 259n3; illegitimate births by, 136, 137; in Kinsey abortion study, 305n15; married, 135–36; maternity homes for, 28, 306n21; self-induced abortions of, 43; sterilization of, 207, 208; therapeutic abortion for, 204–5; traditional roles of, 163; use of abortionists, 326n18; use of black physicians, 286n10; use of midwives, 296n117; use of Planned Parenthood, 231. *See also* African Americans
Women, married: abortion practices of, 11, 20, 23, 58, 152–53, 277n42; in abortion raid cases, 165; abuse of, 41, 59, 273n102; African American, 135–36; childless, 152; discrimination against in workforce, 133, 162–63, 194, 230; during Depression, 135; and "race suicide," 92, 102, 104; reasons for abortion, 38–40, 104; reproductive rights of, 102, 104; self-induced abortions of, 312n89; use of physicians, 73
Women, middle-class: abortion practices of, 11; demand for abortion, 290n54; psychiatric symptoms of, 201; reproductive rights of, 13; therapeutic abortions for, 203, 207; use of contraceptives, 40–41; views on childbearing, 38, 40
Women, poor: in abortion clinics, 306n19; abortion funding for, 251;

abortion reform proposals for, 142; activism of, 336n72; contraceptives for, 134; during Depression, 134–35, 241; effect of illegal abortion on, 193; fertility of, 231; forced cesarean sections for, 250; importance of abortion to, 37, 40; legalized abortion for, 236, 246; reproductive rights of, 248; self-induced abortion by, 43, 119, 137–48; sterilization of, 231; therapeutic abortion for, 144, 205; use of midwives, 76

Women, unmarried: abortion practices of, 23, 31–34, 58, 60, 69, 136, 202, 268n15, 327n32; in abortion raid cases, 165; African American, 306n21; coroners' inquests on, 128–30; counseling for, 84; dying declarations of, 126; exposure of sexual activity, 28, 200, 269n36; independence of, 109; legal abortion for, 221; marriage following abortion, 303n58; postponement of marriage, 133; prosecution of, 122; punishment for, 221, 249; rape of, 33, 270n61; reasons for abortion, 33–34; reproductive rights of, 108; self-induced abortion by, 312n89; sexual danger for, 102, 293n84; students among, 195; suicide of, 185; testimony in abortion trials, 184; therapeutic abortion for, 202; as victims, 23, 32–33, 59, 92, 102, 249. See also College women; Mothers, unmarried

Women, white: access to therapeutic abortion, 205, 207; college attendance, 194; in coroners' inquests, 119; fatal abortions of, 211, 213, fig. 6; and feminism, 228, 236; illegitimate births by, 136–37; pressure for marriage and

motherhood directed at, 163; as private-paying patients, 205; and self-induced abortions, 137; as ward patients, 207; and welfare, 249

Women, working-class, 2; abortion practices of, 20, 23, 27, 31, 141, 152, 153–54; abortions by physicians, 70–71; contraception for, 6, 36; in coroners' inquests, 119; during Depression, 135; of England, 140; family planning by, 230; history of, 259n3; reasons for abortion, 33, 40; in Sanger clinics, 23; sexual freedom for, 92; use of midwives, 73; views on abortion, 6, 29–30; wages of, 29, 163, 270n41

Women's Christian Temperance Union, 297n3

Women's Ephemera Collection (Northwestern University), 256

Women's history, 2, 3, 259n1; poststructural analysis of, 262n21

Women's liberation, 228, 333n35

Women's movements: and antiabortion campaigns, 14; and legalization of abortion, 15–16; move from left, 142, 309n48; nineteenth-century, 11, 12, 264n39; public-health work of, 96, 291n60. See also Feminists

Women's National Abortion Action Coalition (WONAAC), 232, 257

Women's suffrage, 237

Woof, Dr. Joseph T., 19–20

World War II: abortion during, 162–63, 325n8; effect on gender identity, 141, 163, 309n45

Wynn, Dr. Ralph M., 238

Zuspan, Dr. Frederick P., 238

Compositor: G & S Typesetters
Text: 10/13 Galliard
Display: Galliard
Printer and binder: BookCrafters